The Forgotten Plague

The Forgotten Plague

How the Battle Against Tuberculosis Was Won — and Lost

Frank Ryan, M.D.

Little, Brown and Company

Boston   Toronto   London

First American Edition

First published in the United Kingdom as
Tuberculosis: The Greatest Story Never Told

Library of Congress Cataloging-in-Publication Data
Ryan, Frank
    The forgotten plague : how the battle against tuberculosis was
won — and lost / Frank Ryan. — 1st American ed.
        p.   cm.
    Includes bibliographical references and index.
    ISBN 0-316-76380-2
    1. Tuberculosis — History.   I. Title.
RC310.R9   1992
614.5'42'09 — dc20   92-46893

10 9 8 7 6 5 4 3 2 1

MV-NY

Published simultaneously in Canada by
Little, Brown & Company (Canada) Limited

Printed in the United States of America

For my daughter, Catherine

Acknowledgements

I CAN hardly express my gratitude to the many people and organizations who so generously helped me during the research for this book. Where indicated, I have enlarged upon this in the sources and reference section. My special thanks are due to the following, all of whom were either original participants in the story or close relatives: Frederick Bernheim, Sven Carlsten, Sir John Crofton, Götz Domagk, John Grange, Betty Gregory (nee Bugie), Åke Hanngren, Norman Heatley, H. Corwin Hinshaw, Rollin Hotchkiss, Michael Iseman, Karl Jahnke, Hans Larsson, Hubert and Mary Lechevalier, Maja Lehmann, Orla Lehmann, Doris Ralston (nee Jones), Karl-Gustav Rosdahl, Albert and Vivian Schatz, Jan Sievers, John Stanford, Gunnar Vallentin, Britt Håkansson (nee Vallentin) and Byron Waksman.

The following people assisted me greatly during my researches: Dr Jack Adler, Dr M Aoki, Dr Erik Berglund, Dr Bernard Dean, Michael Dixon, Jarl Ingelf, Professor Johannes Köbberling, Professor Sven Lindstedt, Carol Moberg, Kevin Murray, Clark Nelson, Stig Nylén, John Roddom, Michael P. Russell, Professor Hans Schadewaldt, Dr Gisela Schector, Christina Sehnert, Michael W. Starn, Andrew Tait.

I was fortunate that a number of institutions and pharmaceutical companies provided me with invaluable help and reference information: in particular I would like to acknowledge the help of the Bayer Pharmaceutical Company, Ferrosan and subsequently Kabi Pharmacia, Merck Sharp & Dohme Ltd, Hoffman-La Roche, Farmitalia Carlo Erba, E R Squibb and Sons Ltd, the Historical Unit of the Mayo Clinic, the staff of the pharmacy information service and the department of medical illustration at the Northern General Hospital Sheffield, the Rockefeller archives, the archives of The Duke University, North Carolina, the Dept of Oral History at Columbia University New York, the archives of the University of Philadelphia, the Bloomsbury Science Library of the University of London and The Wellcome Institute for the History of Medicine.

In researching the modern story, I had invaluable help from Dr Annik Rouillon, of the International Union Against Tuberculosis and Lung Disease, Dr Philippe Sudre and Dr Mario Raviglione of the World Health Organization, Dr Walter Ihle of the Centre for Disease Control, Atlanta, Dr Jack Adler of the New York Bureau of Tuberculosis Control, Dr John Stanford of The Middlesex Hospital London, Dr John Grange of the National Heart & Lung Hospital London, Professor R Ferlinz, Deutches Zentralkomitee zur Bekämpfung der Tuberkulose, Dr Masakazu Aoki, director of the Research Institute of Tuberculosis, Tokyo, Japan, Dr John Domenet of CIBA–GEIGY Ltd.

For help with the palaeontology details I am indebted to Dr Keith Manchester and Dr Charlotte Roberts of the Calvin Wells Laboratory for Burial Archaeology, Bradford University, to my surgical colleague Mr John Rowling, of Sheffield, and Dr Stephen Webb of the Bond University, Queensland.

The following kindly helped with the translations from German, French and Swedish: Maria Bajaria, Traudi Crane, Professor Götz Domagk, Anna Hart, Alec M Horsfield, Jarl Ingelf, Professor Karl Jahnke, Agneta Magnusson, Dr Helga Buecker and Claudine Murrell.

Finally, I owe a special thanks to Monica O'Hara, my agent Bill Hamilton, my friends Norman and Valerie Treby, Cynthia Williams, my brother Anthony, my editors Sara Kerruish and Lyn Taylor, the indexer Karin Woodruff, and especially to my long-patient wife, Barbara.

The following sources very kindly allowed me to quote from their copyright material. More precise details are to be found in the appropriate reference sections.

Professor Götz Domagk and the Bayer archives at Leverkusen, Germany, for permission to quote from the unpublished diary of Gerhard Domagk. Dr Byron H. Waksman for permission to quote from Selman A. Waksman's, two seminal books: Selman A Waksman, *My Life with the Microbes*, Robert Hale Ltd, 1958; and Selman A Waksman, *The Conquest of Tuberculosis*, University of California Press, 1964. The State University of New Jersey (Rutgers) Special Collections and Archives, for permission to quote from many references to Waksman's life and work and to use the illustrations derived from the collection. The Rockefeller Archives, Tarrytown, for permission to quote from their many sources on René Dubos and Marie Louise Dubos (née Bonnet) – also for permission to reproduce their illustrations. The Rockefeller University Press and Rollin Hotchkiss for permission to quote from the chapter, FROM MICROBES TO MEDICINE: GRAMICIDIN, RENÉ DUBOS AND THE ROCKEFELLER, in *Launching the Antibiotic Era*. The Department of Oral History of the Columbia Library, Columbia University, New York, for permission to quote from the Oral History of René Dubos. Ferrosan Pharmaceutical Co (now Kabi Pharmacia) for permission to quote from the Observanda Ferrosan magazine articles on Jorgen Lehmann. Professor Thomas D Brock and Science Tech Publishers for permission to quote from *Robert Koch – A Life in Medicine and Bacteriology*. Professor Albert Schatz for permission to quote from his extensive biographical references at the University of Philadelphia. Professor H. Corwin Hinshaw for permission to quote from his extensive writings, including the unpublished, *Conquest of a Plague*. Doris Ralston (née Jones) for permission to quote from her unpublished paper, *A Personal Glimpse at the Discovery of Streptomycin*. Professor Johannes Köbberling for *125 Jahre: Ferdinand Sauerbruch Klinikum* – the history of the Wuppertal-Elberfeld Hospital. Harcourt Brace Jovanovich Inc for *Quest: Reflections on Medicine, Science and Humanity*, by Jean Paul Escande, trans Patricia Ranum. Dr Philip Onyebujoh (through the intermediary of Dr John Stanford) for permission to reproduce the illustration of the African woman with the TB-AIDS syndrome. The International Union Against Tuberculosis and Lung Disease for permission to refer to many of their publications. The library of University College London for details of George

Orwell's illness. Dr Arnold Bentley of Royal British Legion Village, Aylsford, Kent, for access to the Preston Hall medical records concerning George Orwell. Jeff Miller of the UCSF Magazine for permission to refer to and copy the illustrations from the magazine article "TB Bounces Back" in the June 1991 edition of the UCSF Magazine. The copyright for the illustrations are acknowledged with the appropriate illustration.

Personalities

Avery, Oswald: doctor and scientist, The Rockefeller University, New York.

Behnisch, Robert: research chemist, Bayer Pharmaceutical Company, Elberfeld, Germany.

Bernheim, Frederick: biochemist, Duke University, North Carolina, USA.

Bernstein, Jack: chief chemist, E.R. Squibb & Sons, New Brunswick, New Jersey, USA.

Crofton, Sir John: consultant physician, Edinburgh, Scotland.

Domagk, Gerhard: experimental pathologist, Bayer Pharmaceutical Company, Elberfeld, Germany.

Dubos, Marie Louise: wife of René q.v.

Dubos, René: research scientist, the Rockefeller University, New York.

Ehrlich, Paul: German doctor who invented the theory of drug treatment for infections.

Feldman, William: veterinarian, the Mayo Clinic, Rochester, Minnesota, USA.

Fox, Herbert: senior chemist, Hoffman-La Roche Pharmaceutical Company, Nutley, New Jersey, USA.

Hinshaw, H. Corwin: consultant physician, the Mayo Clinic, Rochester, Minnesota, USA.

Hotchkiss, Rollin: organic chemist, The Rockefeller University, New York.

Klarer, Josef: research chemist, Bayer Pharmaceutical Company, Elberfeld, Germany.

Klee, Philipp: chief of the department of internal medicine, the Wuppertal-Elberfeld Hospital, Wuppertal, Germany.

Koch, Robert: German doctor who discovered the bacterial cause of tuberculosis.

Lehmann, Jorgen: chief of the department of clinical chemistry, Sahlgren's Hospital, Gothenburg, Sweden.

McDermott, Walsh: American physician and tuberculosis expert, the New York Hospital – Cornell Medical Centre, New York.

Merck, George W.: owner and director of George Merck & Co Pharmaceutical Company, Rahway, New Jersey, USA.

Mietzsch, Fritz: research chemist, Bayer Pharmaceutical Company, Elberfeld, Germany.

Offe, Hans: research chemist, Bayer Pharmaceutical Company, Leverkusen, Germany.

Rosdahl, Karl-Gustav: senior chemist, Ferrosan Pharmaceutical Company, Malmö, Sweden.

Schatz, Albert: post-graduate student, Rutgers Agricultural College (subsequently Rutgers University), New Jersey, USA.

Sievers, Olof: bacteriologist, Sahlgren's Hospital, Gothenburg, Sweden.

Vallentin, Gylfe: chief clinician, Renstrom sanitorium, Gothenburg, Sweden.

Waksman, Selman: professor of soil microbiology, Rutgers Agricultural College (subsequently Rutgers University), New Brunswick, New Jersey, USA.

Contents

PART III – THE GREAT CURE

PART IV – THE TIME BOMB

Introduction

ON 31 August, 1991, the *Lancet*, published an article by three eminent bacteriologists, Stanford, Grange and Pozniak. The title of the article was "Is Africa Lost?" It ended with the extraordinary statement: we are facing one of the greatest public health disasters since the bubonic plague. The focus of this article was a curious and deadly synergy between the new menace, AIDS, and a disease which would have been all too familiar to Hippocrates, a disease which many believed dead and buried – tuberculosis.

For me it came as no surprise. For four years I had been travelling in many countries, researching the human story behind the discovery of the cure for tuberculosis. It had proved a fascinating mission. Tuberculosis was well-known as the greatest killer in history. It was more feared than bubonic plague, more written about, even speciously glamourized in nineteenth-century literature and art. It had inspired great literature such as Mann's Nobel Prize-winning novel, *The Magic Mountain*, great opera such as *La Traviata*. It had robbed humanity of many famous people. Up to the time when the cure was discovered, a dreadful pessimism gripped the public and medical profession alike: doctors worldwide believed that tuberculosis would never be curable. There can be little doubt that the discovery of the cure for tuberculosis changed human history. To me, however, tuberculosis has always had a more personal fascination. My maternal grandfather, a naval survivor from the first world war, had died from pulmonary tuberculosis in a Dublin hospital, three years before I was born.

As a medical student, I was intrigued by a simple statement in a pharmacology textbook: "Streptomycin is obtained from *Strep-tomyces griseus* which was cultured by Waksman in 1944, from a heavily manured field and also from a chicken's throat."[1] There was no further explanation. In 1977 I became a consultant physician, dealing with many serious medical conditions. In 1982 I returned from holiday to find a nineteen-year-old woman had been admitted to my ward. She had taken her own discharge six months earlier against medical advice while running a fever. Now she was back with a recurrence of that same illness, gaunt and wasted, with a temperature of 104 Fahrenheit. As I examined her, she asked me if she was dying. Indeed she was. She was suffering from miliary tuberculosis, the most deadly form of the disease, where bacteria are spread to every organ in the body through the blood stream. I am glad to say that, given the cure, within three days her temperature was normal and she went on to make a full recovery.

I can remember this young woman very well: I presented her case at a medical meeting in the hospital. During the discussion afterwards, I asked my colleagues if they knew how that cure had become possible. "Who," I enquired, "was Waksman?" A chest physician told me Waksman was "an American". In fact Waksman, who was Russian, was the only central figure in the story to publish his autobiography.[2] People had either neglected to read it or they had simply forgotten. I went on asking questions, accumulating little morsels of information. More importantly, I was discovering silences.

A friend, the journalist and writer Monica O'Hara, helped me during the early researches. She placed a notice in the *Liverpool Echo*, asking people who had suffered from tuberculosis in the 1940s and 1950s to write to her. I read what they had to say: I would spend hours talking to my own patients who had previously suffered from the disease. But by now I had come to realize that, wonderful though Waksman's contribution undoubtedly was, there were other remarkable personalities involved, other mysteries.

Who was this German doctor called Gerhard Domagk? There were intimations he had been arrested by the Gestapo when he had been awarded the Nobel Prize for the discovery of the first antibacterial drug long before Fleming's penicillin. Who knew anything of a Scandinavian called Jorgen Lehmann, a deductive genius as brilliant as a real life Sherlock Holmes? Who was this Frenchman, working in New York, called René Dubos, a scientist-philosopher, who as a young man had confirmed the thinking of Louis Pasteur, making an historic medical breakthrough based upon one of the fundamental truisms of the Bible? There were others too, every one of them an unheralded mystery. Each tantalizing whisper suggested that the story of the great cure would prove to be extraordinary.

An accurate impression of how the disease was regarded by its sufferers emerged from a questionnaire sent to the respondents of the *Liverpool Echo* article. We asked them what they expected would happen to them when they were told they were suffering from tuberculosis: without exception, they regarded it as a death sentence. They very often elaborated, giving harrowing details of just how little time their doctors gave them to live. One respondent, a girl aged nineteen at diagnosis, gave a typical reply: "I was the only one in my ward that survived." This was the background against which I viewed this curious silence. And from it I realised that there was only one way in which I could answer that silence: no matter how difficult, no matter how long it would take, I would have to find out what inspired these remarkable people to make such wonderful discoveries. I would write their book for them. It promised to be one of the greatest true sagas of our century, globally set, sweeping in scale – the discovery of the cure for the greatest killer in history. Some undertaking! The title would be the easiest thing about it: it would be called *The Greatest Story Never Told*.

But how should I discover the intimate details of how the cure was found? The silence was truly deafening.

I believe that scientific inspiration is as much a reflection of the personality of the individual as the visual creativity of Van Gogh or the musical genius of Mozart. I needed the intimate details of their lives. To achieve this I had to find a way of getting inside their heads.

I had more than my share of good luck. H. Corwin Hinshaw, Albert Schatz, Karl Rosdahl, Åke Hanngrenn, John Crofton and Rollin Hotchkiss, to name but a few, were still alive. What a pleasure actually to meet and interview these fascinating people, all of whom had played their parts in the cure! Jorgen Lehmann was also alive when I began the book, but sadly he died as I was writing it. Frederick Bernheim too was alive, but elderly and rather ill. Perhaps my single greatest stroke of luck was in finding the hitherto unpublished and forgotten diaries of Gerhard Domagk, all 700 pages of them, with the help of the Bayer archives. They tell a remarkable story. If this book fails in its purpose, the fault is mine alone.

I have not written this book as a scholarly work, intended only for the eyes of other doctors or scientists. I have written it for everybody, for the ordinary man and woman, regardless of whether they know a jot about medicine or science. It deserves nothing less. Most surprising of all, and of very great relevance to our world today, the story is not over.

Quite a shock awaited me when I visited New York in October 1990. I was sitting with my wife in the famous Rockefeller dining room, enjoying the courtesy of lunch with Carol Moberg. I had just interviewed Carol, who had been a friend and assistant to René Dubos. Outside the window, which was close to our table, was the spectacular townscape of Manhattan. Carol, in passing, mentioned the current tuberculosis epidemic in New York City. I knew nothing about this. Initially somewhat sceptical, I rang Dr Jack Adler, the director of the New York Bureau of Tuberculosis. He confirmed it. New York was gripped by the worst outbreak of tuberculosis since the 1960s. When I spoke to his nurse, she was frankly terrified.

That was my first intimation that all was not quite as I thought it to be. I put down the telephone in a genuine state of shock. How could this be happening? I had thought my story neatly parcelled up and brought to a satisfying conclusion. I think my first reaction was anger. How could the world have let them down, after they had sacrificed so very much to find the cure? But when I cooled down, I knew I would have to think afresh about the whole venture.

I began a series of new researches, aimed at finding out what was really happening in the world right now. I received every cooperation from the World Health Organization, from the International Union Against Tuberculosis and the Centres for Disease Control, in Atlanta. Although I could hardly believe what I was reading and hearing, I had to open my eyes to an even more horrifying realization. The new danger was not confined to New York. The entire world was facing a new and very frightening tuberculosis threat. And, in some strange way, it was linked to the AIDS epidemic. How utterly incredible to discover that the new virus of AIDS was coming together with this equally dangerous if more ancient enemy, in the most sinister alliance imaginable. Publication would have to be delayed. I wanted very much to understand what had gone wrong, even if this meant I would have to write a new and fourth section to this book.

Could it be that part explanation for the new threat still lay with the lives of those extraordinary few who had found the cure? That was an extremely important question I asked myself again and again. If so – and I believe now that this is in fact the case – then the telling of their story might help the millions who are still suffering a very real reign of terror.

PART I

AMERICA

1

The Reign of Terror

I am ill because of wounds to the soul, to the deep emotional self.

D.H. Lawrence[1]

i

I T SEEMS almost incredible that during this century and the previous one, a single disease, tuberculosis, was responsible for the deaths of approximately a thousand million human beings. There can be little doubt that the discovery of the cure for tuberculosis changed human history. Yet the story of the cure has never previously been told. Why this should be the case is a mystery – though it seems linked to a widespread belief that tuberculosis is a ghost from the past, something we do not wish to know about, a terror that is over. Nothing could be more mistaken. As our world today faces one of the most dangerous epidemics in all of history, no story could be more relevant.

This is the story behind the discovery of the cure for tuberculosis. It is one of the most important struggles in history, re-markable not only in the great suffering caused by the disease but also in the triumphs and tragedies the quest brought to the lives of those who played their parts in it. Obviously it is very much a human story. There is, however, a second and equally powerful presence in this story, a personality which is definitively non-human – the extraordinary nature of the disease itself. Tuber-culosis is much more than a medical affliction caused by a specific bacterium. It is by turns a strange, a terrible and a fascinating

3

entity, like the multi-layered mystery of the famous Russian doll. No sooner do we think we understand it, than a new form, as baffling and menacing as ever, appears to confound us.

We can hardly pretend to grasp the real meaning of those thousand million lives: how can we stretch our already over-burdened imagination to encompass the fact that it did not stop there, the terror went on and on, back over centuries and even millenia, casting its awesome shadow over four continents and beyond written history. Perhaps we should make a start with the outermost layer of the doll, and the first of its mysteries. When did the disease we now call tuberculosis first infect a human being?

ii

THE PALAEONTOLOGICAL RECORDS tell us that our human ancestry goes back a mere three to five million years. We were preceded by many eras, the best-known of which was that of the dinosaurs, which spanned 180 to 60 million years ago. Before the dinosaurs there was, however, a much vaster age, so primordial and distant that it is only poorly traceable in fossil records, when the earth was colonized by the earliest and simplest of all life forms, single-celled organisms that were the first bacteria. These curious bacteria have been found in South Africa and Rhodesia, in Precambrian rocks estimated at more than three thousand million years old. Surviving in a primitive landscape of spuming volcanoes and an atmosphere devoid of oxygen, at a time when the earth itself was no more than a thousand million years old, bacterial forms have been found inside the simple cells of the first animal and vegetable life, the blue-green algae, which appeared on the earth at much the same time. It would appear that the first infections began co-incidentally with the beginnings of life itself.

There is evidence of a viral infection in the fossil of a bird dating from ninety million years ago.[2] A dental abscess was found in a fossil skull of *Homo erectus*, between one and two million years old.[3] In the 40,000-year-old skull of Rhodesian man from Broken Hill there is the cavity of a mastoid infection that would be familiar to the ear, nose and throat surgeon of today.[4] None of these infections was tuberculosis, but if these common infections are so ancient, the parallel is suggestive.

Tuberculosis has the grim capacity of gouging large holes in bones, especially the spinal bones, or vertebrae, destroying their bodies and causing the spine to collapse in the upper back. This "hunchback" is very suggestive of tuberculosis, particularly if it is caused by an ulcerating destruction of the spinal bones. Tuberculosis also ulcerates the ends of the long bones, causing painful and disfiguring changes which are easily recognizable in skeletons. By searching for these signs we can recognize the disease in the skeletal remains of people who died a very long time ago and changes such as these have been found in the spines of Egyptian mummies – they were confirmed by the paintings of Egyptian artists who drew hunchback figures on the walls of tombs – so we know that tuberculosis was a common disease in ancient Egypt, even as early as 4,000 years BC. One famous mummy of a high priest of Amon still has the track of pus discharging from a spinal abscess along the course of the psoas muscle, a finding which only occurs in tuberculosis.[5] If, as some authorities speculate, the epidemic form of tuberculosis really began in the first cities of the ancient world, then the ancient Egyptians may, in addition to civilization, have bequeathed the world this malignancy.

The earliest suggested evidence for tuberculosis dates from a neolithic grave near Heidelberg, dated at 5,000 BC,[6] where the skeleton of a young man showed destruction of two vertebrae from the thoracic spine. Dr Keith Manchester, an expert at Bradford University and a world authority on ancient tuberculosis, is not convinced the disease in this case really was tuberculosis, but there is general agreement on the evidence of tuberculosis of the spine found in a skeleton during the excavation of burials in the Arene Candide Cave in Liguria, Italy.[7] Once again, the remains were those of a youth, about fifteen years of age, where the spine showed massive destruction of two vertebrae and partial destruction of two others. This unfortunate young man died about 4,000 BC, during the Stone Age. Similar evidence has been found in graves dating from prehistory in Denmark[8] and from the Bronze Age in the Jordan valley.[9]

It is disturbing to imagine our Stone Age ancestors suffering from the telltale chronic cough and emaciating fever and, like the poet Keats, coughing up bright red arterial blood.

Tuberculosis infects many different mammals, especially cattle, and there are varieties of the disease that infect birds (the avian strain) and even fish and small reptiles, such as frogs and turtles. The bacterium that causes tuberculosis dies in direct sunlight but survives in dust for several weeks or even months. Taken with the fact it cannot be killed by many harmful chemicals, this suggests that the bacterium may have evolved as a micro-organism that once grew in the soil. Dr John Stanford, who has spent his life studying tuberculosis, believes that the tuberculosis germ is very ancient, and may well have fought for its survival in the primaeval mud of the earth at the very beginnings of time.[10] The disease may have first infected animals which would have inhaled or ingested it from the soil during browsing. It might then have been passed on to humans through their flesh or more likely their milk.[11] This would plausibly fit some of the known facts, notably the form of tuberculosis caused by the bovine strain, which is contracted through drinking milk from infected cattle. If this theory is true, then time should demonstrate typical changes of tuberculosis in the bones of cattle much earlier than those found in human skeletons.

From the Danish evidence, the disease was already established in mainland Europe by 2,500–1,500 BC, but it probably came to Britain a thousand or more years later. According to Manchester, the earliest definite evidence of the disease in Britain has been found in Cirencester in graves dating from the Roman occupation.[12] Tuberculosis is a remarkably enduring disease and once it arrives in a community, it stays. Throughout succeeding centuries, the prevalence of the disease increased markedly. Since the reign of Clovis, in the fifth century, the kings of France were believed to receive healing powers from God and, in England, during the reign of Edward the Confessor, a ritual was introduced for the cure of The King's Evil, a colourful description for the swollen and discharging tuberculous lymph glands in the neck, called scrofula. Legend has it that . . .

A young woman had married a husband of her own age, but having no issue by the union, the humours collected abundantly about her neck, she contracted a sore disorder, the glands swelling in a dreadful manner. Admonished in a dream to have the part affected washed by the king, she entered the palace, and the king himself fulfilled this labour of love by rubbing the woman's neck with his fingers dipped in water. Joyous health followed his healing hand; the lurid skin opened, so that worms flowed out with the purulent matter, and the tumour subsided. But as the orifice of the ulcer was large and unsightly, he commanded her to be supported at royal expense until she should be perfectly cured. However, before a week had expired, a fair new skin returned, and hid the scars so completely that nothing of the original wound could be discovered; and within a year, becoming the mother of twins, she increased the admiration of Edward's holiness.

Since this "cure" was free, painless, instant and miraculous, it soon became very popular. The practice of "touching", inherited as part of the divine right of kings, evolved into a ceremony of fantastic proportions, made all the more attractive when it came to include a gold piece which was hung about the neck of the sufferer. Louis XIV of France is said to have touched 1,600 persons one Easter Sunday and Charles II, when in exile in the Netherlands, was in such demand that a number of potential patients were trampled to death in the rush to get to him. Samuel Johnson was one of the last sufferers to be touched by Queen Anne, who was also the last of the English monarchs to believe in the practice. Just four years old at the time, it would appear, both from Rowlandson's drawings as from Boswell's biography, that Johnson did not benefit from the experience.

By the mid-seventeenth century it was recorded in the London Bills of Mortality that one in five of the deaths in the city was due to consumption, the older and rather more descriptive name for the pulmonary form of the disease. From the seventeenth to the nineteenth century in England, like the other great towns and cities of Europe and America, it swept on in a continuing epidemic of such monstrous proportion, the disease was called The White Plague of Europe.

Many people assume that tuberculosis first came to America,

as a secondary spread from the European epidemic, in the wake of Columbus. While this is believed to be true of other diseases, such as smallpox, measles, mumps and chickenpox, it is not true of tuberculosis. We know this because American Indians collected the bones of their dead in huge ossuaries making it easy for archaeologists to examine whole communities of skeletons. From these it is clear that the disease already affected Pre-Columbian America, with epidemics raging through the Huron Indians of prehistoric Ontario and the native Indians of New York State.[13] Human figures with the typical collapsed spines decorate the art of the Maja, and tuberculosis germs have been found in a Peruvian mummy dating from before Columbus.[14] The disease extended to the furthermost reaches of prehistoric Asia, as was seen in a skeleton of the Ainu of protohistoric Japan,[15] and in animal remains such as the Indian elephant from before 2,000 BC.[16]

Haltingly, over those two and a half millenia, a painfully slow progress did take place in our understanding of tuberculosis. We learnt that the disease that ate away lungs was the same disease that caused children to die in convulsions; we learnt that the mysterious ague that caused spines to disintegrate and collapse into hunchbacks was the same mystery that caused a grotesque thickening and reddening of the skin of the face, leading to a wolf-like appearance, called *lupus vulgaris*. We learnt it was contagious. By the later years of the nineteenth century a French army doctor called Villemin had gone so far as to show it could be transmitted from infected human tissue to animals. Yet no treatment could possibly cure the disease while its real cause remained a mystery, and this mystery still eluded the most knowledgeable of doctors, as it had for several thousand years.

About the turn of the nineteenth century, the death rate worldwide was estimated at seven million people a year with fifty million openly infected and London and New York two of the worst affected cities. At least half the world's population had come into contact with it, often unaware of the fact they were harbouring living germs in their lungs. During the late nineteenth century, there was a growing fear that the disease might destroy European civilization.

It seems hard to believe that such a desperate situation could be changed by the determination of one man – yet this is precisely what happened. The manner in which he did so, and the lecture in which he announced his discovery to the world – a lecture which is generally accepted as the most important in medical history – would become the first step in the twentieth-century search for the cure.[17]

iii

In Berlin, on the evening of 24 March 1882, a feverish excitement surrounded a small bespectacled man, who was about to address the Physiological Society. Not many years before, Robert Koch, then a totally unknown country doctor, had draped a sheet across his living room to fashion the makeshift laboratory in which he would study bacteria under the microscope his wife, Emmy, had bought him for his birthday. Today, the tiny lecture room, though small and plain, was filled with the most eminent men of science in Germany. Paul Ehrlich was amongst them, a fun-loving extrovert with a reputation for chain-smoking cigars and heavy beer drinking. In stark contrast to this colourful young man was the most distinguished member of the audience, the famous pathologist, Rudolph Virchow. Virchow, regarded as the Czar of German medicine, was the reason why Koch was delivering his presentation in a physiological institute and not in the school of medicine. Medical research throughout Germany was so dominated by this man that his word was taken as gospel; and only recently he had rejected Koch's theories of the bacterial cause of disease. The very establishment of the Imperial Health Office, which employed Koch, was regarded as a personal affront by Virchow, and Koch and all of his work since his employment there had been shunned by Virchow and his school. Now the "Czar" sat grimly waiting, prepared to pour scorn on the young speaker.

Koch rose, he was seen to fumble nervously with his papers as his face wrinkled with concentration. Short sighted, he had to peer closely into those same papers as he began to read. In the words of his friend and colleague, Loeffler, present in the audience and later to become a world famous bacteriologist in his own right: "Koch was by no means a dynamic lecturer who would overwhelm his audience with brilliant words. He spoke slowly and haltingly, but what he said was clear, simple, logically stated – in short, pure unadulterated gold."[18]

His nervousness would not prevent Koch presenting his argument, and he had prepared his ground with a thoroughness that predicted the scientific methods of the twentieth century. It would take some time. He began with the title of his lecture: *Die Tuberculose* – On Tuberculosis. A vague title – it would hardly have attracted such a distinguished audience had it not been for Koch's reputation, added to which there was some curious sense of expectancy. The real subject matter of his lecture had been deliberately kept secret and many of his audience were ignorant of the work he was about to describe since not a word of the experiments which Koch had been conducting since the 18th August of the previous year had been leaked to the public.

He began by reminding them of the terrifying statistics. "If the importance of a disease for mankind is measured by the number of fatalities it causes, then tuberculosis must be considered much more important than those most feared infectious diseases, plague, cholera and the like. One in seven of all human beings dies from tuberculosis. If one only considers the productive middle-age groups, tuberculosis carries away one third and often more of these."

His audience hardly needed reminding. They had been fighting a hopeless battle against tuberculosis all of their working lives.

Koch moved on to acknowledge the debt he owed to earlier researchers, in particular the French army doctor, Villemin. But Villemin, like Klebs, Cohnheim, Salomonsen – indeed every single previous investigator – had failed to find a bacterial cause.

"The nature of tuberculosis," he murmured gruffly, "has been studied by many, but this has led to no successful results. Those staining methods which have been so useful in the demonstration of pathogenic micro-organisms in other diseases have

been unsuccessful here. Every experiment devised for the isolation and culture of the tuberculous infective agent has also
failed. In my own studies on tuberculosis I began by using those
same methods, without success. But several casual observations have induced me to throw away these methods and to
strike out in a new direction – " his voice, though never raised,
was insistent, "which has finally led me to positive results. The
proof was possible through a certain staining procedure which
has allowed the discovery of characteristic, although previously
undescribed, bacteria in organs which have been altered by
tuberculosis."

His presentation must have been interrupted by a rush of
excited murmurings. Both Loeffler and Ehrlich would later describe the increasing excitement with which the audience
followed every step of his work.

Koch well realized the enormity of what he had just disclosed. Yet Ehrlich, describing the speech later, would remark
on how Koch's face remained impassive throughout. He had,
he continued calmly, been forced to invent a new manner of
staining. There was something very unusual about the
bacterium which needed a totally new method of staining or
else you couldn't see it. The eyes of his audience followed
Koch's directions, to the table immediately in front of him on
which, before the lecture, he had painstakingly set out more
than 200 of his preparations. He had brought his entire laboratory with him: his microscopes, test tubes with cultures, Erlen-
meyer flasks, small square glass boxes containing cultures, slips
of dead human and animal tissue preserved in alcohol. He was
quite happy for them to check his findings for themselves. He
expected them to do so – as indeed, these formally trained
scientists would.

This was clearly the most vital step in Koch's discovery and
they listened very carefully to what he was telling them. He had
selected freshly developed abscesses, called tubercles, in
human beings who had died from tuberculosis. He had
removed some of the pus from the abscesses and smeared it
over glass cover slips. Next he stained the smears on the glass
with dyes to see what was visible. A dye developed by Ehrlich,
methylene blue, was his first choice, and he stained numerous

smears using this. Everybody was familiar with methylene blue. But methylene blue just coloured everything with the same deep blue stain, making it very difficult to pick out any fine detail, such as a tiny bacterium. Yes, this was a problem, as he admitted. But he had overcome the problem by pouring over his glass slides a second counterstain.

"When the cover slips are removed from the methylene blue, the adhering film is dark blue and strongly overstained, but the treatment with vesuvin removes the blue colour and the films were now seen to be light brown in colour." At this point in his speech, Koch failed to mention something very important in the subsequent search for the cure for tuberculosis. In the words of Loeffler:

"However, the brilliant research talent of Robert Koch was soon to be illuminated in even greater degree. After he had used his new technique to demonstrate the characteristic rods (bacteria) in all possible tuberculous tissues and fluids, he considered it necessary to repeat the whole experiment with freshly prepared dyes. But when he examined his new preparations, which had been stained for twenty four hours in fresh methylene blue solution and counterstained with vesuvin, he sought in vain under the microscope for the blue staining rods . . ."[19]

A minor diversion for Koch, yet it would later assume great significance.

It was absolutely necessary, he explained, not only to add the vesuvin but to heat the slide thoroughly and for what seemed a long period of time. Otherwise you had to wait for an entire day. They followed the movements of his hands as he indicated the two bottles, one the blue of midnight and the other the brown-black of liquorice. "Now – under the microscope the structures of the animal tissues, such as the nucleus and its breakdown products, are brown, while the tubercle bacteria are a beautiful blue. Indeed, all other bacteria except the bacterium of leprosy assume a brown colour. The colour contrast between the brown coloured tissues and the blue tubercle bacteria is so striking that the bacteria, although often present in very small numbers, are quite easy to find and recognize."

His audience gazed at Koch in unconcealed amazement. Every one of them was a doctor or scientist for whom the cause of tuberculosis was the greatest mystery. Pressed against the sides of his lectern, Ehrlich was close enough to see the darkly wrinkled skin of Koch's fingers, a consequence of so many antiseptic washings with bichromate of mercury. You were careful with disinfecting your hands when you were working with tuberculosis. Ehrlich would later confess that he could barely contain his own excitement: "I hold that evening to be the most important experience of my scientific life."[20]

Koch had arrived, in his slow and painstaking way, at the explanation for the difficulty with the new counterstain. There was something special about the covering of the bacterium: "It seems likely that the tubercle bacillus is surrounded with a special wall of unusual properties . . ." In this very first presentation of his findings and after just eight months of research, he had put his finger on the key factor in the global quest for the cure.

Only three weeks later his speech would be enshrined in a Berlin medical journal,[21] yet the message would already be old news – for tonight the telegraph wires would be humming. By tomorrow morning the name of Robert Koch would be a sensation throughout mainland Europe.

He continued his patient argument: to show the presence of his beautiful blue bacillus was not enough. His audience should note how the bacteria were always present in tuberculous infections; how if you took particles of lung from an animal which was infected or had died from tuberculosis, you could grow the bacterium on solidified serum slopes; how the bacterium of tuberculosis only grew very very slowly, first appearing to the naked eye about the second week, as dry scaly dots; how patient you needed to be with these cultures, which grew so very slowly, yet could be readily transmitted from one culture to another, and then reinjected into animals.

Under the yellow glow of gas lights, he picked out some dissections of tissue amongst the hundreds that crowded the table: guinea pigs inoculated with tuberculous material from the lungs of infected apes, from the brains and lungs of humans that had died of blood-borne tuberculosis, from the cheesy masses in the lungs of chronic human sufferers, from the abdominal cavities of cattle infected with tuberculosis. In all cases the disease which developed in the test guinea pigs was the same. The cultures of bacteria obtained from the guinea pigs was identical on the serum slopes . . .

His audience no longer murmured. They watched him with a fixity that was unnerving. Koch himself wondered if the long sequence of proofs had been too much for them. Perhaps even worse still, confirming the pessimism he had confessed earlier that day to Loeffler: "It will take a year of hard battle before the world will be convinced."[22]

In London John Tyndall, an eminent physicist and scientific educator, waited impatiently to receive the written transcript of this lecture. Twelve days after receiving it he would publish an English summary in the London *Times*,[23] a summary which would be copied unaltered a few weeks later in the *New York Times*,[24] when the editor would rail at the delay in America's receiving the news . . . "it is safe to say that the little pamphlet which was left to find its way through the slow mails to the English scientist outweighed in importance and interest for the human race all the press dispatches which have been flashed under the Channel since the date of the delivery of the address – March 24. The rapid growth of the continental capitals, the movements of princely noodles and fat, vulgar duchesses, the debates in the Serbian Skupschina, and the progress or receding of sundry royal *gouts* are given to the wings of lightning; a lumbering mailcoach is swift enough for the news of one of the great scientific discoveries of the age . . ." American doctors would rush to get a copy of the article, to study with minute detail every word of this methodical little German doctor, Robert Koch, who continued with his patient explanation, laying proof upon proof, attempting to confound his own findings, probing his own conclusions from every possible angle. But no matter what the permutation, no matter how the inoculation, no matter what animal he inoculated, the results were always the same. The animals injected with those gracefully curved blue-staining bacilli subsequently developed the typical features of tuberculosis. With his work-shrivelled and blackened fingers, he marshalled his papers together.

"All of these facts taken together can lead to only one conclusion: that the bacilli which are present in the tuberculosis substances not only accompany the tuberculous process, but are the cause of it. In the bacilli we have, therefore, the actual infective cause of tuberculosis."

Not bad air, not just a weakness of the infected human being's immune system, not any of the myriad theories that had filled the puzzled heads of his audience all of their working lives . . . but a bacterium. Not just a bacterium – but a bacillus the like of which had never been even suspected before, a most singular life form, with a frightening propensity to infect every cat and chicken, pigeon and guinea pig, the white mice and rats, oxen and even the two marmosets, into which Koch had injected it.

The reaction at the end of his speech was strange, baffling to Koch himself. Where one would have expected applause, congratulation, at the very least some heated questioning, in fact there was a complete silence. Virchow put on his hat and stormed from the room without speaking a word.

2

The Lines of Battle

The Lord shall smite thee with a consumption, and with a fever, and with an inflammation . . . and they shall pursue thee until thou perish.

Deuteronomy 28:22

i

WITH HIS DISCOVERY of the bacterial cause of tuberculosis, Robert Koch had brushed aside the encrusted cobwebs, old superstitions and misconceptions that had taken doctors and their patients down blind alleys ever since the dark ages. Yet vital questions about the disease remained unanswered. Most vital of all – how could a tiny living organism develop such a terrible pedigree?

The bacterium that causes tuberculosis, *Mycobacterium tuberculosis*, is barely three millionths of a metre in length and so slender as to be practically meaningless. It grows very slowly, at barely a thirtieth the rate of normal bacteria. It divides and reproduces equally slowly. Perhaps there is something in this reluctant growth that makes it virtually indestructible?

When Robert Koch first saw it down his microscope he remarked two things: using his stain it was a beautiful and brilliant blue; and it reminded him of another terror, the bacterium that causes leprosy. He was right. They are indeed first cousins, both members of the same genus, the *Mycobacteria*. The germ that causes tuberculosis is very difficult to grow in laboratory cultures. It is the most difficult of all to stain for viewing on a

16

microscopic slide. When Koch attempted to confirm his initial staining of the bacterium using a new solution of methylene blue, counterstained with vesuvin, the swarms of bacteria had disappeared. He repeated the stain using the old methylene blue and they appeared again. Something had happened to the old dye solution that made it peculiarly suitable for staining the bacterium. But what? Koch concluded that it must have absorbed some chemical from the air of his laboratory and the most likely choice was ammonia. He then added small amounts of ammonia to his new test solution and immediately the bacteria became visible again. The ammonia contaminating the stain had somehow damaged the surface covering of the bacterium and it had been this damage that had enabled the methylene blue to stain it. Within months this technique for staining tuberculosis bacteria would be improved by the colourful young man who had listened with such rapt attention to Koch's lecture, Paul Ehrlich. Ehrlich so perfected it that the technique we use today is a modification of that devised by him more than a hundred years ago.

Just five years after he had invented the stain, it would come to have a more personal significance. In 1887, he noticed a mild persistent cough, soon developing into a resistant fever with night sweats; he began to lose weight at an alarming rate, his health declining so rapidly that his friends feared for his life. Ehrlich used his own stain only to discover, to his horror, that he himself was suffering from tuberculosis. Fortunately his disease was mild and he survived.

ii

WE ARE INFECTED by the germ that causes tuberculosis in two ways, either by inhaling it in the air we breathe, or by swallowing it in food or drink. Inhalation is the commonest way in which it gets into our bodies, taking in bacteria which are suspended in dried dust or in tiny droplets. If a tiny colony on a culture plate contains in excess of a billion tuberculous germs, consider the numbers of germs flung into the air by the single cough of an infected patient. Unlike AIDS, which is spread only by sexual penetration or by intravenous injection of blood products, tuberculosis is contracted simply by the act of breathing. Everybody is therefore susceptible. The dangerous ease with which it infects people even today in the United Kingdom can be seen from these typical examples.

In July 1978 in Uppingham, England, a nine-year-old girl developed a skin rash over her legs, with painful raised red discs the size of a pre-decimal penny. A skin test was positive (indicating she had come into contact with tuberculosis) and this was enough for her to be treated as a presumptive case of tuberculosis. In December of the same year a second child was seen with the same skin rash and a strongly positive skin test. In mid-December a third child became unwell, developed a cough, his illness developing into a fever, tiredness and finally full-blown tuberculous meningitis. The headmaster at the school all three had attended informed the authorities and a screening programme was set up involving all the adults and children at one primary school. Of a total of 215 children attending the school, 43 had strongly positive skin tests to tuberculosis, 25 of whom had abnormal chest X-rays, two of them with tuberculous meningitis: all 43 required antituber-culous drug treatment. The outbreak was traced back to a single female teacher, whose chest X-ray showed multiple small cavities.[1]

In 1984 there were two similar outbreaks, one in an Ox-fordshire school, traced back to a single infected teacher,[2] and another in Barnstaple, North Devon, where 32 children were infected by a mother who had only come into contact with the children at two Christmas parties.[3]

Over the last three or four decades, a myriad of similar epi-demics have been reported from other parts of the developed world, including the United States, Germany, Sweden, France, Japan, Canada, Ireland, Australia, New Zealand, South Africa, Switzerland, Italy, Norway and the Netherlands. While many originated in schools, others resulted from chance contacts at parties, restaurants, visiting friends and relatives at Christmas, indeed any activity that brought a single sufferer with an infec-tious cough into close contact with a large number of uninfected people.[4]

We can screen people for infection by injecting into the skin a protein derived from the tuberculosis germ. A positive reaction means either that the person is openly infected or, more commonly, has had an infection with tuberculosis in the past. Some idea of its remarkable infectivity will be gathered from the fact that one thousand seven hundred million people in the world today are positive on skin testing, a third of the earth's population.

The second main way to contract tuberculosis is by drinking milk from an infected cow. One of the great public health measures which helped in the war against milk-borne tuberculosis was the skin testing of cattle with tuberculin, which enabled farmers and health authorities to eliminate infected animals. Tuberculosis from milk or milk products usually causes disease in children with scrofulous glands in the neck, which ulcerate and discharge pus. The infection may spread to cause a very painful form of ulceration of the throat, making it difficult to speak, or more dangerous still, a potentially fatal ulceration throughout the intestines. The lung infection can also spill into the intestines because the sufferer swallows infected sputum. But it is the pulmonary form of the disease which is by far the commonest and it was in this form that tuberculosis blighted the lives of billions of people.

What happens is basically simple if dreadful. The bacteria inhaled in water droplets settle in the periphery of the lung and grow very slowly until they form a small local collection, like a cheesy boil. From this boil, the continuing infection spills over into nearby small airways and forms more of these tiny boils. It was the appearance of these small cheesy collections (like little tubers) which, in the early nineteenth century, gave rise to the modern name, the disease in which you find tubercles in the lung, or tuberculosis. This replaced the much older and more descriptive name, *consumption*. What terror this word must have brought to the hearts of so very many people!

From this first or primary infection in the lungs, several things may happen.

In many, the first infection is fought off by the body. The white cells mop up the bacteria and the abscess is walled off from the rest of the lung by a fibrous shell. But our white cells have difficulty disposing of these ingested bacteria. That waxy shell can be as impervious to the digesting chemicals of our white cells as it is to acid, and tuberculosis has the horrifying ability to eat our white cells themselves from the inside and to grow and multiply while actually within the cells. In order to contain the disease, our body decides to accept stalemate and just wall it off. If we succeed, we lull ourselves into a false sense of security: we tell ourselves that we are cured. But tuberculosis remains alive within that fibrous shell and can burst out into life-threatening virulence at any time in the infected person's subsequent life. Relapse is always a possibility, even forty years later, and tends to occur at a time when our physical or mental health is low.

So what was it like to be told you were suffering from tuberculosis? The writer, Betty MacDonald, described this experience with poignancy and humour.

A working divorcee with two small children, she was told bluntly, "You have pulmonary tuberculosis and will have to go to a sanitorium." That feeling, the flickering nightmarish fear, suddenly mushroomed in her. Tuberculosis . . . sanitorium . . . a place where people go to die! She could only sit in front of this doctor, her gaze momentarily fallen onto her gloves and purse, which lay passively on the desk in front of her.

> For somebody who had just pronounced my death sentence, the doctor seemed singularly untouched. He was whistling "There's a small hotel" and looking up a number in the telephone directory. It was nearly five o'clock and the September evening fog had begun to drift up the waterfront. In the lighted windows of an office across the court I watched the girls jam things quickly into drawers, slam files closed and hurry into their coats and hats. I said to the doctor,
>
> "What about my job?"
>
> He had hung up the phone and was leaning back in his chair, suntanned and handsome. "Oh, you won't be able to work for a long time. You're contagious too," he said comfortingly.
>
> "How long will I have to go to a sanitorium?"
>
> "At least a year – probably longer."
>
> I picked up my purse and gloves and said goodnight. As I went through the waiting room I could hear him whistling "There's a small hotel".[5]

iii

WHERE TUBERCULOSIS IS common, most of the population will encounter germs when they are children. Yet here we discover another of its mysteries: the majority wall it off when it is still just a spot in the lungs and they never know they were infected. But if the body fails to contain it, which is the case in about ten per cent of people, then the disease continues to invade the lung tissue about it. This slow spread throughout the lungs, scarring and ruining them by infiltration, is the common pattern of tuberculosis, taking years to kill its victim. This was how it acquired its ancient name, consumption, which aptly described the progressive wasting of the body and the final consuming high fever. This almost primaeval term is the same in many of the old and great languages of the world. The English word was derived from the old French, *consomption*, itself derived from the Latin, *consumptio*: we find that identical meaning in the Hebrew of the Bible, *Schachepheth*; in the ancient Greek, *phthisis*; in the Urdu, *tabey diq*; and the eloquently descriptive Hindu *xoy*, which signifies the waning of the moon. Even the little community of Pathans, who inhabit the North-West Frontier, bordering the present day Pakistan and Afghanistan, had their age-old name for it: *Nare maraz*, the thinning fever.

Nowhere in these ancient communities of the Eurasian land mass, where it was so common and feared, is there a record of its beginning. Throughout history, it had always been there, a familiar evil, yet forever changing, formless, unknowable. Where other epidemics might last weeks or months, where even the bubonic plague would be marked forever afterwards by the year it reigned, the epidemics of tuberculosis would last whole centuries and even multiples of centuries. Tuberculosis rose slowly, silently, seeping into the homes of millions, like an ageless miasma. And once arrived, it never went away again. Year after year, century after century, it tightened its relentless hold, worsening whenever war or famine reduced the peoples' resistance, infecting virtually everybody, inexplicably sparing some while destroying others, bringing the young down onto their sickbeds, where the flesh slowly fell from their bones and they were consumed in the years-long fever, their minds brilliantly alert until, in apocalyptic numbers, they died, like the fallen leaves of a dreadful and premature autumn.

Why should tuberculosis move in such timeless epidemics? We simply do not know. Why should it follow such a malignant course in one person while sparing another? Chance, timing, circumstance, age at exposure, duration and severity of exposure, natural powers of resistance – all of these and more are known to play some part. But often there is no apparent reason: it is simply a mystery. In most of us who have lived through a time when the disease was common, all that remains is a few calcified spots on our chest X-rays, a telltale evidence of a battle fought out in the blissful ignorance of childhood – yet a battle that decided if we would live or die.

If a baby or very young child inhales the germs, or ingests them in milk, there may be very little immunity. Indeed in babies there may be nothing at all to see in the chest X-ray, even when they are in the terminal coma of tuberculous meningitis. Yet up to ninety per cent of babies and young children survive. One link is however absolutely certain. If the infected person is undernourished, if their immunity is depressed (as in the modern example of AIDS), then the disease erupts with an explosive virulence.

For the less lucky amongst us, the disease cannot be controlled by the body's defences. They discover a cough which refuses to go away; perhaps there is a sudden agonizing pain on breathing that marks the beginning of pleurisy; sooner or later will come the gathering exhaustion, the unrelievable breathlessness, the appearance of bright red arterial blood in the persistent foul sputum. In others, death arrives in one fell moment, for example when an abscess in the lung or intestine erodes into a major artery. When this happens the bleeding may be so torrential that the victim dies from exsanguination or from drowning in his own blood. Alois Hitler, the father of Adolf, died from such a haemorrhage on 3 January 1903. He was stricken while taking a morning walk and died a few moments later in a nearby inn in the arms of a neighbour. "When his thirteen-year-old son saw the body of his father, he broke down and wept."[6] Adolf Hitler also developed an illness which is believed to have been pulmonary tuberculosis when he was fifteen-years-old, though he evidently survived.

Often the germs invade a smaller blood vessel, resulting in the repeated coughing of bright red arterial blood, which may signal the final relapse. This was the distressing omen for John Keats, who died aged twenty five in 1821. His dying face was captured in sepia wash by his friend, the artist Joseph Severn . . . "3 o'clock morning, drawn to keep me awake. A dreadful sweat was on him all this night". More recently a lung haemorrhage caused the death of Vivien Leigh, wife of Laurence Olivier and heroine of *Gone with the Wind*, who had suffered from pulmonary tuberculosis for many years of her life. One of the most lethal complications of tuberculosis occurs when pus spills into a small blood vessel, from where it quickly spreads by the blood stream to every organ of the body. This is the condition called "miliary tuberculosis", because the tiny shadows in the lungs appear on the chest X-ray like scattered millet seeds.

Over the long years in which tuberculosis causes the typical slow decline in health, evoked by its ancient name, the disease has a tendency to spread from the lungs or bowel and cause great pain and suffering elsewhere in the body. In the skin and soft tissues it causes disfiguring sores and abscesses; in the internal organs such as the bladder and kidneys it causes an agonizing inflammation. The pain associated with bladder tuberculosis was so severe that earlier in this century surgeons would transplant the ureters into the skin to bypass the bladder in a desperate attempt both to relieve the suffering and delay the development of the kidney failure that would eventually kill the patient. In bones it settles into a protracted and gnawing destructive cavitation, called osteomyelitis, its pus eventually finding its way through the surrounding soft tissues until it erupts onto the skin, where it continues to discharge until the sufferer eventually dies from it. The surgical treatment for osteomyelitis of the tibia was to lay open the bone from the knee to the ankle to allow free drainage in the hope that this might allow a small percentage of the sufferers to heal. Tuberculosis has the capacity to infect every internal organ, from liver to brain, from the fingertips to the delicate structures of our eyes.

Even today, without effective treatment, sixty per cent of

sufferers will be dead within five years of the onset, their bodies wasted to skeletal proportions, their minds lucidly aware of the life that is being taken from them.

This was the fear of the writer Betty MacDonald, as for the composers Chopin and Paganini. It was the secret sorrow behind the pallid beauty of Simonetta Vespucci, the model for Botticelli's Venus, who was painted after her death by Piero di Cosimo, a serpent curled about her breast to signify the disease that would kill her at the tender age of twenty-three years. Jean Jacques Rousseau suffered lung haemorrhages in childhood, as did Goethe. Anton Checkov had his first haemorrhage at the age of twenty-five and for the next fifteen years was hardly ever free from fever and sickness. The great German poet and dramatist, Schiller, who wrote the "Ode to Joy" in the choral of Beethoven's ninth symphony, suffered his first attack when he was thirty-three years old. The remainder of his life was a tragic tug-of-war between the peaks of his genius and the depressive relapses of the disease that would end his life at the premature age of forty-six. Cardinal Richelieu, Sterne, Shelley, Edgar Allan Poe, Eugene O'Neill, Sir Walter Scott – these are just a tiny fraction of an endless litany of artists, writers, composers, statesmen who died from the disease.

There seemed such a common association between tuberculosis and great art that the disease was invested with a specious romanticism and glamour. It was believed that tuberculosis could inspire genius, the so-called *spes phthisica*, as if the bacterium infused into its victims some ambrosial stimulant.

Real life consumptive beauties inspired the arts. Mimi, of the opera *La Bohème*, was based on the true story of a beautiful flower girl of humble origins who deserted her shoemaker husband to glitter fleetingly in the wild demimonde of 1840s Paris, falling in love with Henri Murger, who wrote her story after she had died from the disease. Alphonsine Plessis, another doomed consumptive beauty, was Verdi's model for his great opera, *La Traviata*. Poetry fell into an enchantment with autumnal images. The disease was the inspiration for many a Gothic Victorian bestseller. *In David Copperfield*, Little Blossom dies gracefully, without the distressing imagery of true physical suffering. In this midnight sky, the brightest star was undoubtedly Emily Brontë, throughout whose writing there is a calm acceptance of this dreadful mortality of mere children, which mirrored the reality of the village of Haworth, where the writer lived. Emily's great novel, *Wuthering Heights*, explored with a tormented passion the forbidden love between Cathy and her turbulent adopted brother, Heathcliffe. The novel became a tragic prophecy of real life when, following the death of her wayward but deeply loved brother, Branwell, Emily developed symptoms of consumption herself and, refusing to rest or to see a doctor, she died just three months after Branwell.

It would be all too easy to forget that for the vast majority of its victims, poor and without artistry, the reality of tuberculosis was a distant cry from the pampered invalid of Edwardian paintings: it was the young boy or girl unable to take part in sports at school, too breathless to enjoy life, or the wasted adult driven to poverty by the inability to work, the intermittent years-long separations from family and friends while incarcerated in the sanitoria, the final months of consuming fever, the skeletal weight loss, the coughing of bright red arterial blood into the lonely night-time pillow. Perhaps the most haunting image of all is that of the baby, hidden behind screens in the remotest corner of the hospital ward, where the fatal agony of tuberculous meningitis could be hidden from sight.[7]

iv

IN 1908, Robert Koch made a monumental error when he told a meeting of eminent doctors in New York that bovine tuberculosis was not a source of infection to humans. His American audience were in no doubt that he was mistaken. "On a correct solution of this question depends the health and lives of many children." When Koch left America, his reputation was in tatters.

On his return to Berlin, he immediately threw himself into new studies on tuberculosis. But he never completed them. His health was rapidly failing and he died, aged sixty-seven, on 27 May 1910, at Baden-Baden from a heart attack. For tuberculosis sufferers throughout the world, it was a major setback. The search for the cure fell into a decline that would last more than thirty years. Yet, simultaneously, in Germany a new concept in treatment was beginning to find followers – a philosophy that was regarded with as great a scepticism in orthodox medical circles then as holistic medicine is regarded by those same authorities today. This was the sanitorium movement.

The inspiration for this breakthrough began with an eccentric English doctor, George Bodington, who travelled his rural rounds on horseback and who noticed that country people were much less prone to tuberculosis than those who lived in the crowded towns and cities. He advocated a revolutionary new treatment, notable for its charity towards the suffering patient: "A pure atmosphere, freely demonstrated without fear."[8] Before he died, in 1882, the very year of Koch's lecture, Bodington had set up a small nursing home based on his ideas on open air treatment. Nobody took the slightest notice, apart from a single German doctor, Hermann Brehmer, who was sufficiently impressed to build a small sanitorium at Görbersdorf in 1859. Brehmer added regular exercise to pure mountain air, a not unpleasant cocktail which really did appear to help sufferers; patients flocked to try his treatment, causing other doctors to sit up and take notice, and soon more sanitoria were opened throughout the world.

Unbelievable as it might seem, the great sanitorium movement which grew from such humble beginnings, with its massive utilization of public and private funding, was never subjected to a scientific trial of its effectiveness. But there is an abundance of indirect evidence to suggest that such general measures would not cure a patient who was seriously infected.[9] In mild and early cases, it seems likely that life could be prolonged and that the course of the disease could be slowed down, allowing the body's natural defences a better chance of healing. The ambience of the more exclusive private sanitorium was elegantly captured by Thomas Mann in his Nobel Prize winning novel, *The Magic Mountain*. But Mann's mountain was an idyll, catering for a prosperous elite and supplying a comfort quite unlike that of the public sanitorium. Many ordinary people in the real world were offered no treatment at all. The spartan conditions of the more enlightened American sanitoria, were vividly described by H. Corwin Hinshaw:

The majority of patients were in the age group 20–35 years. The basic remedy was "bed rest" in its most stringent form: 24 hours flat. Meals were spooned to each patient by registered nurses, bed baths and the universal bedpans were imposed on these youngsters who looked and felt normal but who had shadows – even small shadows – on their chest X-ray films. All this in an effort to halt the persistent and almost inevitable trend for such small lesions to advance and destroy the patient. The average patient spent more than a full year in bed, many others much more. Careers were abandoned, marriage was discouraged and pregnancy virtually forbidden. Stress in any form and to any degree must be avoided.[10]

It is a sad fact that in the overburdened clinics attended by the poor, the sheer volume of patients, coupled with the depressing outlook of a disease that killed more than half of its victims within five years of the onset, could sometimes lead to the sufferers being treated with an unthinking cruelty. While the majority of doctors and nurses – who had often chosen their vocation after surviving tuberculosis themselves – were selflessly devoted and caring; nevertheless, the very inflexibility of the sanitorium regime, its wearisome duration and the tender age of so many of the patients, left them desperately vulnerable to tyranny. One eminent physician in Edinburgh, harbouring the common notion that the working class did not have feelings, would declare to his ward full of sick girls: "Here you are, a collection of rosy apples, all rotten at the core!"[11] In the municipal clinics and sanitoria, fighting an unwinnable battle against mass poverty, suffering and looming mortality, the kindly regimes of Bodington and Brehmer could all too readily degenerate into a monotonous cycle of psychological and physical torment, heart-breakingly evoked by A.E. Ellis in his novel, *The Rack*.[12]

The most famous sanitoria in Europe were in Davos, Switzerland, the setting for Thomas Mann's *The Magic Mountain*.[13] Robert Louis Stevenson spent two winters there before travelling to Samoa, where he died from tuberculosis at the age of forty-four years. In the United States a young doctor called Edward Livingston Trudeau, himself a survivor, set up the first American sanitorium next to the beautiful Saranac Lake in the Adirondacks, north of New York.

The single most important achievement of such institutions – a very real and dramatically effective one – was the isolation of the infected from other potential victims. Another major benefit was the improved nutrition which bolstered the immune defences of the sufferers and helped to prolong their lives. But for the great majority of sufferers, we might best compare the treatment of tuberculosis in those days with our sometimes heroic methods of treating the less curable forms of cancer. "It was the fortunate patient who might qualify for surgical treatment"[14], where the operations devised were aimed at resting the affected lung or lungs by reducing the patient's ability to take a full breath. This was achieved in various ways, for example by crushing the nerves to the diaphragm (phrenic crush), by repeatedly injecting air into the potential cavity between the lungs and the chest wall (artificial pneumothorax), by inserting synthetic balls or other bulky solids into the chest cavity at open thoracotomy, or most desperate and destructive of all – and usually performed to try to close cavities in the lungs – thoracoplasty, or excision of whole portions of ribcage, leaving the unfortunate sufferer permanently deformed and with a defective breathing capacity. Such however were the experiences of the "lucky ones".

The surgeons were, after all, fighting an heroic battle against a death sentence – indeed, we should not underestimate the effectiveness of such general measures. The sum effect of the isolation of infective cases in the sanitoria, the rest and the operations, the reduction in milk-borne spread of the disease and the improved nutrition of the nation, was a remarkable reduction in the mortality throughout the Western World. Nevertheless, by 1930, 90,000 people a year still died from the disease in the United States, 66,000 in France and 50,000 in England and Wales. In the United Kingdom it accounted for almost half the total deaths in the population affecting men and women between the ages of twenty-five and thirty-five years. Governments throughout the civilized world brought together doctors, nurses, and lay workers to coordinate nationwide anti-tuberculosis campaigns, often under the tutelage of royalty. In Britain the disease was declared notifiable "among poor persons" in 1908.[15]

Programmes of public education were undertaken, fuelled by the enthusiasm of public spirited volunteers. In Britain, for instance, this took the form of "pilgrimage exhibitions" – the quaint title for a collection of diagrams, pictures and leaflets which was sent around the country in a horse-drawn vehicle. This was subsequently upgraded to a Morris van, its sides bedecked with promotional posters, which toured the length and breadth of the island, transporting a cine-camera with which "the historic saga of John McNeil" could be projected onto a screen. A Bunyonesque morality tale, this depicted the progress of a patient, who gamely endured the privations of the Edinburgh dispensary, before moving on to the salvation of the sanitorium. In the words of Harley Williams, one of the doctors involved: "Though full of laudable instruction this film was a little too good to be human. Soon the costumes of the wife and the nurse became out of fashion and raised loud hilarity. The fact is that health propaganda was in its infancy, and health education hardly born. Looking back, I am astonished at our faith in the advice which was all we could offer, for there was no X-ray diagnosis, no artificial pneumothorax, and no drugs, while TB clinics were hard to find. Often, members of the audience fainted, and there were angry questions at the end. I remember vividly occasions at the Speakers Corner at Marble Arch, London, where talks were given among political agitators, temperance lecturers and cranks of all kinds."[16]

While it might be a little grandiose to call this a war against the disease, behind the well-meaning and quintessentially British pantomime, there was a fierce determination to reduce the appalling death rate. The voluntary organizations were just a part of a much larger initiative, which was government inspired and which included the sanitoria, cheap health insurance, regular national medical conferences, the appointment of regional "tuberculosis officers", and county borough and city tuberculosis dispensaries for the poor, where X-ray investigation and artificial pneumothorax were provided free of charge. By 1936, as a result of an Act of Parliament, if a British tuberculosis sufferer lived in an insanitary house, he could get help from the Ministry of Health for improvements and even rehousing, and his family could obtain a small amount of assistance in food and clothing. Many such charitable benefits were distributed under the tuberculosis officers and their health visitors, from loans of beds and mattresses, free railway fares to and from institutions, even to the extraordinary lengths of retraining and permanent resettlement of sufferers and their entire families in tuberculosis colonies.[17]

Yet, more than fifty years after the introduction of the sanitoria, and despite all such well-meaning measures, the typical sufferer spent his or her shortened life shuttling between rest at home and the long queues at the clinic for medical attention, intermittently went back into the sanitorium, was shunned by most erstwhile friends and even relatives often just to suffer a more protracted form of the illness, eventually to die from the disease. In a medium sized city such as Edinburgh, as recently as 1954, a thousand new cases of tuberculosis were registered in a single year. Worldwide, in that same year, the death rate from tuberculosis remained an appalling five million.

The sanitorium doctors and nurses were dedicated and had amassed a formidable expertise in bacteriological and X-ray diagnosis of the disease in all its manifold presentations, and in the management of its life-threatening complications, but they lacked the single most vital weapon in their war against the disease. A desperate world looked to medical science for the cure.

3

New Jersey

Every morning, the vision of home and the moors rushed on her, and darkened and saddened the day. Her white face, attenuated form and failing strength threatened rapid decline. I felt in my heart she would die if she could not go home.

Charlotte Brontë, writing about her sister, Emily

i

THE SEARCH FOR the cure for tuberculosis was the most urgent medical problem that faced the entire world in the twentieth century. But how should anybody go about this search? Nobody had the slightest idea where to start. At this time, not a single medication had been invented to cure any known infection. Everybody seemed to have a different notion. While some, like Koch himself, believed that the answer lay with improving the natural defences of the human body, others were inspired with a messianic zeal for internal disinfection, rather along the lines of external disinfection as pioneered by the famous surgeon, Joseph Lister. Of course, the answer did not emerge from anything so simple, and after half a century of utter failure, this early optimism was replaced by pessimism. By the 1930s, few people worldwide believed that such a cure would ever be possible. Even those who still had faith in the cure knew by now that the struggle would be titanic.

The cure for the greatest killer in history would not emerge from the great centres of medical learning. No more would it arise from the collective efforts of the tuberculosis experts toiling away in the great sanitoria complexes. Instead it would come from the genius, courage and selfless devotion of a tiny handful of men, often the most unlikely of champions, working alone in disparate countries, yet every one of them gifted in his own unique way. Their involvement would need more even than creative genius. In a curious way, all the torment and turmoil of the most troubled century in history, with its wars, revolutions and its tidal wave of suffering and inhumanity, would prove as formative in this story as the intellectual forces of creation or the twentieth century explosion of technology. In the lives of each of these extraordinary men a moment would arrive, a single convergence of time and circumstance, which would initiate the train of events that would change history.

The story of the cure begins, for no reason other than it is a convenient place to start, with the birth of a child in the little town of Novaia-Priluka, 200 miles from Kiev, the capital of the Russian Ukraine.

ii

ZOLMAN ABRAHAM WAKSMAN – his name was later changed to the more Americanized Selman Waksman – was born, according to the old Russian calendar, on 8 July 1888, just six years after the famous lecture by Koch in the Physiological Institute in Berlin.

His father, Jacob, a city man from Vinnitsa, wove textiles for a living, and his mother, Fradia London, was a native of Priluka. The "Novaia" prefix to the town's name means new – there are other Prilukas in Russia – and the name Priluka means a fertile alluvial plain within the bend of a river.[1] In Waksman's own words, "The town would hardly impress a visitor as worth a second glance."[2] It had few comforts, a small dot on the boundless fertile plain of the Ukraine, where despite its great fecundity, life was little more than a bare existence, based on hard work and struggle. Spiritually however, "it was rich beyond description" and the little boy had a happy childhood, punctuated by periods of unrest when Cossacks attacked the villages in the area, using Jews as scapegoats for the social unrest.

Intelligent and precocious, the young Selman was very attached to his mother, who doted on her only son in a household of women. Fradia was an enlightened woman, who did her best to give him a good education against the odds of a tiny town that was little more than a collection of mud brick terraces in the huge backward land that was the late nineteenth century Ukraine. There is nothing unusual in a son loving his mother. But the relationship between Waksman and his mother was more intense than usual. "My mother loved me dearly, with an unselfish and devoted love. I knew how much she missed me when I had to leave home to complete my education. She led me on the path of righteousness, she counselled me, cautioned me, watched over me, took pride in my attainments, and listened to my ambitions; she encouraged me, when she felt that my own courage was beginning to fail at times. I was devoted to her. I repaid her love with a pride in her, with a desire to live up to her expectations."[3]

Selman's relationship with his father was a good deal less intense. "He was full of stories of wise men, who lived mostly in ancient times, and also of important historical events in the long life of the Jewish people. He and I were good friends, but not comrades. We seldom played games or engaged in activities that would bring us close together. But my father filled a certain place in my life, without which it would have been much poorer. He made it broader and richer, but not deeper or wiser. He was always in the shadow and did not play that profound part in the life of my boyhood that fathers usually do in the lives of their sons."[4]

If there was a passion second only to his mother, this was for the land itself. "The odour of the black soil so filled my lungs that I was never able to forget it: it was later to lead me to the study of the natural processes that are responsible for this aroma."[5]

Waksman grew into a shy youth, who would blush to his roots at the sight of a pretty girl, his high intelligence and imagination finding an escape in books. He craved the kind of adventure he read of in *Robinson Crusoe*, the stories of Jules Verne and *Life along the Mississippi* by Mayne Reid. More than anything, he would have loved to travel. He dreamed of becoming a great explorer, of discovering new tribes of Indians, new herbs, new remedies for curing human ills. He was well on his way to becoming "a dilettante, with a cursory knowledge of many things and without a fundamental background in anything," when a social turmoil shook old Russia and its society to its roots. Defeat at the hands of the Japanese in the war of 1904–05 threw the nation into consternation. Ordinary people awoke to the misery of their existence. They demanded change. They held meetings and discussions, condemned the government, built barricades, organized general strikes. Russia was already on the path towards revolution.

Even the little town in the Ukraine was drawn into this mood of disaffection. The young men knew that life could not continue as it had previously. You got nowhere without a formal education. With the sad acceptance of his mother, who realized that this meant she would lose him, he began the long struggle to get a university education in a country and political system which was implacably opposed to him because he was Jewish.

In April 1908 fate would intervene to save his life. On a clear night, the twenty-year-old Waksman set out in a horse-drawn sled to travel home to Priluka from the city of Vinnitsa, where he spent the weekdays studying. "We left the city in a gay mood, tuned to the peaceful earth, covered by the bright, freshly fallen snow, the well-illuminated sky. The horse knew the way so well that neither the coachman nor I was much disturbed by the road conditions. I recall now, forty-five years later, the bright moonlight and the limitless snow-covered fields, which glistened in the moonlight. Here and there we passed a sleeping village, with its snow-covered, straw-thatched adobe houses."[6]

By eleven o'clock they were approaching the river Bug, only six miles or so from Priluka, traversing a steep hill which led down to the frozen river. In the heady excitement of homecoming, neither driver nor rider paid any attention to the bunches of twigs tied to the telephone poles along the road, a peasant code for the fact that the icecap over the river was melting.

"I jumped off the sled and ran after it, keeping up with its speed, although at some distance behind it. The sled was just about in the middle of the river and I was approaching its shore, when the ice broke. Down into the icy waters went the sled with the driver and the horse. By some miracle, the horse managed to keep its head above water and the driver held onto the horse for dear life."[7]

The young man ran up the hill and alerted the sleeping peasants, who rescued the sled and driver. Later that same night, while recovering on a simple bed over the innkeeper's clay oven, Selman Waksman must have asked himself a very interesting question: why had he jumped from the sled at that critical moment, saving his life and perhaps the lives of very many more by doing so?

We could hazard guesses . . . youthful exuberance, simple joy instilled by the beauty and the peace of the scenery, together with the anticipation of warm firesides. Yet in his otherwise lucid recollections, some forty-five years later, the pragmatic scientist would offer nothing.

iii

AFTER A YEAR'S intensive private tuition, he tried the entrance examination for a gymnasium, or grammar school, but was failed by a bigoted examiner because he could not tell him the name of the river that flows through Berlin.

"It was a hard cruel system, which made easy prey of a boy who tried to beat it. I must have appeared in their eyes a provincial yokel, a simpleton who did not know what he was up against."[8] What was he to do now? Others might have been daunted but his mother understood him perfectly. "She asked me no questions . . . She only looked at me. Her eyes were full of disappointment but they also spoke of courage."[9] It would be this enduring aspect of his character, laid down in this long hard fight for an education, which would later prove important. Earning money by tutoring, he spent it on better teachers. In this personal struggle, surrounded by others engaged in that same struggle, and at an age to be profoundly influenced by the tidal wave of political discontent that was sweeping the country, there was little time for romance. The few girls that formed part of his circle of friends were considered comrades, with one notable exception. "Thus Masha, a girl with strivings similar to our own, was also shaping her life in terms of current problems facing the world rather than of boys as such. Most of the members of my close circle of friends fell periodically in love, one after another, with Masha, and even had ambitions of becoming her husband."[10]

In the September of 1908, he moved to Odessa, almost 400 miles from Priluka, where it was easier to prepare for the gymnasium examinations. His friend, Peisi, and two others travelled with him, "four provincial youths, ranging in age from eighteen to twenty, with healthy pink cheeks barely covered with a thin bloom of hair." The effects on their families, and in particular Waksman's mother, can well be imagined. Distances then were formidable barriers. Four hundred miles would take them nearly a day and a night to cover by train. Sprawled on an upper shelf of a fourth class carriage, packed with peasants, the four excited youths sang revolutionary songs and at each station would rush out to the dining room to fill their kettle with boiling water so they could make fresh tea.

It was finally in Odessa, the famous old seaport, with its sprawling boulevards, its quays, its port thronged with boats arriving and departing from all over the world, that the dreams of a new world, of travelling, of making a different life for himself, once more took fertile root in Selman's imagination. Rather than engage a single teacher, he joined an evening school, where teachers from a gymnasium were holding classes. The fees were high but the instruction was excellent. He devoured the teaching at night and studied all day. Making time, with his friends, to visit libraries, museums – where funds permitted even the theatre or the opera – they also attended political meetings, although Waksman was more interested in the intellectual challenge of his studies than politics. Among the teachers, two in particular impressed him deeply.

One was a giant called Kingi, who had a huge head with a thick beard and a mane of blond hair, who taught Russian literature. The other was Tarnarieder, a hunchback, who taught mathematics, physics and chemistry. Waksman now had real heroes to admire and to learn from. Tarnarieder in particular fulfilled this role, a Jew who was barred from a position either in a university or a gymnasium, yet who, despite the lack of a laboratory, communicated his great enthusiasm for science with the simple aid of a blackboard. He would stay behind with his students long after the classes were ended, talking enthusiastically of foreign universities, communicating as only a great teacher can, the mysteries and the joy of knowledge.

Selman passed his examinations with flying colours, his happiness tempered with sympathy for Peisi, who had failed abysmally. On his return to Priluka, he was seen as a hero, the first of its sons to pass the gymnasium examinations. He had an entire summer at home in which to enjoy his family once again and to earn money from more advanced tutoring that would help pay his way through the long years of higher education that lay ahead of him. But he would not be permitted long to savour his success.

"That summer, I was smitten by the greatest misfortune that could have befallen me – my mother died."[11] It came as a complete shock, without a single premonitory warning. One day, while he was home, she developed an acute blockage of the bowels. The local doctor was absent and Selman was forced to rush her by wagon to Vinnitsa, where a doctor was called to see her. He was unable to help, advising an immediate operation which could only be performed in a first-class hospital. Selman had to take her by train the 200 miles to Kiev, an overnight journey which was very hard on her. By the time she reached Kiev, it was too late. The doctors refused to operate with the result that she suffered a lingering and painful death over two weeks with her son day and night by her bedside. Her last words to him were, "My son, now that you need me most, I am going to leave you. Who will help you in your need!" That night, Waksman stayed with her body in the morgue but he offered no prayers before the burning candles. As Selman in his anguish declared – "That was the end!"[12]

Her loss was unbearable to him, throwing his life into turmoil and causing him to leave Russia for good. His last act before leaving was to visit Kiev, where she was buried, and place a monument on her grave. About the middle of October, 1910, a group of three men and two women left Priluka by train for the German border, accompanied to the nearest station by friends and relatives. They were happy to leave. As they crossed the border, they began to sing the revolutionary song, "We have shaken the shackles off our feet. We are entering upon a new world, a free world, where Man is free." A week later, Selman Waksman stood on the deck of a ship, travelling steerage from Bremen, and taking him to a new and fateful destiny in America.

iv

IT WOULD BE convenient for this story to claim that from his first arrival in America, Waksman was determined to find the cure for tuberculosis. But this was not the case. Writing his own account of his feelings at the time, some forty years later, he wrote: "One of the most interesting potential approaches to the tuberculosis problem was completely overlooked by experts. That approach came about through the study of lowly microbes by investigators who usually had little interest in or knowledge of the medical care of patients with tuberculosis."[13]

The young man making his difficult way in the New World was small and finely handsome with a passionate intensity to his brown eyes behind wire-rimmed spectacles. From his first arrival in the United States, he seemed to burn with an obsessive conviction of his destiny. Only if we understand just how close he had been to his mother, how she nurtured his childhood promise, can we even begin to understand the real nature of the fire that burnt in the heart of the young immigrant, who was so astonished by America that he would stare speechless at black people, whom he had heard about but never seen before.

The small immigrant group landed on a bright autumn afternoon, 2 November, at Philadelphia, where Selman was met by Mendel Kornblatt, a farmer who was married to his cousin, Molki. The Kornblatts lived near Metuchen, New Jersey, and Selman now went to live on the farm, where he helped in the poultry plant and laboured in the few acres that were used to grow truck vegetables. This could hardly continue indefinitely and so, although he was penniless, he knew he had to make a decision on his future.

"Why don't you go to Rutgers College?" was Kornblatt's suggestion.

Rutgers was the agricultural college at New Brunswick, just a stop down the line of the New Jersey railway. Selman duly paid a visit, where he met Dr Jacob G. Lipman, the Professor of soil microbiology, who was also a Russian immigrant, and a man who would help to guide Waksman's future. Lipman was clearly impressed with the young man and offered him a place at the college but Selman was divided in his own mind. "I had a general interest in the problem of chemical reactions of living bodies, but I had only a vague idea of how to go about such a study." He wondered if he should become a doctor. He had even been accepted on the basis of his gymnasium diploma for entry to the College of Physicians and Surgeons at Columbia Medical School, New York – but he couldn't afford to keep himself alive while studying. But Waksman would never forget the black earth of Priluka. Influenced by his childhood memories as much as by Lipman's practical encouragement, he enrolled as an agricultural student at Rutgers, on a free scholarship, where he graduated with a BSc in 1915. An eventful year for a young man who was impatient for progress, he changed his name from the Russian Zolman to Selman, became a naturalized American citizen, and married Deborah Bobili Mitnik, the sister of his best friend, Peisi, who had accompanied him to America and settled down in Philadelphia.

College life must have felt very strange after his somewhat bohemian tuition in Russia. He was twenty-three-years old in a class six years his junior. Uninterested in sport and in a state of culture shock with the New World, he felt very much out of place amongst the young Americans. His classmates would mock his ineptitude with the English language – "Who could blame them for roaring when I pronounced the letters OL in a mathematical formula as 'Oh hell!' "[14] At the same time, his high intelligence and dedication were beginning to show. In return for working his way as a night watchman in the college, they paid him twenty cents an hour and allowed him free board in a house in the centre of the grounds, where his light was seen to burn day and night. Even the spare time job, helping Dr Halsted, was seen as an opportunity. "On cold or rainy days and in the evening I helped with laboratory experiments. This turned out to be one of the most important decisions in my life."[15] Halsted was a master botanist from whom Waksman learnt the first principles of plant heredity, structure and the way in which a complex life form lived and worked.

Within a year he had added a masters degree, which soon caused him to leave New Jersey for Washington.

A simple incident from his early years in America is instructive. On a bright September morning in 1915, newly armed with his degree from Rutgers, he arrived at the old Department of Agriculture building in Washington, carrying a bag full of bacterial cultures. Doctor Charles Thom, who ran the laboratory, was a mature scientist and somewhat sceptical of the young graduate who spoke with a heavy Russian accent. Sizing up the intense expression in those sparkling dark eyes under the as yet unlined brow, he told Selman to close his bulging satchel.

"Look here – you're not planning to spend a lifetime here."

To Selman's surprise, Doctor Thom proposed a trip into the Washington fruit market.

"And what do I do when I get there?"

"You examine any fruit you can find that has gone rotten. And then you report your findings back here to me."

So he went, first thing the next morning, to examine lemons, oranges and other citrus fruits and take an interest in rottenness. To the disgust of the stallholders, he made a minute examination of the bad fruit and reported back to Thom that in his opinion there were two types of mould involved, one producing a wet rot and the other a hard dry rot. There was also a difference between the shades of green of the spores formed by these two moulds.

Thom gazed at him assessingly. There were indeed two moulds, one called Penicillium italicum and the other Penicillium oxalicum. "You will do. Now let's get down to work!"[16]

v

IN SPITE OF Thom's cautious reception of him, Selman Waksman came to admire his new tutor. "Puritanic in nature, strict in his relations with people, he was a true scientist. He was willing to battle for an idea he believed was sound and for the man he believed to be honest. I spent many an hour with him, listening rapturously to his discussions about moulds, about people, of whom he was for the most part highly critical, and about scientific developments in this country and abroad."[17] Selman Waksman was just opening his eyes to a science at that wonderful stage of ignorance when virtually at every turn there are new discoveries to be made. The young man born in the fertile black earth of Russia had fallen in love with these most humble forms of life, the micro-organisms that lived out their lives in the soil. It is not as preposterous as it might first appear.

Take a glass plate with a perpendicular rim and pour into it a hot liquid formed from a jelly-like substance called agar. You may mix up other substances in the agar, such as ox-blood, which gives it a brilliant scarlet colour. When it cools, the agar forms a glassy smooth gel which covers the bottom of the plate in a thick nutrient layer. Now you should take a tiny loop at the end of a wire and heat it until red hot in a Bunsen flame. After cooling, this is then dipped into a solution of soil taken from any location you choose at a certain day of the year and from a very precise depth. The tiny wire loop is now covered with the bacteria that live in this soil sample. This is now stroked very delicately, in a zig-zag motion over the entire surface of the agar gel. The plate is covered with a similar slightly larger glass plate and put upside down in an incubator at the desired temperature. The next morning, taking the plate out of the incubator, you notice first that the covering glass is coated with a dense condensation. Lifting the cover, what you see is magical . . .

Over the surface, following precisely the non overlapping zig-zags from the day before, is a myriad of little beads, pearls, miniature cotton wool balls, sprouting star-shapes of every delicate shade and brilliant colour. Each miniature wonder is a pure colony of a micro-organism that lives in that soil sample. Now, if you wish to study any one of these micro-organisms further, you can take that same wire loop, repeat the manoeuvre taking only a single colony and stroke it over its own private plate of gel, perhaps even to several different gel plates containing different kinds of nutrients, chemicals, vitamins, and so on. The following day, you have a large number of plates over each of which there is only one type of micro-organism growing. This experiment was invented by the famous Robert Koch, who performed it on the cut surface of a boiled potato. Now you can have fun rubbing a colony of bright scarlet over a microscope slide, or a dense little pearl, or the growing edge of a series of concentric flowers, like the lichens you see on old walls.

What you are doing in effect is what the young Waksman did with soil samples, no matter that he performed his work in much greater detail and his examinations down the microscope took a great deal longer. It is easy to see why it should have fascinated him. He was discovering new forms of life.

If, when you coat the microscope slide with a pure colony, what you see down the lens are clusters of little round bodies like grapes, this is a staphylococcus, similar to the type of bacterium that causes boils and abscesses. If it comprises lots of little elongated bodies, tied together in threads, it is a streptococcus, the type of bacterium that caused amongst other things the terrible infection of childbirth fever. If it is a branching wonder, comprising a myriad dividing threads, like coral, you are dealing with a mould or fungus. What Waksman had discovered is that there were a great many living organisms in soil that had never been described before and a lot of them looked like fungi. But they weren't quite typical of fungi, more a halfway house between the fungi and bacteria, and to these had been attributed the name *Actinomyces*. When, in the autumn of 1915, Waksman, then working for his masters degree, had isolated numerous moulds from the soil, nobody at Rutgers knew how to classify them. This was the reason he had carted all those plates full of newly discovered micro-organisms to Washington: he wished to put names to those which had already had names and invent new ones for those which were hitherto unknown – and there were a great many of the latter.

The threads of a fungus as seen down a microscope are called mycelia and the prefix *myco* or the suffix *myces* attached to a micro-organism's name means it looks like or has some relationship to fungi. The soil is seething with the strange family of microbes to which tuberculosis and leprosy belong.

The proper name for the bacterium that was discovered by Koch as the cause for tuberculosis is *Mycobacterium tuberculosis*.

vi

WE MUST TRY to imagine the world in which the young Waksman now moved. A modern student would scarcely recognize it as science, it was so primitive and basic. One only has to compare it with the world of medicine about the turn of the century when the formulary, or standard book of medical treatments, had changed little since medieval or even classical days.

But it would be wrong to think of this driven young man entering a black and unformed void. A closer comparison would be with a cloudless night sky, mysterious and brilliant with stars. We all dream. There may not have been much difference between a more ordinary graduate and this man in the desire to bring such stars, one at a time, into focus, to study them, to come to even a slight understanding of their mystery. The gulf between Waksman and the ordinary lay in the confidence that he could do it.

After learning as much as he could from Thom, Waksman moved on to become a research fellow at Berkeley, California, studying under Professor J.B. Robertson. Two years later he had added a PhD to his two earlier degrees. The doctorate was not in bacteriology but in biochemistry, studying the ability of fungi to produce chemicals, or enzymes, which dissolve proteins. He was now armed not only with a growing original knowledge of bacteria but the as then rudimentary understanding of their life processes. Soon this young man who had only recently arrived in America as a penniless Russian immigrant would be ready to challenge world knowledge.

Immediately he had taken his PhD, he returned to Rutgers, as a lecturer in soil microbiology. He tried the commercial approach for simple want of money, working for two years with a Japanese industrial company, but he realised it was just keeping him from his true destiny. Within just three years of his return to Rutgers, he had written numerous papers, discovered many new bacteria and fungi and, together with a colleague,

Jacob Joffe, described for the first time bacterial forms that were capable of oxidizing sulphur. His first book, *Enzymes*, was written jointly with W.C. Davison in 1922. He became assistant professor in 1926. One of the new life forms he discovered, as early as his student days and in association with another student, R.E. Curtis, would later assume huge importance in his work. This was an organism halfway between the fungi and true bacteria, which grew in delicate grey colonies, giving it the name *Actinomyces griseus*. Photographs of this organism taken down the microscope show a strange and beautiful lifeform, erupting into a liquid medium in a tracery of dividing filaments like the most delicate of winter trees.

In 1919 his only child, a son, was born. Typical of Waksman, he named Byron, not after the poet, but after Dr Byron Halsted, a teacher who had impressed him and who would go on to distinguish himself as a professor of pathology at Yale.

Discovery after discovery, step by step, he expanded, found new ground, expanded again, restlessly active. By 1930 he was made professor at Rutgers, which he had, in the short space of nine years since his return from California, helped to evolve from a simple agricultural college to a world famous institution. In the middle of this storm of achievement, in 1924, he found time for a world tour, funded at his own expense, knocking on famous doors in Berlin, Paris, London, Moscow, expecting the famous to talk to him and critically evaluating their expertise, their opinions. During the tour, he and Bobili went to some pains to visit Priluka, stopping first at Vinnitsa, where they witnessed the effects of Stalin's oppression on the once lively and prosperous little city.

> We finally met two of our childhood friends, Meier Steinberg and his wife Masha. She was the flame of most of our youthful hearts, notably that of Peisi... They both made upon us the terrible impression of people who had finished living and were now dragging out an existence. They had no spark of hope left; only complaint.[18]

The following morning they left for Priluka. They had to wait two hours before the narrow-gauge train for Turbov finally got started. There were beggars of all description at every turn.

There were waiting lines of human misery everywhere. It took nearly three hours to make the twenty mile journey. They were scrutinized by everyone on the train and at the various railroad stops, as if they had just dropped down from Mars.

A young graduate from the agriculture school tried to explain what was happening with the grain harvest. "The peasants are poor to an extreme; this year they will not get back enough grain to equal the planted seed." Through the window of their train, Selman and Bobili witnessed ravaged fields, with more weeds than oats or buckwheat. Finally they arrived at Turbov station, the point where not too many years before, Selman had departed Priluka for America . . .

"With mixed feelings of joy and despair, we saw a large crowd waiting to meet us. Bobili's parents, brothers and other relatives and friends were there to meet us. We were placed in a wagon, driven by that same coachman who used to drive me in my youthful days, when I would depart Priluka for the great world beyond. Along broken roads, we proceeded to our home town.

"Finally we perceived the straw-thatched houses of Priluka! What a picture! Many were in ruins, most were shabby, and only a few in fair condition. The people were in rags. There were large numbers of dirty children and elderly people; very few young and middle-aged men. Our entrance was like a triumphal procession. Everything alive poured out to meet us. I felt like falling to the ground and weeping, not sentimental tears but the bitter tears of a son coming back to his motherland and finding her destroyed, her children reduced to the lowest state of degradation, their means of livelihood gone. I have seen here in the town where I was born and brought up, among the people whom I loved, human misery as it could only be imagined. The first impression was as if I were walking through a cemetery, with a few living ghosts wandering among the ruins."[19]

vii

TWELVE YEARS AFTER meeting Dr Thom, this intense young Russian would establish himself as the world authority in his science with a 900-page textbook, *Principles of Soil Microbiology*.

Within a year of its publication, it was established as the Bible on the subject. A remarkable publication in many ways, the most inspired chapter, vitally important in retrospect, was devoted entirely to the actinomyces. Meanwhile, this dynamic man had made the little agricultural college at Rutgers a focus for newer and even younger recruits to the rapidly expanding science. Students were flocking to New Jersey from all corners of the United States and even further afield, to study under him. One of these aspirants, who arrived in New Jersey in 1924 after graduating from the Agronomical Institute of Agriculture in Paris, was a young Frenchman called René Dubos.

In his stolid initial assessment, Waksman appeared just as dubious about his French student as Thom had been about Waksman himself twelve years earlier. Waksman, who early in his life had eschewed the emotional in favour of the intellectual, may have been suspicious of the young Dubos' tendency to romantic generalizations where he should have been probing discrete scientific fact.

For the first year and a half after his arrival at Rutgers, while working for his masters degree, Dubos had been given a project by Waksman, "the catalytic properties of soil". It would be very useful if a simple method could be devised for counting all of the micro-organisms in a soil sample and this was what Dubos' project aimed to do. He would take soil samples and measure the liberation of oxygen from chemicals in the soil, in the hope that this would be a measure of the activity of all the micro-organisms in that soil sample. In Dubos' own recollection, "it was a most uninteresting concept."[20] He made little attempt to hide his boredom from Waksman. Then, his masters degree complete and working for his doctorate, Dubos picked his own project, something that did interest him. It concerned itself with humus.

Every gardener and farmer was very familiar with this prosaic substance, a conglomeration of soil and organic refuse which had such a magical effect on growing crops. Humus was of course far from the simple material it seemed. It was a complex universe, seething with minuscule life. Waksman's predecessor, Lipman, had already shown that the organic matter itself was quite useless. It was not until those same microbes broke down this complex refuse into the very atoms that made it, that the cycle of life could begin all over again. Exactly how this happened was of great interest to agriculture, and Waksman, like Lipman before him, had been investigating it in a systematic way for years. Now Dubos asked Waksman if he could investigate how bacteria in the soil broke down cellulose. Waksman agreed . . . and suddenly he noticed a change in the young man's attitude.

Dubos had a remarkable originality, yet this seemed to go entirely unnoticed by his colleagues at Rutgers. At this time, between 1927 and 1929, Waksman had collected about him an outstanding group of young scientists, either working towards advanced degrees or carrying out post-doctoral research. The group included Elias Melin from Sweden, later to become Carl Linnaeus Professor of Botany at the University of Uppsala, Tovborg Jensen and Jacob Blom from Denmark, the former who would become Dean of the College of Agriculture and chairman of the atomic energy group in Denmark while Blom would become chemist to the Tuborg Brewery group in Copenhagen, Hans Jenny of Switzerland, later to become professor of soils at the University of California, Harold Sandon from England, later to become professor of zoology in the Sudan. Dubos was the youngest and the quietest of all. "As we gathered around a table at our weekly Friday laboratory luncheons, discussions ranged from politics to science, from agriculture to zoology; Dubos always listened attentively. When he had something to contribute, it was well thought out and logically presented."[21]

Only by degrees did Waksman come to appreciate that there was something out of the ordinary in his young French assistant. He noticed that Dubos read more extensively than most other graduate students, not only in his field but throughout a wide range of allied subjects. Meanwhile Dubos' understanding of the science of bacteriology grew at a rapid pace.

"I shall never forget a chilly morning, early in 1926, when I arrived at the laboratory, somewhat ahead of my usual early schedule, to find Dubos excitedly holding up a plate in which cellulose was being disintegrated by a bacterial culture that he had recently isolated. His eyes were shining. His face was intense."[22]

For Waksman, thinking like a scientist, this intense moment could have only one meaning: Dubos would one day make an important contribution to science. He had not the slightest inkling that for Dubos the significance was hardly scientific at all, but deeply philosophical. For René Dubos did not think like any other scientist. Indeed his was such an unusual turn of mind that it would, given time, change not only the history of medicine – but it would also change the course of Waksman's life.

4

The Philosopher-scientist

At the midpoint of the 20th century, tuberculosis was recognised by all as the "White Plague", undeniably the most dreaded enemy of the human race by any measure. Whether measured by prevalence, cost, social consequences, sheer misery or any yardstick, I believe that any observer of the time would consider the bacillus of tuberculosis as the enemy number one of the human race. None of us – myself included – believed that its control could be attained by medical means within this 20th century.

H. Corwin Hinshaw[1]

i

RENÉ JULES DUBOS was born in Saint-Brice-sous-Forêt, a village near Sarcelles just North of Paris, on 20 February 1901, and spent his childhood on a series of farms in the small towns of the Île-de-France. In 1913, his father, Georges André, bought a butcher's shop in Paris and René's education began in a one-roomed school across the street from the shop. Discipline was spartan and the pupils had to teach one another. A tall, broadly-built boy, who loved sport, especially bicycle racing and tennis, at the age of eight René suffered an attack of rheumatic fever which left him with a damaged heart. To make matters worse, he discovered that he was near-sighted and had to wear spectacles with thick corrective lenses all his life. These twin adversities terrified the youngster though he told nobody about this at the time. One day he was quite sure he would go blind, provided his heart let him live long enough for it to happen.

49

Within just eighteen months of moving to Paris, his father was called up for service in the first world war. After suffering a serious head wound in action, Georges Dubos died from its effects, in 1918. Their grief was all the more since it happened after his return home, discharged from active service.

René now helped his mother, Adéline de Bloëdt, with raising the family of three children, working part-time with her in the butcher's shop. This big-hearted and sensitive boy, bewildered by the loss of his father and resentful of the impact that infectious disease was already having on his own young life, found comfort and escape in reading. At the age of fourteen he was astonished to read Hippolyte Taine's essay on the French fabulist writer, La Fontaine. Taine believed that if La Fontaine had been born in the forests of Germany, the deserts of the Sudan, or a Mediterranean country, he wouldn't have written his fables in the same way. What else but the setting of the French countryside could have given the fables their form! This was a subtle and very important observation. He had realized that the environment was a moulding force not only on historical events but also, and particularly, on the human mind.

After another attack of rheumatic fever had quite convinced him that he would soon die from heart failure, he decided he would have to forgo becoming an historian. Determined to find a job that would help his family, after studying at the French National College of Agriculture – where he found scientific research so boring, he told his mother he would never put his foot inside a laboratory again – he found a job in Rome as a minor member of staff at the agricultural institute, a branch of the League of Nations.

Science was as boring as ever and he toyed with the notion of becoming a translator. For two years he was associate editor of the *International Review of the Science and Practice of Agriculture*. He learnt to speak Italian, English and German well, in addition to his native French. A handsome young man, more than six feet tall, with a bushy head of blond hair, pale blue eyes and a robust sense of fun, he looked more like a Viking than a Frenchman. He had taken a liking for English girls, cajoling them into helping him with his language skills, while he enjoyed the somewhat dilettante life Rome had to offer.

As part of a routine translation, he was reading a journal, while sitting in the beautiful Palatine Gardens. It was a warm May day, and the journal was the French magazine, *Science et Industrie*. René flicked through the pages, from a mundane article about fertilizers to make a discovery that would transform his life.

He found himself reading an article written by a famous Russian soil microbiologist, Sergei Winogradsky, who had fled Russia after the revolution and was now working at the Pasteur Institute in Paris. Winogradsky was studying micro-organisms in the soil. In this article, he made a controversial statement: it was a waste of time just observing how bacteria grew and divided in the artificial world of the laboratory. The place to study them was in their own world, in the fields, the woods – in nature![2]

For René Dubos, it was a revelation. Sitting back against the bench seat in the lovely sunshine of a Roman May, a window of universal vision suddenly burst open in his mind. What if this hypothesis was not a hypothesis, but a law, a pure and self-evident natural law – what if it applied not only to these humble forms of life but to man himself!

ii

SUDDENLY HE WAS so intensely interested in science that he promptly signed for a course in microbiology at the University of Rome. The fact he had no money didn't even enter his head. He was prepared to do any kind of work that came his way. With his language skills, he knew he could earn some money as a guide for foreigners. Nothing mattered any more but the future waiting for him in the science of microbiology. There was such an aura about him these days, a heady mixture of enthusiasm and intelligence, that it impressed an American called Asher Hobson.

Each country sent a delegation to Rome, presided over by an eminent figure, and Hobson, who was a professor of agricultural economics at the University of Wisconsin, headed the American delegation. "Almost all of them wore top hats to official dinners, but Hobson would appear for dinner without one. I used to meet him on the way to the office because we often arrived a bit earlier than the others. Our paths crossed a few times; he soon recognized me and greeted me with a casual wave, and I would reply with an equally casual gesture. That's how we became friends!"[3] In those days young men did not wave to important men – the French representative for example entirely ignored him. René was impressed. Americans, it seemed, did not give a damn for protocol. One day Hobson asked René about his future plans.

"I want to go to the United States."

"Well, why don't you?"

"Because I don't have the money."

Hobson offered him the money. "Go on!" he waved. "Go to the States. If you get into difficulties, just let me know and I'll help you."

Keen as he was to go there, Dubos wouldn't accept Hobson's charity. Instead he was determined he would earn his passage by translating books on forestry and agriculture. But another of Hobson's remarks in that same conversation impressed René so much he would never forget it. "I know how to pick a winner!"[4]

Later on Dubos would laugh: "That's America in a nutshell. Of all the young people there, I alone had dared to wave casually to an official delegate, so he had concluded I must have some originality."[5] Then in 1924, fate intervened once again, to play an even more decisive role. At a conference on soil science in Rome, Hobson introduced René to Selman Waksman, who was by now a world authority. René had the duty, as technical assistant at the conference, of showing Selman and his wife, Bobili, around Rome. Waksman remembered that they first met in the picturesque setting of the Borghese gardens, on a lovely May day. It was a minor duty for Dubos who knew nothing about Waksman and thought nothing at all of it. He was more interested when Hobson also introduced him to Dr Lipman, then director of the New Jersey Agricultural Experiment Station. Dr Lipman was one of those men who had found sanctuary in America as a Russian immigrant some fifty years before and was convinced that anything was possible in this wonderful country. "Come and join us at Rutgers," he urged René. "There will be something for you."[6]

It was a vague commitment, but René was sure that Lipman meant it. As soon as he had gathered some money together, he travelled to London for six weeks, perfecting his English by attending lectures in museums. There was time only to dash back to Paris to see his mother before he was leaning on the rail of the steamship, SS *Rochambeau*, sailing out of Le Havre on a crossing that would take eleven days. Watching the French coast recede into the distance... "I wasn't homesick, but I really didn't know what I was going to do. I had just enough money for maybe three or four months. I was standing there, lost in thought, when I felt a tap on my shoulder ... A strange man and woman! Well, not total strangers – I'd seen them somewhere before. But where? They knew exactly where."[7] By a complete coincidence, Selman Waksman and his wife, Bobili, were returning to America on the same ship and they recognized the young man who had been their guide in Rome. At this time anti-Semitism was strong in America, and the Waksmans had been acidulously snubbed by the other passengers. "So I became very close to them and found out he was a professor of microbiology at that same agricultural college as Dr Lipman, Rutgers in New Brunswick, New Jersey, not far from New York City."[8]

During the long crossing, Selman Waksman and Bobili were often entertained by the enthusiastic ideas of this large bespectacled young Frenchman. Dubos must have pointed out what he had learnt from Winogradsky, a Russian that Waksman knew personally and admired greatly. When Waksman asked René what he was planning to do in America, he told him about Dr Lipman's vague offer of a job.

"Forget it," cautioned Waksman. "There's nothing. However, since you have no plans, come and work in my laboratory and I'll arrange to get you a small fellowship so you can live."[9]

In René's own words: "So shortly after I set foot in New York – about five o'clock the very first afternoon – I left for New Brunswick. Soon enough, of course, I discovered that Dr Lipman had arranged nothing for me, indeed had forgotten me. He had only had confidence that something would happen. Something did happen in the sense that a small fellowship of twenty-five dollars a month was made available to me. As a matter of fact, Dr Lipman also gave me a room in his house, provided that I acted as a tutor for his children. My first year in America was very happy and very successful. I washed dishes, entertained the children, and baby-sat. I also worked in Dr Waksman's laboratory and registered as a student at Rutgers University for work towards an advanced degree in bacteriology. I worked very hard. I can hardly see how a person could work as hard as I did. Of course I looked for other work straight away, in order to earn money. I did all sorts of things, even taught German. But above all, I specialized in microbiology."[10]

iii

FOR RENÉ DUBOS, hoping that his new learning would open his eyes to the mysteries of nature, the formal courses at Rutgers College inevitably proved disappointing. But there was a single consolation. In marked contrast to the highly organized, almost primary kind of teaching he was receiving at the college, the training he received away from the college campus at the Agricultural Station was under the personal if somewhat idiosyncratic direction of Selman Waksman.

"His course was in many ways an inspiring one, even though I now realize how inaccurate, how careless, how poorly documented it was. Nevertheless, he had a very broad view of the field of bacteriology which contrasted in an extraordinary manner with what I was receiving on the college campus. . . From breadth of view, I did learn a great deal from Dr Waksman. I did not learn any laboratory operations from him, and I left his laboratory, as did practically everybody who trained there, without any mastery of technique. Yet, working with Dr Waksman, one had, all the time, an awareness not only of the very complex relationships between one microbe to the other, but also the relationships between microbes and man."[11]

The influence of Waksman's brilliant perceptions upon Dubos' own subsequent philosophy can hardly be overestimated. One particular observation of Waksman's greatly impressed his French student.

"Dr Lipman always used to tell us that he thought it might be useful to introduce this or that kind of bacteria to the soil. Dr Waksman would try to emphasize that it served no purpose at all to introduce this or that kind of bacteria in soil; what mattered was to provide in soil a proper environment for those bacteria to multiply and operate in. Now at this time, Dr Waksman's concept wasn't a terribly obvious one and few people shared it. But Dr Waksman saw very clearly that it was much more important to create in soil an environment in which this or that kind of bacteria could proliferate and carry out reactions that could be useful than to hope that one could do something by introducing bacteria that would not be active if the proper environment were not provided for them."[12]

Now suddenly, with the new research he was performing under Waksman's guidance, those tantalizing mysteries of nature had taken a step closer.

"I really don't remember what decided me on the subject of my doctor's degree. (Only that) it too played a great part in Dr Waksman's broad projects: namely the attempt at discovering what kind of soil bacteria, fungi, or other micro-organisms are responsible for the decomposition of organic matter that finds its way into the soil. Dr Waksman had many of his students write theses on bacteria that decompose proteins, bacteria that decompose amino acids, as well as bacteria that decompose cellulose. It was my lot to work on micro-organisms that attacked cellulose. It was a good project because it had sense. It made one enquire into what kinds of micro-organisms are important in life processes."[13]

So here was the explanation for that chilly morning, when Waksman arrived in the laboratory to find the young Frenchman examining a plate, with his eyes shining. Dubos was gazing down on a strip of cellulose-based paper, which had been incubated with a plate containing soil micro-organisms. Here, before his very eyes, the cellulose was being dissolved. From a practical standpoint, it was a small section of a much larger scientific investigation, begun by Lipman and continued by Waksman – the evaluation of how organic refuse in soil is broken down into humus. But of course for the philosopher-scientist, there was a wider dimension, more deeply illuminating.

In 1927 he attended the International Congress of Soil Science in Washington, where he presented the cellulose work at a meeting chaired by the eminent English scientist, Sir John Russell. After René had delivered his paper, Sir John pointed out the ecological significance of Dubos' findings so clearly that René felt thrilled. He had clearly hit upon an idea that other people could respond to.

This confirmed in his own mind his deepest convictions since reading Winogradsky's paper. Surely now there must be even greater possibilities from this type of research. "After I had finished my thesis, I became interested in those problems dealing with the most fundamental biochemical phenomena of life, which I like to call the biochemical unity of life. I wished I could go somewhere else to receive further scientific training that would permit me to cope with these problems."[14]

When he applied for a National Research Council Fellowship, his application was turned down because he wasn't an American citizen; but the rejection letter was cushioned by a handwritten message on the margin. Dubos would later reflect upon the fact that it was written in a female hand, almost certainly added as a kindly afterthought by the official's secretary. "Why don't you go and ask advice and help from your famous fellow country-man, Dr Alexis Carrel, at the Rockefeller Institute?"[15]

Carrel was a French surgeon noted for his work on the surgery of blood vessels. "Now it sounds incredible, but at that time I did not know Dr Carrel's name, even though he was an important and famous man. Neither did I know anything of the Rockefeller Institute. I knew, of course, that the Rockefeller Institute was the Rockefeller Institute for Medical Research, but I had never had the slightest thought that I would ever be connected with medical research. Nevertheless, in those days I was rather a bold person and I wrote to Dr Carrel asking to come and visit him."[16]

In this way a simple act of kindess on the part of an unknown secretary initiated a train of events that would change history.

iv

THERE CAN BE no doubt that it was a naive if brilliant young man who travelled by train from New Brunswick into New

York to visit Carrel at the Rockefeller Institute, on nothing more substantial than the handwritten suggestion of an unknown secretary. It seemed a stroke of luck that Carrel even took the time to see him: Carrel after all was an extremely busy surgeon and had never in his life worked in the field of microbiology. He could just as easily have suggested that René should try his luck elsewhere. Carrel saw René in his office but there was nothing he could do for the young man. He was not in the field of microbiology and René understood nothing of what Carrel was really involved in. All he could offer were some words of advice:

"Don't accept an appointment, a teaching appointment, in a small college or an out of the way school, because if you begin that way, you'll never get out of it."[17]

He was about to say goodbye, but it was already noon and, out of courtesy towards a fellow countryman, he invited René to join him for lunch. They descended the building and went directly to the dining room of the Rockefeller Institute, sitting down at a table by a small gentleman who turned to René and, speaking with a gentle Canadian accent, said, "How do you do!" The small gentleman was Dr Oswald Avery, a medically qualified scientist, with a lifelong interest in disease-causing bacteria. René Dubos had no inkling that Avery was the man with whom he would spend the next twenty years of his life – who would become "the greatest person in my life except my mother."[18]

You would never have guessed that Oswald Avery was already a world famous figure. "He was small and slender, and probably never weighed more than 100 pounds. In behaviour, he was low-voiced, mild-mannered, and seemingly shy. His shirts, suits, neckties, and shoes were always impeccable, but were as subdued as his physical person."[19] Intensely intellectual, with a domed bald head, the Canadian doctor appeared the film cartoonist's model of the eccentric scientist. But in time this lunch-time discussion in the Welsh Hall would become legendary. Oswald Avery would one day, and partially with Dubos' help, make one of the most revolutionary breakthroughs of science: the discovery that DNA was the wonder chemical of heredity and life.[20]

After lunch, during which René had explained what brought

him to the Rockefeller, Avery invited him back to his office, where they could discuss things further. In René's own words, "I believe this meeting took place in April of 1927. I, fortunately, remember each and every detail of this event. I say 'fortunately' because I have no doubt that it was the most important event in my life."[21] Avery was the most gracious human being he had ever encountered, immensely charming. . . "I sat at his desk, in his small office, and he began pretending, as he always did, to be very interested in what my problem was, asking me about the decomposition of cellulose, and soil microbiology. After I had told him my story, he said in a very – how should I say – timid and most shy manner, 'My goodness, but that's similar to something we've been trying to do in the lab here.' "[22]

The young man, desperate for further work, was of course pleasantly surprised.

"Yes indeed! Your work is fascinating because in our department we are interested in a certain substance that is chemically like cellulose."[23]

Dubos was now given a resumé of Avery's preoccupation. He had already demonstrated that a bacterium called the pneumococcus, which caused epidemics of pneumonia that killed tens of thousands of people, survived against the body's defences because our white cells could not destroy the capsule that surrounded the germ. That capsule, as they had demonstrated, was composed of a polysaccharide, or very complicated sugar molecule, remarkably similar to the structure of cellulose. In this respect, Dubos's PhD thesis, based on the destruction of the cellulose by soil micro-organisms, might be relevant. Dubos would later laugh at the way Avery had brought the topic of conversation round to his own interests.

Then Avery added, in that quiet, shy voice: "For many years now we have been trying to decompose that capsule. It is resistant to every enzyme that we know of, and yet if you would help us to decompose it, that would permit us to do some other experiments, interesting experiments."[24]

"Immediately at that, I remember how he opened his right hand drawer, taking a little tube about two or three inches long, containing that polysaccharide, shaking it in front of me and telling me, 'We have a substance here that makes up the capsule that surrounds the pneumococcus. It's called type 3 polysaccharide. If we ever could find an enzyme that would decompose that substance, we would be very far ahead. That would open up all sorts of possibilities." '[25]

René Dubos took the vial containing a white powdery substance from Avery, read the label which was handwritten in Avery's flowery script. It contained pure concentrated polysaccharide from the capsular coating of billions of pneumococcal germs. They discussed it at length, well into the afternoon. It wouldn't be enough for him just to find a serum that would destroy this very capsule. He must find a serum that would destroy it effectively and yet be safe enough to give to human beings. Now – did he really believe he could manage to do that?

Avery cautioned Dubos with the difficulties he himself had already experienced in this quest: "It won't be at all easy, you know. That's why I need somebody bright, René. Somebody who can work a miracle with my little kitchen chemistry."[26]

With all of the audacity of his twenty-six years, René replied, "I'm convinced that a microbe exists in nature that will attack those polysaccharides. If such a microbe didn't exist, polysaccharides would cover the earth, which they don't. Somewhere that microbe must exist!"[27]

Avery seemed pleasant enough but promised René nothing. He took him to see two other men who worked at the Rockefeller, Dr Rufus Cole, who was director of the hospital, and Dr Simon Flexner, who had met Koch on his ill-fated final visit to New York. Cole had in 1900 discovered the bacterium which causes dysentery. This same man had also led the Rockefeller team that found the virus which causes the paralysing disease, poliomyelitis. Flexner was director of the institute. René Dubos spoke with these men for a couple of minutes and that was it – he returned to New Brunswick.

By this time he was so desperately short of money that he was forced to become a summer guide, assisting foreign participants at an international soil science congress that was meeting in various places about the United States. On a train out of Chicago, he met the director of the agricultural experiment station in Fargo, who offered him a job. He went so far as accepting this offer and in August 1927, planning to settle in

North Dakota, travelled to Fargo. However, during those three months since he had visited the Rockefeller, the slow wheels of academia had begun to turn in an alternative direction. In a letter dated 7 June 1927, Selman Waksman supplied the Rockefeller Institute with the following reference:

Dear Dr. Avery,

Replying to your letter of June 4th concerning Mr René J. Dubos, I want to say that Mr Dubos has been with us for the last three years. He has made very rapid progress in advanced studies in bacteriology. He is a very keen student and is capable of grasping a new idea and developing it further very readily. Although he has had to spend a good part of his time in preparatory courses such as biochemistry and physical chemistry, he has succeeded in carrying through a very fine piece of work on the decomposition of cellulose by aerobic and anaerobic bacteria... I recommend him heartily for a position in your department...[28]

On the very day he arrived in Fargo, René received a telegram from the Rockefeller Institute, telling him he had been given a fellowship on the stipend of $1,800 a year. In Fargo he would be earning $3,000. Suddenly, in August 1927, he was faced with the most important choice in his career.

He decided to return to the Rockefeller. As he later explained: "I don't think there was any other institution in the world then – and perhaps there is none now – that would have taken a person like me, knowing nothing at all about medicine, and coming from an agricultural experiment station, and given him a chance to work in a hospital. I came back for two reasons. First, I had become aware of the great reputation of the Rockefeller Institute. Second, I felt right from the beginning that I could make a very important discovery in Dr Avery's laboratory."[29]

5

The Cranberry Bog Bacillus

I have been sick as a dog the last two weeks; I caught cold in spite of 18 degrees C. of heat, roses, oranges, palms, figs and three most famous doctors on the island. One sniffed at what I spat up, the second tapped where I spat it from, the third poked about and listened how I spat it. One said I had died, the second that I am dying, the third that I shall die ... All this has affected the "Preludes" and God knows when you will get them.

Frédéric Chopin: Mallorca

i

WHAT MUST HAVE gone through his mind when Dubos first found himself sitting alone in a small laboratory on the sixth floor of the Rockefeller Institute Hospital, gazing at a wooden desk in a large room full of a motley collection of notebooks, simple laboratory instruments – test tube racks, glass Mason jars, droppers for various dyes and chemical agents, tin cans holding pipettes and platinum loops? Avery's laboratories were housed in a former hospital ward, still ornamented with its quaint marble fireplaces. The individual laboratories were a conglomeration of rooms of different sizes, high-ceilinged, and served by simple wooden desks that had been designed originally for office work. Avery's laboratory was the smallest, formerly the ward kitchen, and next door to it was his equally tiny office, spartanly bare of the photographs, pictures and mementoes that most office workers find essential for sanity.

René Dubos knew absolutely nothing about medicine or medical microbiology, or even what a pneumococcus was. "When Avery described the pneumococcus with its capsule of polysaccharides that prevented phagocytosis, he was using words I didn't even understand."[1] Why on earth had this young man agreed to take on what Avery himself knew was a task of Herculean difficulty?

Incredible as it might seem, the reason was not scientific at all but philosophical. At that moment he had had an inspiration as ambitious as ever fuelled any experiment in medical science. Every substance of living extraction was broken down in soil. It was a self-evident truth, based upon one of the best known precepts of the Bible: dust thou art and unto dust thou shalt return. Now he was faced with the much more difficult task of making that philosophy work.

The first act on arriving in the morning was to put a match to the Bunsen burner. There were indeed plenty of common kitchen utensils. Against one wall in each laboratory was a single large porcelain sink that was used in any operation that needed water, from staining slides to preparing extracts of bacterial cultures for testing. As he would subsequently confess, he hadn't the slightest idea of what he was to do or how to go about it.

"My first impression was that the atmosphere of Dr Avery's laboratory was so peaceful that I even doubted that there was much eagerness among the workers in the laboratory. I believe it took me at least one or two months to realize the manner in which Dr Avery conducted his department. What was peculiar to it was the fact that Dr Avery never asked anyone to do anything. In fact, he almost urged people not to do too much. Of all the persons I have known in science, he certainly was the man who most was concerned with thoughts, long thoughts and meditations, before doing experiments, instead of the usual manner of rushing in and doing as much laboratory work as possible."[2]

Although charming in conversation, Avery was extremely secretive about his private life and his family background. It would be many years later, after Avery's death, that Rene Dubos would discover some rudimentary facts about him.[3] Oswald Avery was born on 21 October 1877, in Halifax, Nova

Scotia, where his parents had arrived from Norwich, England. His paternal grandfather had made paper for the Oxford University Press and his father, imbued with a divine purpose, had emigrated to Canada with the specific mission of Baptist evangelism. The second of three brothers, by the age of eight he witnessed his mother being rescued from the brink of death at the call of Jesus. The young Oswald was brought to New York at the age of ten years when his father accepted the office of pastor of the Mariner's Temple, situated on the lower east side of the city, an area notorious for its poverty and violence. His ambition was to save the immortal souls of Jews and Catholics, no small task in the environment of the Bowery. In the words of Oswald's mother:

> "People, people everywhere. Crowded into the lofty tenement houses, burrowing in basements, packed in cheap lodging houses, and swarming on the streets. To the casual observer the picture is bewildering. Even to the ordinary Christian worker the situation is one that would seem to defy all effort to improve it. Vice in a hundred repulsive forms holds many in its iron grasp. Relentless lust and passion hold captive many who long ago have lost the power to resist. . ."[4]

At fifteen, Oswald lost his much-loved elder brother, Ernest, who was intellectually gifted and who would, as a toddler, step up on a stool, arrayed in his father's white collar and tie, and preach sermons. It is believed that Ernest died from tuberculosis.[5] This was the undisclosed background of this shy, courteous Canadian, a background that must have made Avery painfully conscious of the dread terror of epidemic pneumonia – and tuberculosis too – in those squalid, overcrowded blocks. But he never talked of this even to his friends, despite the fact that what Dr Avery liked to do most of the time was to talk.

He would invite each of the workers in his laboratory into his office and review – "not in the form of a systematic review, but in the form of a conversation" – the problems he had dealt with the year before and the problems he had thought about during his recent vacation, which he always spent on Deer Isle in Maine. The young and impatient René hardly understood a word of all this, yet Avery was slowly and subtly expanding René's horizons. To the non-scientist it might seem surprising that a change from one bacteriological laboratory to another should create such a confusion but the world of medical microbiology was light-years from the preoccupations with soil and agriculture at Rutgers. Later on René Dubos could hardly remember anything of what was discussed in these frequent and endearingly sociable conversations. "All the occupations, preoccupations of the laboratory ... were so completely different from that with which I was familiar that everything seemed strange."[6]

Even more fundamentally: "I had to learn the very words that were being used, because essentially they were meaningless to me."[7] He found a practical outlet for his enthusiasm in the difficulties Avery was experiencing in cultivating the pneumococcal germ in the laboratory.

The bacterium that so interested Avery was hard to grow in artificial cultures and this was creating difficulties with the various research projects already under way. Here at last was a problem Dubos was familiar with. For no other reason than it was the only experiment he knew how to perform, he started to investigate the media they were using for culturing the pneumococcus. Very quickly, using the crudest of techniques, he made a surprise discovery: the pneumococcus grew much better when oxygen was removed from the medium in which it was growing than when they bubbled oxygen through it. This was the mistake they had been making. These researches took him about eight months to complete, during which he learnt a good deal more about bacterial biochemistry. More importantly, his constant rubbing shoulders with medical scientists opened his imagination to a new world, and the world that most interested Avery: immunology. Like most of his contemporaries, Avery was convinced that the cure for bacterial infections would come from a natural substance, like an antibody, that would fit the pneumococcal capsule like a key in a lock. So it was, after his eight months of acclimatization to this alien world of medical research, René Dubos was guided back to the very problem for which Avery had selected him in the first place.

The problem was as follows. The pneumococcus was a killer because the human phagocytes could not digest the tough capsule that coated the germ. In this way it bore a curious resemblance to the much more dangerous germ that caused tuberculosis. This was especially disastrous when the pneumococcus gained access to the blood stream, where it almost invariably proved fatal. Avery had gone so far as to show that if you removed the capsule from the germ, those same phagocytic cells easily destroyed it. Another scientist working with Avery, Dr Michael Heidelberger, had, with the assistance of a chemist, Walter Goebel, managed to extract the capsular material from billions of germs and concentrated it in the pure crystalline form that Avery had shown René in the test tube. Also in Avery's department, they had developed an antibody test that would show the presence of this capsular material wherever it might be found even in the most minute quantities. In other words Avery could supply René with the pure substance to be destroyed and he had a measuring technique that would tell him exactly when, where and how successfully he had destroyed it.

Now there was just one almighty problem to be solved: where on earth should he look for the agent that would destroy it?

"The thought occurred to me that polysaccharide produced by the pneumococcus was not unlike other polysaccharides existing in the soil under conditions where organic matter is deposited and has to be decomposed."[8] Maybe the answer lay with that most lowly of materials, so often a subject of derision except to gardeners and soil microbiologists – humus!

He began searching in samples of soil and sewage in the hope that one of these might contain some bacterium or some fungus capable of attacking the polysaccharide. Using techniques that seem closer to gardening than the intellectual exercise of science, he trowelled soil into pots, searched in farmers' fields, manure heaps, lawns and hedges, altered growing conditions, added and subtracted chemicals. This was when he also put into practice the guiding principle he had learnt from Waksman. "I then devised a culture medium in which the only source of carbon was the pneumococcus polysaccharide."[9]

ii

WINOGRADSKY HAD SAID that we must study bacteria not in test tubes but in their natural environment. Now Dubos set out to recreate a natural environment in which one micro-organism fought a struggle for survival at the cannibalistic expense of another.

What he did was to make a very dilute solution, one in a hundred thousand, of that white crystalline bacterial coat, inoculating it with samples of soil or sewage, then incubating these mixtures under different conditions of oxygenation, acidity, alkalinity, any environmental variation he could think of. In every experiment the only source of carbon was the capsule of the pneumococcus. Now he could determine if any living microbe in the soil had destroyed that capsular material, using the serological technique already developed by Avery.

For a little time he had no success at all in finding his likely micro-organism. Then he remembered that just ten miles from where he had lived in New Brunswick, there were cranberry bogs, where a gummy material very similar to the pneumococcal polysaccharide accumulated.

He wrote to Waksman, asking him to send on some soil samples from the cranberry bogs. As soon as he received some, he set back to repeating his experiments. Suddenly there was a dramatic change. To his intense excitement, he found that the pneumococcal capsule material in his bacterial culture media was indeed disappearing. There was only one rational explanation. Some bacterium or fungus from the cranberry bog soil samples was devouring the pneumococcal capsule – but which, of the teeming millions that lived in the sample, was actually responsible?

He devised another series of culture media, still only containing the polysaccharide as the source of carbon, subculturing again and again, eliminating more and more of the micro-organisms that were not what he was after. Within an incredibly short time – the whole experiment didn't take more than three or four months – he had obtained a pure culture of a previously unknown bacterium, the Cranberry Bog Bacillus, that destroyed the pneumococcal capsule.

It was May 1929 and Avery went on his usual holiday in June, thinking there would be little further progress over the summer months. But Dubos, proud that he had proven a theory that had originated with Louis Pasteur – that one micro-organism can be employed to counteract the dangerous effects of another – was now inspired. He worked every waking hour of the day, seven days a week, trying to extract whatever it was in the bacterium that dissolved away the pneumococcal capsule. Within a matter of a week or two, he had his first relatively crude extract of bacterial enzyme, which he now tested for its ability to dissolve the capsule. It worked.

Avery was still on holiday. Dubos decided to go ahead with animal experiments, injecting mice with the deadly bacterium, then giving half their number an additional injection of the enzyme he had extracted from the Cranberry Bog Bacillus. The experiments continued throughout the summer. By the month of August, he had obtained a filtrate which, if injected into a mouse, would protect the mouse from being killed by the deadly bacterium. It was a thrilling achievement. The time had come to let Avery, up in Maine, know what was happening.

Avery immediately cut short his holiday and dashed back to the Rockefeller. Additional animal experiments were set in motion, the conditions of the experiments altered. With Avery's experience, the quality of the experiments was greatly improved. They could calculate the precise timing with which the enzyme must be given, how late into the infection in the mouse, how big a dose was necessary. They went so far as to study how the enzyme really worked. By staining blood samples taken from the mice, they could see that the pneumococci were being attacked exactly as Dubos had anticipated, the capsule surrounding them was disintegrating and then the naked bacteria were being devoured from the very blood stream by the phagocytic white cells. In the unprotected mice, those same phagocytic cells could not take up the bacteria and digest them, the infection spread at a furious rate, and the unfortunate animals were overwhelmed by teeming masses of bacteria and died. They were ready at last to announce their discovery to the world.

The experimental success was reported under the authorship of Avery and Dubos in the journal, *Science*, in 1930,[10] when it created an immediate sensation.

René was deeply disappointed by the fact that Avery put his

name first on the scientific paper. "I think it's absolutely clear that I have an immense and abiding admiration for Dr Avery. Yet I was grieved that he came back from vacation and put his name first to the paper, whereas I had considered that all the work was mine. It disturbed me very much because everybody was convinced that I had just been a pair of hands in Dr Avery's laboratory and that everything had been Dr Avery's work. I resented that very much and was very upset. The endless letters of admiration for the achievement which Dr Avery received from all over the world and which he showed me, were to say the very least, somewhat painful to me."[11] The more mature Dubos would see this differently, but there was no time for René to waste in harbouring resentments. Suddenly his work, and his life with it, was vibrant with excitement: the real love affair of original research, the ensuing years of relentless hard work, was only beginning.

iii

DUBOS WOULD LATER compare the mood of the Institute in those days with the charged spirituality of a Benedictine monastery. The Rockefeller Institute had been founded in 1901 in the mould of the Pasteur Institute in Paris, the Koch in Berlin, the Kitasato in Tokyo. Its purpose was missionary: to enable Americans to play a leading role in the scientific quest for the causes of – and ultimately the cure for – the infectious diseases that had plagued humanity since the beginning of time. Although the buildings themselves were modest in size, the fourteen acre site on the banks of the East River was endowed with a relatively generous garden. Anybody who has visited New York will appreciate just how unique an endowment this is. The founding guardian angels had placed an iron fence about the parkland in which the buildings had first been erected, to make absolutely sure it would save its tree-lined avenues from the encroaching megaliths of Manhattan.

A great deal now hinged on the singular relationship between two very different personalities and their attitudes to work and to each other. For Oswald Avery, hermitically shy, the laboratory was his whole life. In contrast to this delightful scientist with his reserved gentle manner, René Dubos must have seemed a large bundle of raw enthusiasm. Perhaps it was the huge contrasts in their personalities that enabled them to work consummately well together. Any time he wanted, René knew he could just call into Avery's office and they would talk. Later in life Dubos would admit that he was learning far more than he realized at the time: in particular, his eyes were opening to wider issues in medicine and philosophy as well as the more fundamental principles of science. They would try out a new idea, encounter problems, change direction, try something different. Always now there was an excited buzz of expectancy. New discovery charged the air.

It is obvious that René Dubos was in love with America; and Americans, in their turn, loved this larger than life Frenchman, who spoke with an accent like Maurice Chevalier and used his huge hands constantly to express his impassioned thoughts, who, "when he talked to you, he would look you straight in the eye. He decorated every conversation with the most wonderful ideas."[12]

In a series of scientific papers, Dubos and Avery published the results of these further experiments. They described how the enzyme of the Cranberry Bog Bacillus only attacked the pneumococcus capsule: it was as specific as a guided missile. They described how best to prepare it, how to obtain the best possible yield of enzyme for further research. They described how the enzyme cured life threatening pneumococcal infections induced not only in mice, but rabbits, rats and monkeys.

At last they were ready for human trials. "Emotionally," Dubos would later declare, "this was my greatest hour in science." They had drawn up the necessary conditions to test the enzyme from the Cranberry Bog Bacillus in people suffering from epidemic lobar pneumonia when suddenly, without even a tremor of warning, their Benedictine world was shaken to its foundation by the scientific equivalent of an earthquake. This earthquake was a rival discovery of such importance that all further application of the Cranberry Bog Bacillus enzyme became clinically redundant.

To compound his dismay, René had also encountered a

stalemate in his researches. "I realized the implications and pursued them for three or four years. However, I could not carry the work very far because there were serious gaps in both my knowledge of genetics and biochemistry and in the states of these sciences themselves."[13] The technique he was searching for, a means of forcing bacteria to produce a single enzyme, was beyond the biochemical and biological knowledge of his day. It would be twenty years before Monod, Jacob and Lwoff, working at the Pasteur Institute, would discover the technique of adaptive enzyme induction, earning them the Nobel Prize.

René Dubos, still only thirty-one years old, had made a revolutionary discovery. But now all of his pioneering ideas had failed him. His research was in danger of losing all momentum and the world at large was no longer listening to him. In the words of Selman Waksman: "Had the scientific world fully appreciated at that time the significance of this discovery (the Cranberry Bog Bacillus enzyme), the practical development of antibiotics might have occurred so much earlier".[14]

René would continue his researches against increasing complexity and difficulty into 1935 and even 1936. But it was all to no avail. The rival discovery was so simple and yet so powerful, it would prove a much better and safer medical treatment for the pneumococcus than his Cranberry Bog Bacillus enzyme. It would find its way into every surgery, every chemist's shop, and every home. The name of this star was not penicillin, as people might assume, but a different antibacterial agent called Prontosil. It was found by a young doctor called Gerhard Domagk, working in the pharmaceutical research laboratories of the Bayer company, at Elberfeld in Germany.

Never in history had there been a greater need for such a breakthrough. Most of the human race died from infections. On 2 March 1930, the year that Dubos and Avery first announced their discovery of the Cranberry Bog Bacillus to the world, the writer David Herbert Lawrence died of tuberculosis in a sanatorium at Vence, just outside Nice on the French Riviera. He was forty-four years old. All of his creative life he had suffered from the disease. His face with its hollowed cheeks and passionate eyes personified the twentieth-century torment of consumption while with his burning prose, the "Prophet of Love" had fashioned the most brilliantly sensual example of the so-called *spes phthisica* ever to enrich the world of literature. Yet his sad death beyond the shores of his native England would not even be included amongst the fifty thousand of his fellow countrymen who died from tuberculosis in this single year.

PART II

EUROPE

6

One of Three Survivors[1]

The Tsarevitch Nicholas, presumptive heir to the throne of Russia, was
receiving treatment for consumption in Nice. His mother visited him
there on several occasions, and in 1865 the Tsar Alexander II came to
receive his last words and to order the return of his body to Russia on
board the frigate Alexander Nevsky.

René and Jean Dubos: *The White Plague*

i

TAINE BELIEVED THAT human genius is shaped by the
surrounding world. For Selman Waksman, science,
based on the black fecund earth of Priluka, had offered a
lifeline of order and truth in the encroaching chaos and anarchy
of the Russian revolution. For René Dubos, that key moment of
inspiration had come from reading Winogradsky's article, in
the sunshine of the Palatine Gardens in Rome. Gerhard Johannes Paul Domagk would also be profoundly influenced by the
world about him, from its shy mysteries to its darkest hours of
inhumanity and terror.

He was born on 30 October 1895 in Lagow, a small town in the
German province of Brandenburg. With its walls, gateways
and ancient castle, he enjoyed a carefree childhood in this
picturesque little town, wrapped about two beautiful lakes and
surrounded by beech woods. His father, Paul, was a teacher
and organist, and his mother, Martha née Reimer, came from
a farm just outside the town, which had originally belonged to

75

the Knights Templar. Domagk might have been quoting Taine when, many years later, he reflected on those childhood experiences:

"In this landscape of sand and forests and lakes, where everything seems very poor, where nothing is grand or eye-catching, there is an immense variety of beauty. But you need to learn to perceive it. It was my parents who taught me to perceive things in this way and it is to this simple art of perception that I owe much of the important things in my life. I learnt that God and all the miracles of nature are not only felt in the great things, in the snow-covered mountains tops melting down to rush off into the sea, but in our modest home landscape, in the rustling of forests – yes, and in every plant, every blade of grass."[2] The child, sitting on his rocking horse in the schoolhouse garden, dreamed past the round tops of acacias , down to the great lake where he could see the boats go by and where he would soon learn to catch crabs and fish. But it was the woods he loved most of all, where he would hike with his mother and sister, collecting plants and wild flowers.

In the words of his lifelong friend, Ferdinand Hoff: "Domagk was born to see things. But for the scientist it is not enough to dream of the beauty of nature – you need the facility of precise observation, even to the smallest detail. Domagk possessed this gift from his earliest childhood."[3] While out riding his bicycle, he could spot enough four-leaved clovers on the road side to tie them into bunches.

A photograph from this time shows a blond haired little boy in a sailor's suit standing with a protective hand on the lap of Charlotte, his younger sister. It was an idyllic life that would be destroyed, as for so very many of his generation, by the outbreak of the first world war.

ii

WHEN WAR WAS declared, Gerhard was already a first-year medical student at Kiel university. Suddenly all thoughts of his education were abandoned and he volunteered, at the age of eighteen, to join the German army. Without the slightest conception of the real meaning of war or concern with any thoughts of danger, all he could think about was the excitement of meeting up with his old school friends again, all of them wildly enthusiastic to enlist. Keen to get straight into the fighting, they pestered three different regiments until they found one that promised to send them to the front straight away. This was the Royal Infantry Regiment of grenadiers at Liegnitz. Perhaps the most revealing indication of his boyish naivety is the fact that he took his favourite lute with him, a precious possession he was forced to abandon when he was very quickly dispatched to the front. Told he could not send it home because of its size and awkward shape, he cut off the neck and dismantled the rest, packaging it to his parents' home. The reconstituted lute was their present to him on a rather more sober homecoming on his first Christmas home from the fighting.

In October 1914, Gerhard and his young friends found themselves in the German trenches on the battlefields of Flanders, from where, in two letters to his parents dated 24 October and 28 October, he wrote, enthusiastically still. The food was good but the water was getting more difficult and they had to boil everything. He couldn't wait to be sent to the enemy lines.

For the moment, Gerhard and his best friend, Uli, had to content themselves with volunteering for food details. "You had to run above, along a wired enclosure, through the beet fields towards a little forest in the east near Mangelaare, where the kitchen was situated in a little oasis of peace. For this trip, under continuous machine-gun fire called the 'evening blessing', the old experienced 'trench pig' took his time, spending as many hours as possible out of the Flanders mud and fire in a haystack or similar. We war volunteers, in contrast, had the stupid idea in our heads of breaking the speed record, as, loaded with bread, chocolate, tobacco and market produce, we dashed back to our squad. When the 'blessing' started, we jumped with all of our treasures into a water-filled bomb crater, so you can imagine the state of our bread and ships biscuit in thin linen bags. You can also imagine what the chocolate and peasoup looked like, if there was any left in the cooking vessels by the time we got back to the trenches."[4]

Throughout it all, his letters home were still couched in optimism and boyish innocence.

6 November: "If the weather stays like that, we'll be all right.
We can keep going. And we are having fun in the trenches." He
had run out of cigarettes and chocolate and asked his parents
for a food parcel, a side of bacon perhaps. 18 November – in a
long letter, he recounted fourteen hard days in front of Ypres.
They were under constant attack by British planes. All their
companies suffered great losses. Beyond the canal there were
Belgian and English soldiers but when things got a bit hot, "as
usual, the British retreated to safety so we couldn't take many
British prisoners of war."[5] They moved forward into new trenches only to come under heavy attack. The French were known
to rain fire upon them if they saw so much as the top of a helmet
or heard the clattering of food utensils. People no longer volunteered for the food details.

On 10 November, just twelve days after his nineteenth birthday, he had his first experience of what it was like to go over the
top.

"During the night we had to get ourselves ready and wait in
the trenches for the command telling us to jump. Everybody
tries to get out of the trenches as quickly as possible and then
run as fast as your legs will carry you, towards the enemy
regardless of the whistling hail of gunshots. By the time we
reached the French they had retreated to the shelter of their
running trenches. The few who didn't get away surrendered. A
quick respite in the trench and then another jump through a
beetroot field where we dug ourselves in as quickly as possible,
took off the packs and spades and got working. All around us
gunshots were whistling and shrapnel exploding. Here, some
comrades got shot – the land behind us was full of dead bodies
and with injured, who were groaning. As soon as we had finished digging, we dragged the injured, at least those who were
within reach, into it.

"It is unbelievable how pleased they were to hear that I was a
medic. Of course I didn't let on that I was only in my first year,
but wearing my expert expression, I put on temporary band-
ages. This was at least a comfort for the poor soldiers. Towards
the evening they were collected by the ambulance corps. On

this day some of my best comrades lost their lives. Whilst digging in, my friend Walter Schroeder, was hit by an enemy bullet straight through the head and collapsed without saying a word. His parents would receive the official notification from the regiment. A few days later, Siemann, a friend of Papa's, took another head shot. Langisch was slightly injured. Uli had his trousers shot to bits.

"After the storm attack we have been in the front line continuously until the day before yesterday – nothing hot to eat, rain all the time. You have no idea what we look like. We are encrusted in mud a centimetre thick. All our things have been wet for a long time – not a single piece of bread to eat. We dug a water hole and to our horror there was a landslide caused by a grenade and the head of a dead Frenchman appeared in the trench above the hole. The mud in the trenches is so bad that in some places our comrades had lost their boots when they came to relieve us."[6]

In this letter describing his experiences to his family, he thanked them for their earlier letter to him and for the food parcel they had sent him and he asked for biscuits next time. In a postscript to this letter, written many years later, Gerhard Domagk remarked: "That's how we saw things at the time – or that's how the propaganda machine led us to believe. The fact that things turned out differently later on must not detract from how I saw it then."[7]

In December, after a few weeks of resting, his unit boarded a train in Hanover that would take him past his home town towards the Russian trenches and the wintry conditions of the Eastern front. While waiting at the station, in a touching reminder of happier days, he bought himself Leibniz cakes. Immediately they alighted from the train, they fell into the mundane reality of war. "We didn't feel cold as long as we walked or marched and marching was what we did for most of the days and nights." He had barely arrived in Poland, when he was marched into a battle of such ferocity it would subsequently form a part of his regiment's history.

"At four o'clock in the afternoon, before the battle began our commander gave us tobacco and post. A few minutes later he was dead. Lieutenant Schmidt took over the command, waving us onwards towards the Russian trenches. Within minutes, Lieutenant Schmidt was wounded in his thigh and could no longer walk. We spent the night in the trenches defending ourselves, taking a few Russian prisoners. Next morning we were told to attack again. I had just stuffed my pipe when I lost it in the hurry and confusion. During the attack, the officer running beside me was killed. Suddenly my helmet was blown off my head. I felt blood running down my back. I tried to bandage up my own head. I was placed on a Russian farmer's small cart, which was used as sickness transport, and driven to a church where I was operated on and bandaged up. Fourteen days after I had left Lichtervelde in Belgium, I had returned to Lichterfelde near Berlin, with my uniform stuck to me with blood and dirt, as an injured soldier."[8]

In a letter to his parents from the hospital in Berlin, he told them he had lost all of his personal possessions in the battle. He was desperately worried about his close friend, Uli. "I hope Uli is still fit and well. I haven't met any of my friends since I have been injured. I, and many other injured, were brought back to the hospital very quickly. Fortunately, none of us were badly injured. We really showed it the Russians on that day. Our Company alone took 800 prisoners. Please send me a parcel with gingerbread and pancakes, I'm really longing for them and so are my four comrades who are convalescing with me here."[9]

Still there remained an echo of his earlier optimism, but things were about to change. A few days later he was sent on a short course to train as a medical assistant. Then in May 1915 he found himself on board a train taking him back to the Eastern front in this new role. When he heard that his train would take him through Liegnitz, he wrote to his sweetheart to see if they could meet at the station when he was passing through. During the battle, he had lost his only photograph of her, taken in her confirmation dress. Sadly it was not possible for them to meet.

Soon the greatest nightmare of his life would envelop him. Here, in the field hospitals of the Eastern front, the nineteen-year-old medical assistant would see with his own eyes the grotesquely swollen limbs of comrades that were barely older than boys, their wounds black with gangrene and crackling with the putrefying bubbles of foul-smelling gases. It would be these terrible experiences that would both torment and inspire him for the rest of his life.

"I shall never forget the primitive conditions in which we operated in those days, whether on the floor in the barns, or under the open sky, where complicated operations involving life and death had to be performed. Often, we operated under oil lamps swinging from the rafters. One could hardly work for all the flies. If I think about it now it seems unbelievable that such operations could be performed without many bacteria entering the wounds and killing our patients. If we managed to get a few hours sleep, we did so under the open sky and pestered by flies, until we were woken up by rain.

"In the mornings, walking through the barn, we found more and more dead people under the straw. We had to count the number of operated patients in every barn because people who had had head injuries clambered over the others, who could not move, to escape into the open air. Here I learnt all about the dreadful gas gangrene infections which brought death and terrible disfigurement. It is estimated that in the German army, this horrible infection of wounds caused 100,000 to 150,000 deaths. These harrowing impressions as a medical student in my first year have haunted me for the rest of my life. It made me want to do something against this malicious and treacherous enemy.

"I think it was then that I swore to work and work very hard to make a small contribution to that problem if ever I survived and got back to my homeland. Later, before Verdun, it became clear to me that war was the natural enemy of mankind and it became more and more senseless. I swore many times before God that I would help with all my strength and energy to meet this madness of destruction in the small way that I could only do it – to ease the hopelessness and need in which the nations of this world had got themselves entangled. This proved much harder to achieve than the destruction of so very much. Wasn't it possible to be brave without killing? Yes, maybe much more brave. This made me realize what a wonderful vocation it was to be a doctor and what it demanded of you. In our days at the Somme, when we didn't sleep at all and we inhaled more chloroform than any patient, we saw the commitment of our elders and we didn't want to offer any less than they did. That's how we learnt in our young years about the serious business of dying and living, before we had a real opportunity of enjoying the beauty of life."[10]

iii

GERMANY'S DEFEAT IN the war threw the country into a bewildered despair. The country had made vast sacrifices yet there had been no gain whatsoever, only senseless losses. With a heavy heart, Gerhard Domagk surrendered his weapons and began the slow journey home. From his class of friends at school, born in 1895, only Gerhard, Uli and two others had lived. With desperate poignancy, one of this precious few died three years later from tuberculosis, contracted under the conditions of the trenches. Finally there were just three survivors.[11]

What was Gerhard to do with himself now? Even when he arrived home, there was no escaping the morass of despondency, economic disaster and the agony of loss. "It was a terrible thing to meet all those other parents whose sons had not returned." He didn't even stay for Christmas. He was in a great hurry to get back to Kiel to take up his university career once more, a very different spirit from the eighteen-year-old lute player who had left it some four years previously. Those carefree years spent in pranks and fun as a boy belonged to a bygone world of impossible happiness. In its place was a new cold world of pitiless struggle, a world that seemed to have abandoned its former morality and into which this battle-hardened young man carried a sense of mission. Gerhard Domagk, still a mere twenty-two years of age, was determined to prove with his work that he could do more, or at least no less, than the selfless doctors he had assisted during those grotesque war experiences.

"In Kiel, I worked very hard – feverishly. I was very hungry and I wasn't able to keep warm. But this no longer mattered to me. I was determined to achieve my goals." He was tormentedly aware of his own good fortune in surviving. So very few had been as lucky and even these survivors appeared so deeply traumatized, they were like lost souls. "Many were not able to return to their work. They were waiting for another adventure. Others were dancing on a volcano, some of them with broken wings. They were just brooding and under the perpetual influence of alcohol." Now some of these tattered survivors of the great war had to pick up the pieces. His old clothes would no longer fit him and he couldn't afford new cloth, so he adapted his soldier's uniform and wore that to the university classes. Food was scarce and in a physics lecture he fainted from hunger and overwork. But these were minor irritations against the inner furnace of this new driving ambition.

Many of his fellow students worked down the coal mines or in the factories during the holidays to finance their studies. A doctor who was called out in the middle of the night to help his patients earned the same salary as the porter at the station. Studies had to be sacrificed in the interest of earning money – no matter that the money earned was miserably inadequate, barely enough to keep body and soul together for just a week or so, so that for the rest of the month they had to starve. A remorseless determination, born on the blood-soaked fields of Flanders, Ypres and the Russian front, became essential for the young man just to survive. Now, at last he was enjoying his contact with real patients, during the clinical part of his training.

"In a way the best time was when we were assistants in the hospital, when at least we got our board and lodgings free. At least we were looked after as well as the orderlies in the hospital, who could leave after eight hours of work. And they could sleep in between."[12]

After graduation, he moved to the City Hospital in Kiel, working as a junior doctor with the professor he so admired, Hoppe-Seyler. These were exciting early years, during which Domagk developed a close working relationship with a like-minded young colleague, Ferdinand Hoff, who would later become Professor of Internal Medicine at Frankfurt University. Each as dedicated as the other, they bolstered one another's enthusiasm through the penniless days, the long hours of ward duties, encouraging each other's day to day research. It was while working with Seyler and Hoff that Domagk made his first perceptive observations in patients suffering from bacterial pneumonia.

In the words of his friend, Hoff: "Here we saw with our own eyes how helpless the doctors were ... we saw the terrible circumstances on the big wards full of tuberculosis patients."[13]

It was in those desperate clinical arenas that Domagk learnt an extremely important lesson. With good medical care and devoted nursing, many patients with serious infections survived, in time recovering good health again. Why did some people die while others survived? What was it in the human body that fought off deadly infection in this way? Nobody really knew the answer.

All the time he was on the battlefield, Gerhard had been in touch with a "blonde girl who wrote letters to him on blue paper", that same sweetheart he had attempted to meet at Leignitz station. Her name was Gertrud Strübe and he had known her ever since his schooldays. He had gone to war carrying her photograph close to him and it had upset him greatly when he had lost it at the time of his injury. Now there was the temptation of a brief romantic dalliance with a new assistant but he could not forget his former sweetheart, now living in Basle. He knew he had to make up his mind. Suddenly it was all decided. Knowing he had to go to Kiel one more time to buy some glassware for his researches, he wrote to Gertrud to say he would like to meet her at Lake Constance.

On 31 July 1923, he attempted to catch the night train from Greifswald to Munich, but this was crowded and he took a relief train, which left a little earlier. Before his train reached Kreiensen a fault developed with the engine and the train was kept waiting for a replacement engine at the station. Domagk left his compartment in the rear of the train to have a drink. At that moment, the main train went through the stop sign and hit the relief train at full speed, destroying the rear compartment completely. Like Waksman on his snow-bound journey, fate had stepped in to save Domagk's life.

Now he had to stay and help the injured. He lost his suitcase with the precious glass and there were more than fifty dead. The fate that had spared him had also prevented him once again from meeting with his sweetheart. Finally they did manage to meet in Dresden at Christmas, where he proposed to Gertrud, she accepted him and they became engaged.

In 1923, while attending the Pathologist's Conference at Leipzig, this intense young doctor with his pale blue eyes and his close-shaven fair head, attracted the attention of Professor Walter Gross, director of the Pathological Institute of Greifswald University. When he invited Domagk to join his team as an assistant, Domagk readily accepted.

Immediately he arrived within the smoke-blackened stone walls of Greifswald's pathology institute, Domagk began his work, testing how it was that the human body fought off serious infections. In some star-shaped cells, hidden away in the clefts of the liver he observed how old red blood cells were culled from the blood. Rather like amoebae, these stellate cells actively devoured the ageing red cells, a phenomenon called phagocytosis which he traced further until he could witness a wonderful internal economy taking place, with the red pigment containing its precious iron being removed from the destroyed cells and eventually stored within the liver to be reused in the manufacture of new red blood. Domagk felt tears come to his eyes. In his jubilation, he dashed from the laboratory to the library next door, where he discovered that the eminent Professor Karl Albert Aschoff had described this same phenomenon just a few years earlier. But Domagk was not disheartened. "Instead," he remarked, "it boosted my confidence and I told myself: if you have made an identical discovery to some other astute observers, even though you knew nothing of their independent findings, you will discover other things too."[14]

The intense researches continued. In 1924, a year of devastating economic collapse and spiralling inflation in Germany, he was working late into the night and using up so many scarce resources in the laboratory, there were complaints from other colleagues. But when the head of the pathology department, Walter Gross, called him to his office, it was not to reprimand him but to praise the quality of his work. Domagk had already made some interesting new discoveries.

In experiments on mice infected with a bacterium called the *staphylococcus*, which causes abscesses and blood-borne infection, he had shown how, within just minutes of injecting these germs into the blood stream, they were devoured in huge quantities by these curious stellate cells within the liver. Other cells played parts too, some of the white blood cells and a mysterious cell called the monocyte. It was now clear to Domagk, as it had been to Aschoff, that these amoeboid cells in the liver formed part of a galaxy of similar cells, dispersed throughout the whole body, which had this special job of scouring bacteria and foreign material out of the blood stream. This newly discovered system was called the "reticuloendothelial system". It was an important discovery.

Domagk now took this a step further. What if the animals were immunized against the bacteria before injection? He tested this and found that it increased the ability of this marvellous defence system to cleanse the blood. He probed further still: what if the bacteria themselves were in some way damaged before injection? Soon he witnessed the most startling discovery of all. Suddenly the reticuloendothelial system really did go to war. Its stellate defending cells became absolutely stuffed with bacterial bodies and the very spaces all about the cells were littered with the debris of battle. So this was the way the body defended itself against bacterial invasion of the blood stream! Domagk now knew that if bacteria infecting a human being could be damaged in some way, even if still alive, they would be readily cleansed from the blood and tissues by the action of this extraordinary natural system. This was the most vital realization of all.

Gross was very keen that Domagk publish these findings, which he did in this very important year, 1924[15], in the summer of which he qualified as a lecturer. In his appraisal of Domagk's potential, the normally cautious Gross wrote, "The paper shows an outstanding ability to pose fruitful scientific questions and a remarkable independence of thought on generally accepted but poorly proven ideas." Gross, in also noting that

Domagk had already taken his researches beyond the field of pure pathological morphology, realized that there was a wider importance to this work.

When, in 1925, Gross was appointed Professor to the University of Münster, Domagk followed, beginning work at the Institute of Pathology that would one day bear his own name. In Münster, Domagk was able to set up his own laboratories. He was quickly broadening his fields of interests, to include cancer research and research into kidney diseases. He married Gertrud that same year, when she was a secretary on a very small salary, and they lived under frugal conditions in a rented flat. In 1926, their first son, Götz, was born, followed three years later by Hildegard, then Wolfgang in 1930 and the baby, Jörg, in 1932.

Although they remained as poor as church mice, Domagk was never in doubt that he had made the right decision when he had committed himself to a life of research. But now he was inflicting his philosophy of "work, work, and go hungry" on a young wife and family. Still he remained convinced it was the right decision. "To work and to work and to starve and still to get married and to starve together – but also to be happy together. Yes, this was the right thing to do. Things were getting better in spite of storm and rain, the sun kept coming through and eventually we had enough money to take our four children once a year for a holiday on the Baltic. Our youngest two children were christened there when they were already old enough to run because we had had to postpone the ceremony from one year to the next. We had to count our pennies and pay our debts."[16]

In spite of the success of his work, his hopes of progressing to a higher station were very slim. "Fortunately, I had messed up any opportunity to marry into a position and because I couldn't, and didn't, want to rely on paternalism, the only remaining path open to me was one that was ultimately based upon my own performance."

This was his position when, out of the blue, Gerhard Domagk, still aged only thirty-one, was approached by Heinrich Hörlein, head of pharmaceutical research for the Bayer company of IG Farbenindustrie.

iv

WHY WAS BAYER interested in Gerhard Domagk? To answer that question, we must return to that famous lecture, given by Robert Koch, in the Physiological Institute in Berlin.

Sitting in his audience, transfixed by Koch's words, was the young man called Paul Ehrlich. The son of a prosperous Jewish family from Strehlen, Ehrlich was destined to become one of the most famous names in medicine. Koch and Ehrlich would become lifelong friends. But while Ehrlich believed that Koch's theory of immunotherapy was the answer for certain infections, he knew it would never cure the majority of bacterial infections. Even as a child, Ehrlich had been fascinated by chemistry. At the age of eight, he had the town chemist make cough drops according to his own prescription. After Ehrlich had recovered from his mild dose of tuberculosis, Koch had given him work but it wasn't long before Ehrlich was offered his own research institute, where his prolific imagination was soon driving his contemporaries mad with a stream of new, and seemingly fantastical, ideas.

Instead of cutting up dead bodies to peer into whole organs for signs of disease, he invented the notion of slicing tissues into very thin sections, which could then be stained with chemical dyes and viewed down the microscope. A minor digression for Ehrlich, it founded the science of histopathology. Wandering about his institute with his little brown-legged dachshund, Manne, and listening to the man outside in the square, whom he tipped to play barrel organ tunes from *Carmen* and *Die Fledermaus*, Ehrlich spent long hours studying bacteria in tissue slices, occasionally making notes on his detachable shirt cuffs. Soon he had come up with a totally new and revolutionary theory of how to treat bacterial infections.

Essentially what he observed was that certain animal or human cells coloured with certain dyes, while others did not. Exactly the same applied to bacteria, protozoa and the whole range of micro-organisms that caused human diseases. Realizing that this must mean that the surface membranes of the cells, or micro-organisms, had different affinities for different dyes, it must surely be possible to construct dyes, or chemicals, that would kill bacteria while not killing the human being infected by the bacteria. It all sounds simple and logical today but at the time nobody in the world believed Ehrlich. Even Robert Koch found the notion of swallowing or injecting chemicals totally repugnant. But Ehrlich was not the man to be dissuaded by the opinions of others.

The tale of science is very often one of attrition, with heroic endurance against disappointments. Ehrlich devoted the rest of his life to a great programme of experimentation, not hundreds but thousands of experiments, testing one dye after another against infectious diseases. At last, with the assistance of a gifted young Japanese assistant, Dr Kiyoshi Shiga, who had found the bacterial cause of dysentery, he showed that a dye, trypan red, cured a single mouse infected with the fatal tropical disease, sleeping sickness. But when they tried it in human sufferers, it did not work.

Ehrlich now had the most subtle, possibly the most important, inspiration of his life. What if by altering the slightest part of a dye molecule, it dramatically changed the effects within the body? He began a further series of experiments, trying out a great many new chemical substances, all minor variations from one another. On the 606th permutation, with the assistance of another Japanese assistant, Dr Sahachiro Hata, he discovered Salvarsan, the first drug in the world to cure syphilis.

But there was a drawback. People died from the side-effects of the drug. Ehrlich, the lovable scientist, could not face the fact that even wonder drugs will sometimes have side-effects. In spite of his receiving the Nobel Prize for Medicine in 1908, in spite of the fact that vastly more lives were saved than were lost from the side-effects, Ehrlich regarded his life as a failure. Like so many geniuses before him, the stress of it all, his smoking and drinking habits, the never ending struggle against insurmountable odds, all conspired to overcome him. He died, in 1915, convinced that his ideas had failed and that his life's work had been consigned to the scientific dustbin.

Sad as it may seem, Ehrlich was largely right in his despairing assumption. Few believed in his idea of treating infection with man-made drugs. Worldwide medical science still firmly believed that the only effective treatment of bacterial infection must lie with immunotherapy and vaccination. The anti-drug camp had their prejudices confirmed by the failure of any kind of therapy to fulfil its early promise in diseases such as gonorrhoea and the epidemic pneumonia which so interested Oswald Avery. They were a very powerful pressure group and most scientists in the world were persuaded to join them. In Germany however there was a notable exception. His name was Carl Duisberg and he was the president of Bayer, then a factory which, although already producing some very successful medicines, was largely devoted to the manufacture of dyes for the textile industry.

In Germany, at this time, there was a carnival chapter of advance in the understanding of organic chemistry. In 1910 Bayer had created, at Elberfeld, the first drug research laboratory of any pharmaceutical company, in a small single storey house that had been a plumber's workshop. Bayer was already famous. This company had, towards the end of the nineteenth century, discovered the two wonder drugs of pain relief, phenacetin and aspirin. It was no accident that Wilhelm Roehl, who had studied and worked with Ehrlich, wrote in October 1909 to Carl Duisberg, asking for help.

Roehl had left Ehrlich's institute fascinated by the experiment with sleeping sickness. Duisberg saw a new opportunity, engaged Roehl and brought him to Elberfeld. The tiny new laboratory had found its first research worker. Duisberg quickly consolidated his acquisition, putting a chemist called Heinrich Hörlein, in charge of the research department. Roehl knew exactly what to do. Immediately he took Ehrlich's ideas further. How, Roehl asked himself, had Ehrlich managed to cure that single mouse?

Following Ehrlich's precise technique, though without the dog and the barrel organ music, he tested one azo dye after another in animals infected with trypansomiasis, the protozoal cause of sleeping sickness. Almost immediately, he confirmed Ehrlich's much earlier conclusion. The azo dyes, cheap derivatives of coal tar, appeared to glue themselves to living cells, exactly the reason they were good dyes for natural fibres, such as cotton. Now he also confirmed, though more comprehensively, Ehrlich's singular conclusion: they also appeared to cure sleeping sickness in mice. The curative properties of the dyes did not in fact rely on their dye colour: it was a property of the chemical structure of their molecule. The Bayer chemists, under Roehl's direction, could now manipulate the original dye molecule to find uncoloured derivatives which were just as good in curing the disease. After years of laborious research, in 1916, Roehl found what he was looking for, a new drug called Germanin. Humanity had the first treatment in history for sleeping sickness.

Roehl however was not satisfied. From Germanin he went on to discover a new cure for malaria. Quinine, derived from the bark of cinchona trees, had been discovered as long ago as 1820, but it was extremely expensive and there simply was not enough to treat all who needed it. In December 1924, the Bayer chemist, Fritz Schönhöfer, distilled the first golden yellow drops of a new substance, Plasmoquine, which proved to be thirty times better against malaria than any other compound previously made in a laboratory. It was an important discovery and quickly became a standard drug in the treatment of malaria. It is very sad that Roehl did not live to see this happen. In March 1929, after a visit to Cairo to attend a congress on malaria, he developed a carbuncle on the back of his neck and, just forty-eight years old, the doctor who had devoted his genius to fighting infection died from one of the most common and deadly of germs, the streptococcus.

Roehl had been more successful than he could ever have dreamed. Not only had he proved Ehrlich right – more pragmatically, he had confirmed Duisberg's faith in chemotherapy, a critical factor at a time when virtually nobody else in the world believed in it. While other pharmaceutical companies refused to lose money to such fruitless endeavour, Bayer had good reason to believe the rest of the world was mistaken.

It was against this background that Heinrich Hörlein had read Domagk's paper in the Virchow archives, describing the importance of the reticuloendothelial system in the animal's response to blood-borne bacterial infection.

Hörlein was fascinated. Here was a medically qualified man of the highest calibre who was researching why people died from infection. Hörlein, himself a chemist and not medically qualified, considered the fact they had no pathologist on the staff of the Bayer laboratory. Now, reading carefully through Domagk's work, Hörlein became convinced that the study of pathology must be a vital step in conquering such diseases. He offered Domagk a job, working in the company's research laboratories. Domagk accepted. The year was 1927 and he was still only thirty-one years old.

v

GERHARD DOMAGK KNEW that his new task would prove no easy option. When he first came to Elberfeld, he was given a single room over a storage chamber for glass. So he began by gathering together some animal accommodation, no matter that it was off the beaten track. In 1929, significantly the year of Roehl's death, he received permission to build a new pathology institute. He had few personnel, no more than a technical assistant and two washer boys in the beginning, but now things began to grow, quickly, organically. Soon there were five, ten, twenty, fifty workers in his laboratory. He took them from leaving school at the age of fourteen and taught them himself.

In 1911, scientists had discovered that a synthetic derivative of quinine, ethylhydrocupreine, would kill pneumococci in a test tube but its use in human sufferers was abandoned when it was discovered it caused blindness. This calamity was entirely typical of earlier efforts to find anti-bacterial compounds. Although this may seem picaresque, compounds of gold, which had long excited the darker arts of alchemy, now interested doctors. Gold and, as we have already seen, even more dangerous potions such as arsenic, had been evaluated by no less authorities than Koch and Ehrlich. In the 1920s a distinguished Scandinavian veterinarian scientist, Mollgaard, advocated gold for tuberculosis and early studies appeared to show such promise that Ferrosan, a Swedish drug company based in Malmö, invested large sums of money in Sanocrysin, only to make a disastrous financial loss when later scientific studies showed no benefit whatsoever in people suffering from tuberculosis. This experience caused a profound shock to Ferrosan and left the management with a jittery sense of vulnerability which would have important repercussions later.

Hippocrates had treated consumptives kindly, with honey, barley gruel, dark resinous wine mixed with water, and herbs grown in the gardens of temples dedicated to Aesculapius, the God of Healing. But with the passing of the golden age of Greek enlightenment, the Western World had fallen into barbarism, when evil spirits and sin would dominate medical thinking for two millenia. The disease was put down to possession by evil spirits or demons and the folklore remedies often relied on the principle of transfer of evil from the afflicted to animals, plants, or inanimate objects. In China, even into the twentieth century, tuberculosis was still treated with pith balls soaked in the blood of executed criminals. As recently as the nineteenth century in Europe, similar superstitions were commonplace. A living trout was attached to the sufferer's chest, a fresh catskin was wound round the body, a piece of meat moistened with the sufferers urine was fed to a dog. John Wesley recommended suckling milk direct from the human breast, a therapy he believed had cured his father. It was much vaunted by the fashion of the wet nurse sharing the sufferer's bed until the disadvantages for the wet nurse became apparent.[18]

Even now, well into the twentieth century, with the new passion for "inner disinfection", a bizarre litany of poisons were recommended as "cures" for tuberculosis, including iodine, salts of mercury, cinnamic acid, copper, calcium and silica – most exotic of all, responsible workers in Japan, where the death rate from tuberculosis was horrific, advocated an Agatha Christie cocktail of potassium cyanide and copper-cyanourate. Such "treatments" were soon found to have limitations and even more hastily abandoned. Behring, Koch's pupil, who had received the first Nobel Prize for his discovery of the tetanus anti-toxin, expressed the prevailing despair all too plainly: "disinfection is a vain dream."

Bayer might have found a cure for sleeping sickness and malaria, but these were caused by big single-celled organisms, the protozoa. Bacteria, much smaller – perceived at this time in much the same light that we currently view viruses – were a different matter. Many scientists worldwide had come to the nihilistic conclusion that an anti-bacterial drug would never be found.

Domagk was convinced that this polemic of despair was based on false beliefs and misconceptions about the very nature of infection. This climate prevailed . . . "because so many times previously doctors had known only disappointment with such remedies. They all had such preconceived notions about the nature of infection. They had resigned themselves to the fact that in Germany alone two to three thousand young mothers died of puerperal fever every year – and much the same numbers in England too. Instead they tried to save their patients with the operation of a total hysterectomy (which involved the emergency removal of the womb and all of its surrounding tissues). Apart from the fact that this operation meant infertility for every one of the operated women, it also meant that a not inconsiderable number of them died during the very operation. Nobody seemed to consider cutting off this terrible disease before the serious infective complications set in. If we could achieve that, two thousand young women would not need to die from childbirth fever."[19]

It is clear from Domagk's own diaries that he saw his work as a fundamental struggle for integrity and truth through the meticulous observation of science. In all that was to follow, an intense inner faith would buttress the external struggle.

Immediately he began to design the great experiment that would give him the scientific tool he needed.

He was utterly single-minded in his approach. A vast army of bacteria attacked mankind, but he ignored them all except for one bacterium. This single bacterium was the cause of puerperal fever, epidemics of scarlet fever, the dreaded rheumatic fever which damaged heart valves, or which caused so many young lives slowly to fade from chronic kidney damage, a bacterium that induced terror by the bedside where it was all too readily visible in the scarlet wave that ran along the skin in erysipelas and cellulitis. It had a special predeliction for causing blood poisoning, when it was almost invariably fatal, causing great pain, huge discharging abscesses, and invading the heart valves, the liver, kidneys, even the bone marrow and the brain. It was the germ that had killed his predecessor, Roehl.

But a huge systematic search, as pioneered by Ehrlich, needed a suitable experimental model and no animal model existed that was accurate enough for him. He invented his own. First he selected a particularly vicious strain of streptococcus, which had caused a fatal blood-borne infection in a real patient, and he demonstrated how this particular strain invariably caused a similar fatality in his laboratory mice. This bacterium and the response in mice became his test system. More vitally still, he was opposed just to testing chemical after chemical against bacteria in the test tube. Test tubes did not contain those amazing phagocytic cells he had discovered, hidden in the mysterious crevices of the liver and the spleen. Domagk was not just looking for a chemical that killed bacteria, and very likely any other living thing it came into intimate contact with: he was looking for something gentler, infinitely more subtle, a formula that would damage bacteria just enough for those phagocytic cells to do the rest, while not harming the human body at all.

He began a series of experiments in which this deadly bacterium was injected into mice which had been pre-treated with his test drugs. Working side by side with Domagk was an unusual chemist, Josef Klarer.

Klarer was born in Munich in 1898 and, like Domagk, had been seriously wounded in the first world war. On returning to Munich University, he took his doctorate in chemistry, "obtaining the highest honours for his sensational thesis", based on the synthesis of the pigments that colour blood red and leaves green. Intellectually in a class of his own, he turned down the professorship he was offered to join the research team at the Bayer laboratories. At Elberfeld he was given the task of synthesizing compounds that might find uses in the treatment of bacterial infections. An enormously creative man, who eschewed theory for practical experiment, he was tough in his work habits, unmindful of his own health and uncommunicative with his colleagues. Yet beneath this rough exterior, Klarer was "a highly sensitive man" who would, in his later years, disappear for a time to his country house at Tegernsee, where, under the loving care of his two sisters, he would conceive plans for further research while tending the flowers in his garden. "Klarer was the only man to be allowed such freedom for it was known that he would invariably return with new ideas."[20]

In 1927, when Klarer began to synthesize new chemicals for Domagk's research, he took known dyes previously examined by Roehl, introducing new chemical side-chains. By 1931, he had synthesized no less than 300 new chemical compounds which were subsequently tested by Domagk for anti-bacterial properties. In spite of the fact that none of these compounds proved useful, Domagk remained unflinchingly optimistic.

For yet another year, vast numbers of experiments were set up, their results evaluated against the bacterial cultures in test tubes. By December, few of Domagk's colleagues had retained any confidence in the latest test chemical passed on for testing by Klarer, a red dye which had already proved useless against the streptococcus growing in test tubes. If a drug did not kill the germs in test tubes, what was the point of testing it further? But Domagk was insistent. He wasn't just interested in the dye killing germs in test tubes: he wanted to know how this same dye affected bacteria in the tissues of the living animal.

The red dye, numbered with Klarer's initials, Kl-730, had a new chemical side group attached, known as a "sulpho-namide" group. Five days before Christmas, despite the useless results in test tubes, Domagk stayed behind to see what effect the new compound would have in his laboratory mice. What he saw astonished him. Where he expected, as so very many times over the past five years, that the mice would all be dead, as the control animals next to them were certainly dead, instead those test mice were alive and merrily frisky, running about in their cages. There was no longer any notion of normal end of day activity, of travelling wearily home, of going to sleep: they carried on all night exploring the phenomenon further, until everybody was so exhausted their legs wouldn't hold out any longer. Barely able to keep their eyes open, they made tissue sections from the internal organs of the sacrificed mice, stained them for bacteria and inspected hundreds of slides under the microscope, repeating and repeating the tests until their vision blurred over and they were no longer able to make out fine detail.

They were gazing at a miracle. They needed to be sure, to be absolutely certain there was no alternative explanation. Yet here were the test mice in the cage, lively, running about, taking food . . . it seemed, perfectly well.

Every single mouse that had been inoculated with this crystalline chemical, labelled Kl–730, was still alive despite being injected simultaneously with a deadly species of strep-tococcus. Not a single one of the mice given that same bacte-rium but no Kl-730 was alive.

The story down the microscope was the same. In the body tissues of the unprotected mice, the bacteria were found every-where in swarming masses, while in sacrificed surviving mice that had been given the magic drug, there were no living bacteria, only dead bacteria that had been taken up and de-stroyed in that vital and wonderful internal defence galaxy of reticuloendothelial cells.

Domagk described his own feelings. "We stood there astoun-ded at a whole new field of vision, as if we had suffered an electric shock."[21]

The Prontosil Miracle

Then suddenly an illness came to my help and in a few weeks decided my future . . . [1]

Adolf Hitler: *Mein Kampf*

i

W HAT THE CHEMIST, Klarer, had placed in Domagk's hands was more than just a scientific breakthrough: it was exceedingly beautiful. Deeply iridescent crystals, the colour of venous blood and archetypical of life itself, they were given the striking name of *Prontosil rubrum*.

Five dull and repetitive years were now crowned with a wonderful success: but for Gerhard Domagk the hard work was only beginning. Maybe, in his streamlined laboratory test system, mice had been protected from injected streptococcal infection, but this was a very long way from administering the drug in much larger doses to sick people.

In a further series of experiments, he tested Prontosil against many different bacterial infections in animals. While the drug was often miraculously effective, it did not cure every infection. While it wiped out the bacteria that caused many infections, including the pneumococcus that interested Avery, the bacteria that caused abdominal infections – the so-called Gram-negative bacteria – were completely resistant. Most striking of all, in every case where the infective organism was the virulent streptococcus, the new drug showed exceptional promise. It was rapidly absorbed from the bowel after taking it by mouth and was excreted very readily in the urine. It appeared to be well tolerated by the test animals, no matter which species. There was however a major difficulty. The drug was not very soluble in water and since you cannot give something insoluble by injection, this meant it could only be taken by mouth – a great disadvantage in seriously ill patients. Another of the Bayer chemists, Fritz Mietzsch, a quiet, distinguished and scholarly man, the very opposite in personality to the mercurial Klarer, took it upon himself to tackle this vital problem.

Mietzsch now juggled with the atoms that made up the Prontosil molecule, to create the freely water soluble sodium salt – a burgundy red solution. Prontosil was now ready for human testing.

Only two kilometres from the Bayer research laboratories was the municipal hospital of Wuppertal-Elberfeld. This famous old hospital, dating from the nineteenth century, with its hotchpotch of separate blocks abutting against the very streets of Wuppertal, would provide the clinical setting for the first patient in the world to be treated with Prontosil.

Head of the department of internal medicine was an interesting doctor, Philipp Klee, who would subsequently become Domagk's clinical partner. Klee, with his domed intellectual forehead, large piercing blue eyes and a receding halo of pure white hair, bore a physical resemblance to the German philosopher Goethe, with whom he shared a distant family connection. Unashamedly intellectual, patrician in temperament, his very bearing and manner radiated authority. However, behind the impressive public figure, with his upright posture and rigid self control, was a deeply sensitive private man. At a time of growing antisemitism in Germany, he had, in 1921, had the courage to marry Flora Palyi, a gifted Jewish artist from Budapest. Domagk and Klee were already close personal friends and it was to this man that Gerhard Domagk now entrusted those first precious red tablets and ampoules of liquid for trial in human beings.

Where tuberculosis wages a slow war of attrition against humanity, if on a vast and millenial scale, the streptococcus is the microbial *blitzkrieg*. This bacterium can survive for weeks or even months in dust, particularly if protected from daylight. It produces a formidable battery of poisons, which it injects into the body tissues surrounding the site of infection, or more dangerously still, into the blood stream itself. For example these poisons have the property of rupturing the red blood cells, of killing the body's white defence cells, of dissolving away the defence ring of fibrous tissue, thrown up to try to confine the infection into a local boil – and even dissolving away blood clots the body forms in the local veins to prevent the infection spreading through the blood stream.

Before Prontosil, infection with this bacterium so terrified doctors that a surgeon, on witnessing the typical sharp red lines of rising infection along the sides of his accidentally infected finger, would have the finger amputated. This was the bacterium Domagk had chosen for his test system with the mice and it was against the various infections caused by this bacterium that Prontosil was now tested to its limits by Philipp Klee.

In 1933, an eighteen-year-old girl – we shall call her Heidi – was admitted to the Wuppertal-Elberfeld Hospital, suffering from a septic throat infection. Swabs taken from her throat grew the streptococcus germ. Within a day or so, her temperature had risen to over 40 degrees Centigrade and the white cell count in her blood had peaked from a normal of about 5,000 or 6,000 to a staggering 26,000. Huge abscesses built up in the soft tissues behind her tonsils, which had to be lanced open. While this had a dramatically beneficial effect – over a stormy ten days, her high temperature had returned to normal – then, strangely, Heidi fell ill again. Red blood cells and protein appeared in her urine. Fourteen days after the tonsillar abscesses had been drained, her temperature soared again, with tremendous shivering attacks followed by drenching sweats. The following day, her right jugular vein became hardened and exquisitely tender to touch, and was obviously infected and completely blocked by a blood clot. Within another day, her temperature had climbed even further, and her kidney ailment, a dangerous complication called acute nephritis, had deteriorated to the stage where she had virtually stopped forming urine. Klee, with his wide experience of these dangerous infections, had no doubt that Heidi was dying. There was nothing to lose in giving her the new drug and he treated her with repeated Prontosil injections, directly into a vein. Within just twenty-four hours, her temperature had fallen to normal. Her kidneys began to pour out a copious dilute urine. Klee continued to give her Prontosil intravenously and by mouth for a further six days. Four weeks later Heidi was discharged home, completely recovered.[2] Had he just witnessed a therapeutic miracle? Even this time-hardened doctor of the old school thought he probably had, but he went on trying the new drug in many more patients before he was convinced.

Over the following two years, Klee and his assistant, Römer, gave Prontosil to patients who were desperately ill from many different forms of infection. The results were indeed miraculous. To the properly sceptical and meticulous Philipp Klee, who had seen so very many of his patients die from exactly such infections, this was the most wonderful experience of his life. Prontosil cured many people suffering from bacterial infections for which there had previously been no medical treatment available. These included severe tonsillitis, abscesses, infected glands in the neck, even the horrific infections that complicated septic abortions and septic infections of the womb.

Klee's colleague, Schreus, working in the skin department of the Medical Academy at Düsseldorf, found that Prontosil cured serious skin infections such as cellulitis and erysipelas, hitherto very often a death warrant. It even cured infections of the most delicate tissues of the eye. Orthopaedic surgeons gazed disbelievingly at cases of bacterial infections of the large joints cured by this simple medicine. Prontosil revolutionized the treatment of acute rheumatic fever. The dreaded epidemics of scarlet fever had lost their terror. It even cured some, though certainly not all, of the previously fatal infections of the great valves within the heart. But Klee was well aware that it was no panacea. Some of the more advanced forms of infection, for example those that presented very late, with people already dying with circulatory collapse, or those complicated by spread throughout the blood stream – especially the boil-forming staphylococcus that caused abscesses to form in every internal organ – responded little if at all.

Just two years after Prontosil had been discovered, on 15 February 1935, Domagk published the first report of his wonder drug in a German medical journal, under the unassuming title: "A contribution to the chemotherapy of bacterial infections".[3] The same issue carried reports of the clinical trials of Prontosil by Klee and Römer at Wuppertal and Schreus at Düsseldorf.[4]

An antibiotic, as it would be defined more than a decade later by Waksman, is not only a drug that is used to treat bacterial infection, but also one that comes from another living micro-organism. A drug manufactured in the laboratory for exactly the same purposes is, technically speaking, a "chemotherapy". In this strict sense Prontosil was the first chemotherapy for infection. This, however, is a distinction which has all but lost its original purpose for the prescribing doctor as much as for the lay public; and nowadays chemotherapy is more often a term used for the drug treatment of cancer. In essence, therefore, the "antibiotic miracle" began with Prontosil.

Across the world there were millions of people who might immediately have benefited from this discovery. Sadly, few doctors believed the words of Domagk or the German clinicians. This early cynicism would be remembered many years later by the distinguished American physician, Walsh McDermott.

In May 1935, a young woman desperately ill with streptococcal blood poisoning was admitted to the New York Hospital. She was started on the pitiful treatments of the day, none of which had the slightest effect. Her condition rapidly worsened. It was obvious that she was going to die from it. Her family insisted that she should be treated with the new German drug. Her doctors, although openly incredulous, gave her Prontosil on the basis that they had nothing else to offer. She promptly recovered. The doctors however refused to believe it was the drug that had saved her. In the ironic words of Walsh McDermott: "Naturally our staff were pleased, but they were particularly pleased because this happy combination of events had occurred in a university hospital, with its high scientific standards ... 'Isn't it fortunate that this happened here in the New York City Hospital, and not in some small hospital out in the sticks, where they really would have believed this German dye had made her better.'"[5]

ii

ONE OF THE most sinister and tragic of all streptococcal infections was puerperal fever, a condition, following childbirth, when the swollen womb and its luxurious lining becomes a culture chamber for swarms of this terrible bacterium. For a newly delivered mother to develop this complication in 1936 was a catastrophe hardly better in outlook than in the mid-nineteenth century when one in three expectant mothers admitted to a famous Parisian maternity hospital died from the condition.

At the time of Prontosil's discovery, a London doctor, Leonard Colebrook, had known many years of despair in attempting to treat puerperal fever. In 1928, he found that Ehrlich's drug, Salvarsan, had some useful activity against steptococci in test tubes but when, working with a colleague called Ronald Hare, he tried it in a group of twenty-eight patients with blood-borne streptococcal infection, seventeen of the patients died.[6] Colebrook was bitterly disappointed. Colebrook and Hare had no more luck with a mercury derived drug, Mercurochrome in 1927.[7] He was only too well aware that trying the fashionable serum therapy against puerperal fever was a waste of time.[8]

There is nothing more depressing to a doctor than the death of his patients. When, in 1936, Leonard Colebrook, working with his colleague Kenny, decided he would test the efficacy of Prontosil in this dreaded condition, he set out with an understandable sense of pessimism.

Working on the labour wards at the Queen Charlotte Hospital in London, he administered Prontosil to thirty-eight newly delivered mothers, all suffering from puerperal fever. Three died and thirty-five survived. Comparing this with his previous experience, he remarked that of the last thirty-eight patients treated prior to Prontosil, ten had died. Added to this, he had given the Prontosil to many women who were late in the course of the disease and the most desperately ill.[9] Later in that same year, Colebrook and Kenny tested the drug in a further series of twenty-six women, this time administering the drug earlier in the course of the infection, when not a single one of them died.[10] Colebrook did not need any further convincing.

Slowly but surely, in several European countries, those first results obtained in Germany by Klee and his colleagues were amply confirmed. In a dramatic twist of fate, Domagk's own daughter, aged six, developed an infection which threatened her life.

In late November 1935, little Hildegard had been learning embroidery when she decided to play with her brothers, sliding down the bannister in their home. Forgetting that she still had the needle gripped in her hand, she accidentally pricked herself in the soft web of muscle between the thumb and the first finger. This tiny wound became infected with the deadly streptococcus. The bacterial poisons coursed up her arm, in red flares. The glands became very swollen under her armpit and she had to be admitted to hospital for urgent treatment. Conventional treatment at the time was surgical and the little girl suffered fourteen lancing operations, all to no avail. By 4 December, the glands were bursting with pus, her temperature was peaking repeatedly at 39°C and the infection had become blood-borne. The surgeon who was looking after her wanted to amputate her arm to save her life. But Domagk refused. He treated Hildegard with Prontosil and within just two days her temperature had fallen to normal. After repeated courses of treatment, she went on to make a good recovery without amputation.[11]

iii

FOR THE FIRST time in history, without surgery, simply by taking a course of tablets or injections, patients suffering from overwhelming infections could be rescued from the brink of death. It wasn't long before the ordinary man and woman came to realize its miraculous potential. Shunning publicity, Domagk would point out that the discovery had come from teamwork, involving many others besides himself, in particular the chemists, Klarer and Mietzsch, the hospital clinicians in Wuppertal and Düsseldorf, and the Bayer company, with Hörlein behind the whole programme. Nevertheless, to the media and public alike, Gerhard Domagk was now the hero of science. Reports of wonder cures littered the newspapers of every continent and letters poured onto his desk in Elberfeld from grateful patients, from parents of children, and from medical colleagues worldwide.

If that first case treated at the New York Hospital had underlined the sceptical reaction to Prontosil in America, suddenly, a year later, there would be a dramatic change of heart.

In December 1936, Franklin D. Roosevelt Jr, son of the President of the United States, developed a serious streptococcal infection. A previously fit Harvard crewman, he had contracted a very severe tonsillitis, which had spread to involve his sinuses. His condition was grave, with such imminent danger of blood-borne spread of the disease that his mother and his fiancée were constantly at his bedside. His throat had become massively swollen and raw and his temperature had risen to such a "portentous" degree that Dr Tobey, who was alarmed at his condition, commenced treatment with Prontosil, both by intravenous injection and with tablets. Following Prontosil he made a rapid recovery.

On 20 December 1936, *The New York Times*, under the headline, "NEW CONTROL FOR INFECTIONS", reported the successful outcome when the doctors interviewed by the paper were so cautious that the reporter could not resist a wry comment: "This is not exactly wild enthusiasm, yet enough to make energetic and curious physicians rush to the medical library and look up Domagk and his chemicals."

On 8 August 1937, in a letter typical of many hundreds from grateful patients, Hildegard B., aged twelve years, expressed her gratitude:

> Earlier this year I had an infection in my middle ear after I had the measles. This turned into a blood poisoning. After operating on my ear they had to clamp off a blood vessel in my neck. For three weeks my life

was in great danger and my temperature jumped from 35 to 41 degrees. The doctors gave me Prontosil to fight the infection. For weeks I had two injections of Prontosil every day and after that I had to take two tablets every day for a long time. . . I know that Prontosil saved my life so you have been my saviour in inventing it. Thank you.[12]

Domagk would receive very many such letters from grateful patients and their relatives: Klarer never received one. It was a pattern that would be repeated again and again, from country to country, with ever newer discoveries, when the role of the chemists was sadly ignored. Meanwhile the reputation of Prontosil, Domagk and the Bayer research laboratories grew worldwide. But such phenomenal success would inevitably excite professional and corporate rivalry. Within just a few years, its chemical molecule was manipulated by research chemists all over the world. By far the most important secondary discovery was made by two French researchers, Jacques and Thérèse Tréfouël.

In 1935, while the ink was still wet on the patents, Dr Tréfouël and his wife, together with two other French colleagues, Frédéric Nitti and Daniel Bovet, synthesized the drug for themselves to confirm Domagk's initial and very curious finding. If you put Prontosil into a test tube with streptococci, it did not kill the germs. The French doctors now made a simple assumption: it was well-known that azo chemical links were easily split on the chemical bond between the two nitrogen atoms – what if this had to happen *inside* the body before the drug had any anti-bacterial effect?

They experimented with the molecule, broke it across the azo link and tested the chemicals that resulted for anti-bacterial activity. One such product, *sulphanilamide* was every bit as active as Prontosil against streptococci – indeed it was even more potent! They had solved the enigma: it was sulphanilamide which was the real active ingredient of Prontosil, released within the body by natural chemical processes acting upon the drug.[13] This piece of the molecule, a much simpler chemical, had long been manufactured by the ton as a side product in the dye industry and nobody had ever thought of testing it as an antibiotic.

It was now realized that sulphanilamide had been described way back in 1909 by a chemist, Paul Gelmo, then working for his doctoral thesis in Vienna. But Gelmo had no idea of its anti-bacterial properties. Instead the compound was taken as a starting point in the synthesis of dyes by Bayer itself. The Bayer directors were naturally dismayed to find their patent was already out of date. The active principle of their wonder drug could be manufactured by anybody who wanted to do so – and what was more, sulphanilamide did not turn the patient's skin as red as a boiled lobster. The Elberfeld drug company was bereft of any financial compensation for their years of hard research as, suddenly, every laboratory in the world was racing to find its own variation on the sulphonamide theme.

And already the first brave researchers had turned to face the mountain. Would sulphanilamide cure tuberculosis?

iv

IN 1937, ARNOLD R. RICH and Richard H. Follis, at the Johns Hopkins Medical School in Baltimore, tested sulphanilamide for anti-tuberculous properties.

After injecting fifty-nine guinea pigs with a virulent strain of human tuberculosis under the skin they treated thirty-one of them with sulphanilamide, while observing the remaining animals as untreated "controls". The treated animals were divided into three groups of gradually increasing dose of the drug.

By the end of the experiment, all twenty-eight control animals had developed blood-borne tuberculosis. The animals given the lowest treatment dose of sulphanilamide had suffered the same overwhelming disease, with tuberculosis spreading to every internal organ through the blood stream. In the animals on the higher doses, there was a much less extensive spread of infection. This was most noticeable in those given the very highest dose of sulphanilamide, where there was a striking reduction in visible abscesses throughout the internal organs, in dramatic contrast with the untreated group of guinea pigs, where the lymph glands draining the groin were grossly swollen and the internal organs, particularly the spleens were a mass of abscesses, teeming with tuberculous bacteria.[14]

Rich and Follis did not suggest the drug would do the same for human sufferers. To get such beneficial effects in the guinea pigs, such massive doses of the drug had had to be given that, in human terms, the equivalent dose would have killed the patient. Sulphanilamide would never be used in the treatment of tuberculosis. Nevertheless, for the first time in history tuberculosis had been held back, even if only a little, by the use of a medicine.

If the medical profession at large were too prejudiced to take notice, a vital few took heart and inspiration from it. Buttle and Parish in Britain – Grey, Ballon and others in the United States – took the experiment a step further by showing that sulphanilamide also slowed down the growth of tuberculous bacteria in test tubes. The molecule of sulphanilamide was altered again and again, searching for new options with enhanced potential. In 1940, two doctors working at the Mayo Clinic, William H. Feldman and H. Corwin Hinshaw tested a derivative of sulphanilamide, called sulphapyridine, and found that it too slowed down tuberculous infection in guinea pigs. But like sulphanilamide, the doses used were much too poisonous for extrapolation to humans. In the Bayer laboratories at Elberfeld, Domagk had already begun his own search for the cure.

After the discovery of Prontosil, he systematically tested every new drug derived from it by the Bayer chemists for activity against tuberculosis. Impressed by the action of sulphanilamide and the other sulphonamide derivatives against the bacterium in guinea pigs, he knew that further research was vital. But many of his co-workers were sceptical. Because the tuberculosis bacillus was protected with its thick waxy coat, they believed that a curative drug would need to contain high fat residues as part of its molecule. They were so convinced of this that they tried very hard to incorporate such fatty residues into the sulphonamide molecule, but nothing came of it. Domagk disagreed with them and was determined to go his own way. He carried on testing hundreds of sulphonamides, none of which proved to have any better action against tuberculosis, until suddenly there was a more interesting response. In bacterial cultures and in animal experiments, a new sulphonamide, sulphathiazole, showed a much more striking effect. It would be two years later, in 1941, before he felt ready to present his findings to a meeting of chest physicians in Vienna, by which time circumstances were so much changed in Europe that nobody took any notice.

In the early hours of the morning, 15 March 1939, Hitler had given the order for the incorporation of what remained of Czechoslovakia after the Sudetan annexation, into the greater Germany. By the end of the day, the state of Czechoslovakia had ceased to exist. The next country on Hitler's agenda was Poland. For Gerhard Domagk, as for millions of ordinary German citizens, there was little enthusiasm for a second great bloodbath. Yet throughout 1939, all research interest was already switching from the more difficult long-term medical problems such as cancer and tuberculosis to the treatment of infected wounds on the battlefield.

In the eye of a continuing storm of international meetings, lectures and intensive research, Domagk continued his very personal struggle for decency and humanity, a struggle which he recorded in his diary throughout all the cataclysms and upheaval of war. Soon his work, and the international recognition it had brought him, would place his life in danger.

v

DOMAGK WAS PROUDLY German. He also had a deep faith in the essential good of human nature. On many occasions, throughout 1939, he recorded in his diary the grief he felt at this new outbreak of war – and how it would disrupt so much vital medical research in all the great universities of Europe. He could not believe that the wonderful effort previously devoted to furthering progress and humanity would now be devoted to destruction. How could so many scientists, colleagues he knew well – men who had played such a wonderful part in rebuilding Germany after the devastation of the first war – now allow

themselves to contemplate the same all over again? He could
see how even his working companions were allowing themselves to be distracted into a langour of hopelessness. The
shock of impending war was sapping morale everywhere. Even
the chemists at Bayer, previously so hard working and gifted,
were providing him with few new products for testing. Domagk refused to surrender to this war psychosis. In spite of the
fact that so many others appeared to have given in, he insisted
on starting a new line of research, searching out new ways of
treating nutritional deficiencies.

But his heart was laden with foreboding. Only a week after he
had reported his results to the German Natural Scientists and
Doctors Conference in Stuttgart, he was racked by new doubts.
How could he justify even these new experiments to help the
hungry or people sick with cancer, when millions would soon
be torn asunder by bombs and grenades in the best years of
their lives. "What will come of humanity if everybody just goes
along with this war fever?"[15]

On the very eve of war, the world still showered him and the
Bayer team with honours. At the Paris World Fair, in 1938,
Prontosil was awarded the Grand Prix. In March, 1939, he was
invited to Budapest, to receive the Klebelsberg medal. The
University of Edinburgh awarded him the Cameron Prize. The
medical faculty in Leeds, together with the British Medical
Association, voted him the Adingham gold medal. But he could
derive little comfort from the awards. Memories of the killing
fields of the first war had returned to haunt him. He had hoped
to travel to Flanders in the autumn of 1939, on the twenty-fifth
anniversary of the battle, but this proved impossible. In May,
1939, while attending a conference in Rome, he found some
respite from his deeper worries in visiting the Forlanini Institute for Tuberculosis. Indeed, tuberculosis was coming to
occupy more and more of his thoughts.

When travelling to a conference on cancer in June, 1939, the
Belgian passport control stopped him at Lüttich station. He was
surrounded by special police officers, who demanded to know
his reason for coming to Belgium. He had to be rescued by Dr
Thonnard, before being allowed a two days visitor's permit.

During the conference, he was invited by the chairman to say a few words on the growing importance of chemotherapy; he did his best. Afterwards, he could remember little of the medical content – only the atmosphere of tension, bitterness and anger, which seemed universally prevalent. This humane and civilized man was bewildered at the speed with which a malignancy was infiltrating the entire world. When, in June 1939, he wrote a reply to a letter from Philadelphia, describing him as the saviour of mankind, Gerhard Domagk's reply was courteous; but between the lines there was a bitter note of sadness.

"These awards bring me great pleasure after so many years of grinding work. Most rewarding of all are the letters from grateful patients, who could be helped, and particularly the letters from children – and of course the objective judgement of experienced representatives of the medical world. If only for a short time, I can forget all the toil and weeks of disappointment and I feel able to take on new problems. . ."[16]

For Domagk and his family, in August 1939, there was a fleeting reprieve of serenity and peace.

"We are enjoying blue late summer days on the Baltic. There is an amazing cleanness and clearness in those few hours before sunset. We spend our time watering the newly planted shrubs and winkling out the weeds. Wolfgang is Bigears with his amazed big child's eyes. All the grass has been removed between the raspberries. Götz roams the fields, looking for frogs and rabbits."[17]

But Domagk was aware that these balmy days were numbered. He had received a personal invitation to go to New York in September to attend the International Congress of Microbiology, where a formative meeting of minds would take place between Selman Waksman, René Dubos and Alexander Fleming. Domagk would miss the meeting. In spite of his inner hopes, his occasional spurts of optimism, everything continued to point towards war. His mother, who had come to visit him, had to leave in a hurry because so many people in a local factory had been called up for military service. His father, the schoolteacher, now seventy-three, had been forced to return to work. When they drove his father to the steamer, it refused to accept him because all boats had been requisitioned by the authorities.

These were unpredictable days, with rapid swings from high hope to deep despair. In his diary, Domagk noted from day to day and week to week, the inexorable slide towards a war which was, in all but declaration, predetermined.

"The resorts are empty. One telegram follows another. The post office is working overtime. . . On the last morning before our departure, we saw uniforms on the watchtower. They are bringing in the sailing boat which was only newly built by a boat builder in the area. On the way out they found a mine. Mother takes father back to the steamer. The children are more clinging than ever in their cries. Mother is very brave. A beautiful farewell, without tears. Everybody will do their best – even when alone. Remain calm. On the station in Lübeck, we meet many sad wives. We spend the night in Mecklenburg. In the hotel, there are more army officers and wives, with eyes red from crying.

"Officially, mobilization has not been announced, but they are bringing in horses from the surrounding villages. One of the government buildings has a sign, saying: 'We accept volunteers'. Compared with 1914, the mood is subdued. The memories of the dreadful war experiences are still awake in peoples' memories. The cafés and bars are full of young people, too young to go to war. They are playing dance music and hits, unable to hide a subdued determination. What is it all about? Is there no other solution? Does the world still not know any better? Do they still have to use the most primitive remedies, like wild beasts who have plenty of food but still growl to stop each other from helping themselves?"[18]

For a time, he watched the first army officers arrive for breakfast in the dining room. Then he left to spend a few moments sitting on a bench, enjoying the beauty of the countryside, the forest and the peaceful lake, just as it was once in his childhood days. A little dog sat down beside him, rubbing his coat against his shoe. On the bench next to him was a group of women, chatting away.

He read a poster which declared that no guarantee could be given for the transport of civilians. He had to abandon his plans to go to a meeting of the German pathological association and instead decided to take a train back to Ludwigslust, from there an overcrowded train on to Berlin. There was a race to get one of the remaining taxis, fifty per cent of which had been requisitioned for the army. There were very few private cars and the roads were very quiet. Unusually quiet. Hitler was at this very moment in a meeting in the Chancellory. Outside, on Wilhelmsplatz, people hung about, hoping to get a glimpse of him when he came out. There was an unusual seriousness and calm about. No panic. The next and last train from Berlin to Cologne was supposed to leave at eleven o'clock at night and he arrived there two hours before departure. The station was overcrowded. Members of the Red Cross were assisting people, mothers with young children.

"The trains are arriving. The panic starts. I help as much as I can with some children, screaming, whining, sighing. Dust, noise, children crying, marching boots, pushing, screaming, pulling, shouting, a whistle. Everybody sinks into their place on the train, eyelids falling over children's eyes, sitting on boxes and chests. Bigwigs lean back in their cushions and pillows as if they had never been children, never felt childlike innocence. Quarrelsome women in their hordes want to sit more comfortably. They are full of hatred. Mothers and sons leaning head to head, the same profile. The moon is waning yet the night is beautiful in God's stillness."[19]

Soon afterwards, the inevitable: "The campaign into Poland has ended. Hitler marched into Danzig amidst great jubilations. Now England has declared war on Germany."[20]

vi

HE KNEW IT would happen all over again: the obscene wastage of young lives, the field hospitals trying to cope under impossible conditions with wounded limbs grotesquely swollen, black, bursting with pus and foul stenching gas bubbles. Tuberculosis would have to wait while he focused every fibre of his energy on the search for a drug that would cure gas gangrene.

The early days after the declaration of war were difficult days of hard bitter duty. Rationing had been introduced and his local grocer, whom he had known for years, refused to supply him with butter or cheese because he had not yet received his ration card. On many occasions, when he arrived home in the evening after work, he ate dried bread and salt washed down by a thin brew made from the last few coffee beans. A hard note of realism recurs again and again in his diary. "But such things will not change voluntarily. For humanity to triumph it will take energetic and kind hands, open eyes that see and behold".[21]

By September, the Bayer team had discovered a new sulphonamide drug, Mesudin, which was more effective against gas gangrene than anything ever known. In a letter to the army doctors, Domagk gave them details of the animal experiments, urging them to concentrate on drugs that would help combat this dreadful infection. The army doctors took little notice. Mentally he was still in a state of shock with this tragic outbreak of a second world war. "It will be an inhumane war." With touching pathos, he took heart in the fact that on the French-German border, the two armies facing each other were said to have put up posters calling, "Don't shoot!"

His son, Götz, had a bad fall on 30 September, while rolling a wheel up a hill and he was brought home with his bloodied face badly lacerated and contaminated with dirt. By the following day he had become very feverish and his upper lip and face became badly swollen. His father treated him with Prontosil.

Military doctors were arriving at the Bayer institute, to hear more about the gas gangrene work, and Domagk told them as much as he knew. He was no longer interested in publishing his results – his only wish was to help, and as quickly as possible. On 26 October, he fell ill with flu himself and treated himself with Prontosil. In the afternoon, depressed by myriad worries in addition to his illness, he took what appeared a routine phone call from Berlin. A Swedish journalist expressed an unusual degree of interest in his previous researches and discoveries. The same night, Domagk had another call from the same man, with a totally unexpected message of congratulation. At midnight, that same night, he was woken up by a phone call, informing him that he had received an urgent telegram.

Professor Domagk,
  The Professorial Committee of the Royal Caroline Institute has today
decided to honour you with this year's Nobel Prize for Physiology or
Medicine for the discovery of the anti-bacterial action of Prontosil.
Signed,
Gunnar Holmgren,
Director of the Caroline Institute.[22]

vii

FOLLOWING THE DISCOVERY of Prontosil, when one might
have expected all Germany to celebrate this untiring scientist
and his contribution towards humanity, the Nazi party had felt
threatened by his humanitarian pacifism. At a time when Hitler
was asking for blood sacrifices, this dwelling on the sanctity of
life was most unwelcome. Brownshirts spread rumours that all
this fuss about the sulphonamides was just witchcraft and
quackery.

But it wasn't easy to dispel the magic of a wonder drug. They
took their lies and innuendo to the darkest depths. Spreading
rumours that there had been deaths following the administration of Prontosil, they managed to sow distrust where there was
not a jot of evidence to substantiate their allegations. One day
Domagk was called to such a case in Berlin by telegram, ac-
cusing him and his drug of directly causing the death of a
patient, only to find that the postmortem examination revealed
blood-borne tuberculosis as the cause of death. Domagk had
never claimed that his drug cured tuberculosis – quite the contrary. But now, despite his heart-felt German patriotism, his life
and philosophy were under scrutiny. All the more so, it
seemed, as impressive statistics appeared to prove just how
wonderful his discovery had been.

In 1938, without his being aware of it, Domagk had been
nominated for the Nobel Prize by many French, American and
English scientists. The Nobel Committee in Stockholm was well
aware of the dangers this posed.

In 1935 the German pacifist writer, Carl von Ossietzky, had
been awarded the Nobel Prize for Peace, enraging Hitler. But

Hitler's anger did not prevent Goering sending two of his henchmen to Stockholm to ask for the cheque that went with the prize in order to secrete it in the party's own coffers. The Nobel authorities refused. Ossietzky was a journalist who had helped to found the *Nie Wieder Krieg* (No More War) organization in 1922 and became editor of the *Weltbuhne,* a liberal political newspaper. In 1927, following a series of articles in which he unmasked the Reichswehr's secret rearmament preparations, he was sentenced to imprisonment. Subsequently released under amnesty, he was rearrested on 28 February 1933 at Hitler's order and sent to Papenburg concentration camp, where his health deteriorated and he fell seriously ill with tuberculosis. He was still incarcerated in the camp when, in 1935, he was awarded the Nobel Prize for Peace. This caused a major international outcry, which embarrassed the Nazi authorities, who were forced to move Ossietzky to a Berlin hospital, where he died from blood-borne tuberculosis on 4 May 1938.

After the supposed insult of the awarding of the prize to Ossietzky, who had only recently died such a harrowing and notorious death, Hitler himself had decreed that in future the granting of a Nobel Prize to a German citizen would be considered an anti-German act. It was against such perilous opposition that the Nobel Committee in Stockholm considered Domagk's contribution. Yet they thought so highly of his achievements that they remained unanimous in his favour – and it had been a tenet of Alfred Nobel's original will that the prize be awarded regardless of the nationality of the recipient.

At about one o'clock in the morning, he received another phone call from Berlin – this time from Dr Banse of the Reich newspaper press, asking him for confirmation of the rumour that he had been awarded the Nobel Prize. Every office in the country, no matter how prestigious, was by now firmly under Nazi control and the party were suspicious of a political intrigue. The press and national radio were ordered to silence.

On 27 October, Domagk returned to work, to show seventeen military doctors round the institute. He told nobody except the director of the company about the award of the Nobel Prize and he specifically asked the director not to mention anything for the time being until he had had the reaction of the Reich's government. Meanwhile, in an urgent communication, he wrote the following note to the Chancellor of his university, Münster, for advice on whether he should accept or decline the Prize.

> *I received the enclosed telegram and ask you to advise me how best to answer this communication. In so far as I can ascertain, it is forbidden (for a German citizen) to accept a Nobel Prize for Peace. Does the prohibition still stand? Is it also applicable to natural science?*[23]

The Chancellor replied with a telegram: "Wait for further information."[24]

For an agonized week, Domagk was left in suspense without a single word, before receiving some slight encouragement from the University Chancellor:

> *Münster, 2 November, 1939,*
> *Dear Dr Domagk,*
> *Congratulations on the high award that you have received. At the moment, Hitler prohibits German nationals from accepting the Nobel Prize for Peace. I have been in contact by telephone with the Reich's Ministry for Home Affairs and with the cultural political department of the Foreign Office, and have written them an urgent letter, pointing out that major differences should be made between the so-called Nobel Peace Prize awarded by the Norwegian Landtag and the Scientific Nobel Prize awarded by Sweden. As soon as I get more information I shall let you hear of it.*
> *Heil Hitler*[25]

Behind the scenes, the Vice-Chairman of the Nobel Committee, Professor Folke Henschen, tried to persuade the German government to alter its rigid stance in the case of such an outstanding non-political contribution to humanity. He even tried a personal letter to Hermann Goering but received no reply. In final desperation, he turned to the German ambassador in Stockholm, who telegraphed Berlin and two days later received a reply from the cultural section of the Foreign Office, which he read out to Henschen over the telephone:

"Please inform Nobel Committee that the award of Nobel Prize to a German is positively unwelcome."[26]

So far, not a word of the prize had appeared in the German newspapers, while Domagk was receiving telegrams of congratulations from America, forwarded by an acquaintance working for Bayer over there. He was congratulated by the Bayer director, William Weiss. As was his duty, he informed his district military commander, under whom he was a staff doctor. While the government maintained its foreboding silence, the local commander sent him his congratulations.

Still the menacing silence continued. Apart from the director, nobody at the company knew about it. One of the technical assistants got hold of the news from her aunt in Finland, but Domagk asked her not to speak about it. With a growing realization of the difference between the media propaganda and the reality he was now experiencing, Domagk asked himself in an understandable outburst of anguish: "Is this situation worthy of a free nation?"[27]

On 3 November, having received no advice from the Nazi government, he wrote the following lines to Professor Holmgren, Rector of the Caroline Institute.

"With all my thanks, I confirm receipt of your telegram and the subsequent letter of confirmation from Professor Liljestrand, informing me that I have been awarded the Nobel Prize for Medicine or Physiology for the year 1939, honouring my research in the field of chemotherapy of bacterial infections. I was very pleased with the recognition of my work and I would like to thank you and the teaching staff of the Caroline Institute of Stockholm. To the best of my knowledge, as a German national, I am not allowed to accept the Prize. I am still in the process of obtaining detailed information about the legal position. Since this is taking longer than I would have hoped, I have to ask you to excuse the delay in my replying. However, I do hope that I will have the opportunity to talk about my work in Stockholm to any Swedish colleagues who are interested and, in this way, offer a small thankyou for the recognition that you have given to my work. I cannot tell you at this moment in time if I shall be able to come on 10 December to Stockholm. I will let you know as soon as I have further news. With best greetings[28]

On the evening of 17 November, Domagk had just completed his preparation for a lecture he was to give to a Congress in Berlin, when the Gestapo arrived at his Wuppertal home to arrest him.

While they were searching his house, they maintained a two-way conversation with Ober-Führer Müller in Berlin, letting him know of their progress. In Domagk's own words: "I was taken in a car by soldiers armed with rifles and put in cell No 10 of the town gaol for interrogation. No reason was given for my arrest. On one occasion when a man arrived to clean out my cell, he asked me what I was doing there. When I told him I was in gaol because I had received the Nobel Prize, he tapped his head and declared: 'This one is mad'. Only later, during questioning, was it revealed that it had something to do with the Nobel Prize. After a few days of imprisonment, there was still no explanation. Only once was it was mentioned, and then casually, that I had been too polite to the Swedes. For my wife, who was extremely worried about me, these were days of extreme anxiety. I had to be prepared for anything."[29]

He was released, physically and mentally exhausted, after a week, a terrifying experience that would leave him physically and mentally shocked. No explanation for his arrest was ever given. "I kept telling myself this is a war to put injustice right again. The whole horrible affair took its toll on me healthwise. During the arrest I felt severe pains in my chest, something I had never known before. It was hard to overcome the feeling that my attitude to life and its ideals had been shattered."[30]

In spite of congratulations trickling through from many eminent colleagues in the outside world, from Professor Windhaus in Göttingen, Fischer in Copenhagen, Heubner in Berlin, Heymans in Ghent, Zeissler in Hamburg, others in Norway, even San Francisco, the blackout in the German media was ruthlessly propagated. Months later, he still felt unwell. He went to see his friend, Philipp Klee, at the Wuppertal Hospital, for a comprehensive medical checkup. Klee, who was fighting his own desperate battle to keep his Jewish wife, Flora, from being arrested and taken to a concentration camp, told Domagk he could find no physical disorder. From time to time, throughout Domagk's life from then on, these problems would resurface. Although he realized they were caused by stress, he could never again shake himself free of them.

Nevertheless on 28 November, following his release, he was determined to go to Berlin and deliver his planned educational lecture. But when he arrived at Potsdam station, his name was called out over the loudspeakers and he was ordered to go to the exit, where a Gestapo officer was again waiting for him. He was taken back to the offices of the secret police and told he would not be allowed to give his lecture. Instead he was ordered to sign a prepared declaration, addressed to the Nobel Committee in Stockholm, which included the following terse statement:

"In accordance with the law of which I have now been fully advised, I am obliged to decline the Prize offered to me."[31]

8

Visionaries

"Bring me the candle," he called to Brown, with whom he was staying, "and let me see this blood." He looked at the bright red spot on his pillow and then, his excitement and intoxication gone, he said calmly, "I know the colour of that blood. It's arterial blood . . . That blood is my death warrant."

John Keats (aged twenty-six)

i

I N 1921 A YOUNG doctor from Northern Ireland, V.D. Allison went to work in St Mary's Hospital, London. He chose the bacteriology department in this famous if rather dilapidated old hospital, a laboratory which was then run under the brilliant if somewhat dictatorial leadership of Dr Almroth Wright. A pupil of Ehrlich, Wright was a burly man of mixed Presbyterian Irish and Swedish parentage, a brilliant linguist and *confidant* of George Bernard Shaw. Early in his career he had been convinced by meeting a Russian bacteriologist, called Haffkine[1], that the cure for bacterial disease would not come, as his teacher Ehrlich had proposed, from anti-bacterial drugs, but from assisting the body's natural immunity, for instance with vaccination. This idea, in common with Koch and indeed most scientists worldwide, was entirely credible and would prove of importance later but with Wright it assumed infallibility; taken with a personality which had declared his lab "an independent republic", it lent itself to a disastrously negative attitude of mind when it came to considering the potential of antibiotics.

At this time Alexander Fleming was a young unknown Scottish doctor, working in Wright's department. Allison would later tell his own revealing story about working with Fleming.

"Early on, Fleming began to tease me about my excessive tidiness in the laboratory. At the end of each day's work, I cleaned my bench, put it in order for the next day and discarded tubes and culture plates for which I had no further use. He for his part kept his cultures . . . for two or three weeks until his bench was overcrowded with forty or fifty cultures. He would then discard them, first of all looking at them individually to see whether anything interesting or unusual had developed. I took his teasing in the spirit in which it was given. However, the sequel was to prove how right he was, for if he had been as tidy as he thought I was, he would never have made his two great discoveries."[2]

Fleming and Domagk were alike in their curiosity with the seemingly trivial or unusual.

In 1928, a year after Domagk began work with Bayer, another doctor, Merlin Pryce, was working with Fleming on mutant forms of staphylococcal bacteria, the cause of boils. In order to examine colonies of these bacteria on agar in Petri dishes, Fleming had to lift the lids off the dishes, exposing the cultures to contaminants from the air. The room he was working in was small, cluttered with his work and stiflingly stuffy. Not unnaturally Fleming had a tendency to leave his window open onto Praed Street. Pryce turned up one day to see Fleming in the little disorderly laboratory, where he found him as usual surrounded by heaps of culture dishes. With his dry Scottish humour, Fleming pulled Pryce's leg about forcing him to redo much of Pryce's earlier work in order to produce a scientific paper when Fleming, still speaking laconically, took up some old cultures and peered under the lids. Several of the cultures had been contaminated by a fungus. This wasn't at all unusual, given that he left dishes to lie around for such long periods – but now suddenly he stopped talking. Then, after a moment's observation, said, in his usual unconcerned tones: "That's funny!"[3]

On the plate was a thick round disc of greenish mould, with feathery raised surface – one of those tiny fungi, usually green, brown, yellow or black, which proliferate over decomposing organic refuse in damp locations – while all about the mould the colonies of staphylococcus had been dissolved into droplets resembling dew.

Pryce wasn't over impressed by this. Strange things would occasionally get into bacterial cultures and spoil them. Moulds were very commonly found as contaminants in laboratory air. Perhaps the mould was producing digestive acids or some such toxic chemical which seemed of little interest.

But Fleming was a good deal more curious. His eyes glinted with interest as he picked off a scrap of mould and incubated it into a culture of broth. Pryce would later remark: "What struck me was that he didn't confine himself to observing, but took action at once. Lots of people observe a phenomenon, feeling that it may be important, but they don't get beyond being surprised – after which, they forget."[4] This was never the case with Fleming, who had previously instructed Pryce to be sure of gleaning every possible morsel of information from his mistakes.

Alexander Fleming had just discovered the fungus, *Penicillium notatum*, which produces penicillin. In subsequent biographies, people have often criticized Fleming as blundering into his great discovery but this is an injustice. Many of the greatest scientific discoveries have been triggered by a chance observation, or the result of pure luck. In 1877 John Tyndall, the English scientist who first brought Koch's discovery to the attention of the London and *New York Times*, became interested in Pasteur's discovery of micro-organisms that were to be found in "fresh air". In an experiment designed to map out the floating diarama of germs in what had previously been assumed to be good fresh English air, he exposed a series of test tubes, all laid out carefully in rows, to the atmosphere. He made a most remarkable catch. In many of his tubes he found a mould, called Penicillium, which he found "exquisitely beautiful". He even made the observation that . . . "in every case where the mould was thick and coherent (in one of his test tubes), the bacteria (also contained in the test tube) died, or became dormant, and fell to the bottom as a sediment."[5] Unlike Fleming, he made no attempt to take this further.

It was surely in the very unorthodox untidiness of his personality, coupled with a very sharp and original perception,
that Fleming was at his most creative! Had his personality been
more tidily orthodox, he would most certainly have thrown his
cultures away long before they had been contaminated by the
Penicillium mould and he would never have made his great
discovery. Like great artists or writers, scientists too derive
their inspiration from the complex interaction of their personalities and their work. A lesser scientist would have taken
the discovery little further than that empirical observation,
behind which the vital significance was hidden from them in a
chaos of incomprehensible signs. It was again the creativity of
the true scientist that made him carry on in his seemingly wandering and half-hearted way to investigate the curious observation further.

Part of the explanation for the subsequent delay must have
been Wright's influence: Fleming had long been brainwashed
in favour of vaccines. Yet when, in 1934, Lewis Holt, a gifted
young biochemist, came to work in the laboratory on the
cause of scurvy, Fleming proudly showed him the lethal effects
of a crude extract of penicillin on a culture of dangerous
staphylococcal bacteria. Fleming's problem was that he was
unable to extract the penicillin from the mould in a purity or
quantity that would make it useful. Holt was so impressed, he
was determined to help. In a clever intuitive move, he thought
up a way in which they might purify and even extract penicillin
but, for some inexplicable reason, Fleming showed little interest and Wright was opposed to any further research on it. This
unfortunate attitude delayed the production of penicillin until
long after Prontosil had made its global impact. In 1936, one of
Fleming's colleagues, Ronald Hare, became seriously ill after he
had cut his finger on a sliver of glass infected with the streptococcus. Like Domagk's daughter, the infection rapidly
climbed his entire arm and, with his life at risk, he was admitted
to hospital where he was treated by Colebrook with Prontosil.
There was some irony in this since Hare was known to be very
critical of Domagk. Fleming visited him at his bedside and
observing how ill he looked – his skin had also turned red with
the drug – told Hare's wife to say her prayers. When Hare

survived, Fleming, although reluctant to say so openly, was profoundly impressed.

A second incident was to prove even more fruitful in persuading Fleming, with his subsequent colleagues, Chain, Florey, and Heatley, to take penicillin production seriously.

In 1935 Domagk arrived in London to address the Royal Society of Medicine on the subject of Prontosil. Fleming was in his audience and after the lecture remarked to Lewis Holt, who had been fascinated: "Yes, but penicillin can do better than that."[6] He thought the quantity of Prontosil given was high and the results not as dramatic as he would have expected with penicillin. But secretly Fleming was every bit as impressed as Holt, while Wright, needless to say, refused adamantly to believe the German statistics.

During Domagk's London lecture in 1935, a vital cross-fertilization of ideas had clearly taken place. Fleming, a man not readily given to praise, would subsequently confess, with laconic succinctness: "no sulphonamides without Domagk: no penicillin without sulphonamides; no antibiotics without penicillin."[7] In retrospect, it seems unbelievable that when, in 1936, the re-inspired Fleming spoke about penicillin at the Second International Congress of Microbiology, nobody took the slightest interest. The fashion world of science – yes, indeed science is prey to fashion – no longer gave a damn about a discovery made some seven years before and from which nothing useful appeared to be emerging.

Fleming's problem with penicillin was still that same difficulty in mass production of a stable product. It has to be remembered that he was working in a tiny laboratory that was part of a London hospital where Domagk was working on behalf of a giant pharmaceutical company, who saw it as a first priority. This was the situation when, in 1939, Fleming travelled to New York to take part in the Third International Congress of Microbiology.

ii

WE KNOW FROM his diary that Domagk was desperately keen to attend this congress but was prevented by circumstance from

doing so. Selman Waksman was present, and equally importantly, René Dubos. Fleming was already well acquainted with
Dubos, whose work he admired. Dubos at this time was at the
peak of his scientific creativity and was currently working on
something remarkable; he must have given Fleming some inkling of how things were progressing at this meeting – we know
that he asked the laconic Fleming, no doubt very enthusiastically, how he was getting on with penicillin. Fleming
explained that at last the job of purifying and mass producing
penicillin was in the hands of dedicated experts, the Australian
Dr Howard Florey, who had for a time worked at the Rockefeller University, Dr Ernst B. Chain, a chemist of mixed Russian
and German parentage, and Florey's Oxford based colleague,
Norman Heatley. In fact the first intravenous injection of penicillin was still two years away and would be given to a
policeman in Oxford in February 1941. This unfortunate man, at
death's door from blood-borne infection with the abscess-
causing staphylococcus, was initially improved by the antibiotic but died when supplies of penicillin ran out.

For Selman Waksman, something would happen at this
meeting with all the iconoclastic impact of Dubos' revelation in
the Palatine Gardens, or Domagk's vow made before the
carnage of Verdun. A meeting of minds would take place
between Waksman and Alexander Fleming that would change
medical history in not one but in many extraordinary avenues.
Waksman found himself spellbound with what Fleming was
now saying. Here was a discovery of global importance that had
come from a humble micro-organism from the air. Nobody in
the world knew more than Waksman about those humble
micro-organisms that lived in air, soil, water. Suddenly he saw
the implications. Just how profound an effect it had upon his
thinking we can judge from the memory of his protégé, Dr H.
Boyd Woodruff, who was working very closely with Waksman
at Rutgers at this time. "Suddenly ... a turning point
developed. Dr Waksman appeared in the laboratory one day.
He was highly agitated. 'Woodruff,' he said, 'drop everything.
See what these Englishmen have discovered a mould can
do!' "[8] From this very moment, the direction of Waksman's
researches, his entire life, would be radically altered.

Penicillin would soon become one of the most important of antibiotic discoveries, dramatically curing many acute bacterial infections. But would it cure tuberculosis?

Two doctors called Smith and Emmert set up an experiment in which extracts from various strains of Penicillium mould were incubated with cultures of the tuberculosis germs. It had no effect. Next they tested penicillin against tuberculosis grown in eggs and in guinea pigs which had been infected with tuberculosis. But the answers were unequivocal. Penicillin had no significant effect against tuberculosis.[9]

For the myriad detractors, it was just more evidence that tuberculosis would never be cured by antibiotic therapy. Tuberculosis, they argued, was not like the acute bacterial infections. They pointed to the fact that within a week or two at most, an acute bacterial infection, such as that due to the much-feared streptococcus, either killed a patient or the patient got better. Tuberculosis was not like this at all. Once established in the lungs, or the bowel, in the throat, in the kidneys, in the eye, or in the very marrow of the bones, tuberculosis festered on and on, impervious to all efforts to cure it, seemingly indestructible. No antibiotic would ever kill such a germ, protected by its thick impenetrable waxy coat. Their pessimism was very understandable. Worldwide, tuberculosis was a terror on such leviathan scale, its various manifestations, its social implications, its perverse feeding off such human calamities as war, poverty and famine, was of such a Piranesian darkness and complexity, it palled even the most ambitious scientific imagination. More than a mere disease, it brooded in the subconscious of every doctor and nurse, as much as in the anxieties and terrors of the lay population, an impregnable and pitiless shadow. The nightmare had always existed, it would continue to exist, constant yet subtly changing, metamorphosing, as now with the outbreak of a second world war, to hone itself perfectly to this new human disadvantage. Five million people who were suffering from the disease this year would be dead from it by the end of the year. How could human artifice ever hope to defeat it?

Unknown to the antibiotic scientists and working entirely on his own at Duke University, in North Carolina, a biochemist

called Frederick Bernheim had taken it into his head to do
something about it.

iii

FROM THE EARLY days of his university education, Bernheim
had a hearty appetite for scientific adventure. After studying
for his AB degree on the distinguished campus of Harvard, he
moved to Cambridge, Massachusetts, for his PhD, before jour-
neying on to Munich, to continue his fascination with the
chemistry of life. In 1930 his unique enthusiasm and talent were
recognized by Duke University, North Carolina, where, in spite
of the fact he had had no formal training whatsoever in pharmacology, he was appointed assistant professor in this subject. To
the non-scientist, it may seem that pharmacology, which deals
with drugs and drug therapy, is little removed from biochemistry, which is the study of the chemistry of life, but in practice
they are separate, if related, disciplines. The newly appointed
Bernheim, well aware of the gaps in his knowledge, set about
educating himself in all that was known about drugs, their
chemical nature and how they acted within the body. It did not
take him long to realize that the pharmacologists of his day
knew next to nothing. There was only one way in which
Frederick Bernheim would ever obtain answers: he began his
own unique and highly creative series of experiments.[10]

Soon these experiments led him to discover the importance
of a chemical called histamine in allergic processes. This in its
turn led to the discovery of the drugs now used against the
distracting itch of urticaria, which we now call the antihista-
mines. Throughout these researches, what really excited
Bernheim was the realization that nothing was known about
the way drugs affected the vital internal chemicals in living
cells, called enzymes, which controlled the wonderful chemical
balances of the body. During the ten years from 1930 to 1939, he
conducted hundreds of such brilliantly original experiments,
enlightening science again and again. Now suddenly, at the
very time that the international meeting was taking place in
New York, this amazing biochemist, who had never worked

with bacteria in his life, veered abruptly away from the effects of drugs on the body's tissues and turned his sights on tuberculosis.

In a letter to the medical writer, Julius H. Comroe Jr, dated February 1978, Bernheim explained why he did so.[11]

With the outbreak of the second world war, he knew there would be a massive increase in the suffering and death from tuberculosis. He was only too painfully aware that even with Domagk's discovery of the sulphonamides, there was no effective treatment for this terrible infection. Bernheim wasn't just going to sit back and worry about it. He was going to do something about it. But what could he, with no knowledge whatsoever of the tuberculosis germ, really do? He set his mind to discovering what little he could about the living chemistry of the tuberculosis germ itself.

What, he asked himself, did the germ need as food? Bernheim devised a test system in which he added small amounts of interesting substances to a culture of the tuberculosis germs, at the same time measuring the amounts of oxygen that were being used up by the germs. If the oxygen uptake by the germ suddenly increased, he knew that the test substance was being used as food by the germ. To his astonishment, he found that tuberculosis germs did not increase their oxygen uptake when he added ordinary foods such as carbohydrate or the building blocks of proteins, called amino acids. Bernheim had to think again. Then he had a moment of inspiration. During those previous ten years of experiment, he had found that the commonest drug in the world, simple aspirin, had the most curious effects on the chemistry of life. He repeated the experiment with aspirin. There was an extraordinary change.

He found that if he added a tiny amount of sodium salicylate to the suspended bacteria, the oxygen uptake by the bacteria doubled. Unable to believe it, he repeated the test. The results were the same. Next he measured the carbon dioxide production of the germs and found this increased in a complementary way to the decrease in oxygen. This had to be important.

On 30 August 1940, Bernheim communicated his discovery to the world in a tiny paper, contained within a single page of the journal, *Science*.[12] Nobody was more determined than he was that this strange observation must be taken further. Indeed he now planned to make this experiment the first step in the search for a drug that might cure tuberculosis. Sadly, for Frederick Bernheim, his personal search would eventually prove unsuccessful. Yet his key experiment would inspire a friend and colleague. As soon as he received his first copies of the *Science* paper from the publishers, Bernheim entrusted a copy to the ordinary post, braving the Atlantic Ocean with its patrolling battleships and U-boats, on its slow journey to Gothenburg, Sweden. The fragile letter with its single page scientific paper was addressed to a remarkable young man, only recently promoted to Chief of Chemical Pathology at the Sahlgren's Hospital. This man's name was Jorgen Lehmann.

9

One Small Candle

Discoveries are made by men, not merely by minds, so that they are alive and charged with individuality.

J. Bronowski: *The Ascent of Man*

i

NO MEDICAL SCIENTIST of the twentieth century was ever more unorthodox, more impulsively creative, than this charming Scandinavian doctor, Jorgen Lehmann. Gifted with a deductive ability and speed that in his own lifetime became legendary, yet nevertheless handsome and witty – in so many aspects of his life and personality, Lehmann seemed the very embodiment in real life of Conan Doyle's fictitious genius, Sherlock Holmes.

He was born of distinguished parents in Copenhagen, Denmark, on 5 January 1898. His father, Edvard, was a professor of theological history, and his mother, Karen Wiehe, was a gifted sculptor and a personal friend of Gauguin's. The family was already quite famous. His father's uncle, Orla, is a national hero in Denmark, where a public holiday, 5 June, is "Orla Lehmann day". At school however the young Jorgen followed quite a different family tradition. "I graduated second last out of a class of 103 students at a private school in Lund. My father came last in his class. Consequently I am not at all typical of the 'intelligent scientist'."[1]

Jorgen was far from the dunce he seemed at school. Åke

131

Hanngren, who knew him both as a friend and colleague, had no doubt he was a true genius[2] – but his genius inhabited a wild spirit, untamable with the mundane academic conventions. Rebellious, eccentric, brilliant, he didn't care a jot for the hierarchical posturings of his more conventional colleagues. It was a stubborn independence that would soon get him into hot water.

When Jorgen was still a child, his father moved to Berlin as Professor of Theological History at the Kaiser Wilhelm University. Then, just sixteen, he was uprooted once again in a move to Lund, in southern Sweden. He would joke that his father fled Germany in time to escape the first world war while he fled Denmark to escape the second. A rootless childhood, it would mark him for the remainder of his life with a unique way of speaking.

"My parents spoke German and I myself went to school in Denmark. I spoke German at home, but it wasn't good enough; then I spoke Danish but that wasn't good enough and I couldn't get anywhere in Denmark; so I came to Sweden to go to university where my Swedish wasn't good enough neither."[3] Jorgen Lehmann spoke a curious tongue that was a mixture of Swedish, Danish and German, all in the same sentence, which his son, Orla, would describe as "Scandinavian". But this wasn't a form of dyslexia. Lehmann cared nothing for how he spoke. All he cared about was his work – medicine!

Jorgen Lehmann was gifted with a fantastic imagination, which was apparent even as a child. Later on he would joke about his over-developed imagination, realizing how vital a part it would play in his life... "when it comes to creative scientific work, imagination is essential. As far as I understand it, this means fantasy exactly as we think of it with music – it cannot be acquired."[4]

He qualified in medicine at the famous old university of Lund in southern Sweden, where he took his thesis in 1929 on the chemistry of enzymes; in other words he was interested, like Bernheim, in the chemical processes of life. He was lucky in his teacher, the innovative research chemist, Professor Thunberg, who opened his eyes to the wonders of organic chemistry. Over his long and eventful career, he would repeatedly acknowledge the debt he owed to Thunberg, whom he regarded not only as his first but his only real teacher. Jorgen's son, Orla, who was looked after by Thunberg as a child and loved him as a grandfather, was at the bedside of the old professor when he was dying, to hear him exclaim in tears how he felt neglected by his own country. Thunberg believed, with some justification, that his research on enzymes had paved the way for Krebs' great discovery of the citric acid cycle (which reveals how the body makes use of oxygen to generate internal energy). He died convinced that factional jealousies between rival university centres in Sweden had excluded him from the Nobel Prize awarded to Hans Adolf Krebs in 1953.[5]

Two factors played an important role in the early years for Lehmann: his vivid imagination and, like René Dubos, an admiration for America, where bright young men could become professors. What more natural than he should find himself working at the Rockefeller Institute in New York in 1935, where, for eighteen months, he researched nerve conduction under the direction of the Nobel Prize winner, Professor Gasser. Theirs was a curious relationship, as would be explained by Lehmann's second wife, Maja:

"Gasser would arrive very early every morning to find Jorgen the only one there before him. The chief would come across to inspect Jorgen's work and exclaim: 'Lehmann – I don't believe you!' Day after day it was the same story. But Jorgen was not put off in the least. He was so sure of himself he just carried on. When the work was complete, Gasser said it was fine after all and would be agreeable to having his name on the paper. But Jorgen said, 'The name on the paper must be mine alone. I need to say I have done it myself in order to get a job at Aarhus.' Gasser had never believed him anyway."[6]

Even as a young man, Jorgen was quite prepared to upset the establishment if he was sure he was in the right.

In those days the now famous university was still a relatively small institute. We know that the young men working at the institute would take time off at weekends to get together. They played tennis, travelled to Manhattan. Although they had little money, wealthy Americans would treat them to a day out in their limousines. Lehmann, who had to wait until he was nearly fifty-years-old before he owned his first car, would always dream of owning a big American limousine and his first car would be a black Studebaker. While he was in America, his young wife, Marie Louise, and their two sons, Orla and Klas, had to stay behind in Lund but he wrote them entertaining and amusing letters, recounting his American experiences. The separation was particularly hard on Marie Louise de Vylder, whom he had married in 1925. Throughout these difficult years, she was forced to supplement the family income by taking five or six pupils into her home.

Lehmann must surely have met Dubos while working at the Rockefeller. Dubos was by now well established in his researches and was coming to the conclusion of the Cranberry Bog Bacillus experiment in that same year that Domagk would publish his discovery of Prontosil. It is likely that Lehmann would have attended meetings where Dubos would have talked about his researches. What effect this had on Lehmann's thinking is not known. We do know of a certain meeting that did take place, in that same dining room where Dubos had met Avery some eight years previously.

One day he just happened to be sitting next to a distinguished looking middle-aged woman, a doctor, who introduced herself as Alice Bernheim.

"That's interesting," Jorgen exclaimed. "You know, I have been writing for years to a doctor here in America, called Frederick Bernheim. He works at Duke University, North Carolina. We appear to have a lot in common. Maybe you know of him?"

"I should think I do," she laughed. "Frederick is my son!"[7]

Jorgen was invited to go along and meet Frederick at the family's country retreat, a place called Quillery, some miles outside New York. It was the start of a lifelong friendship.

While still working at the Rockefeller, Lehmann received a telegram from Aarhus in Denmark, inviting him to go home as Professor of biochemistry in this distinguished old university. He was delighted to accept the invitation, although his family would have to move to Denmark. In the apartment in Lund, the two boys had kept a menagerie of more than twenty separate animals, including an Irish collie, turtles, fish, a hartsong bird and a canary. During the move the canary died, and Jorgen had to comfort his heartbroken eldest son, Orla, who would always remember how his father patiently explained how a sudden noise might be quite sufficient for a little canary's heart to stop.[8]

Orla, who would remain devoted to him throughout his life, felt in retrospect that the move to Aarhus was misguided. "My father suffered in Denmark because he was grossly underpaid. He had moved back from high-powered research at the Rockefeller to teaching laboratory technicians how to test urine. He felt he would never discover anything here."[9]

In fact this proved unduly pessimistic. Soon after his arrival the first opportunity for his exceptional deductive powers presented itself.

A twenty-eight-year-old woman was admitted to the University Hospital in Aarhus, in a state of severe paralysis. The physicians looking after her thought she had poliomyelitis but there were puzzling features to her case. During discussion at a clinical meeting, one of the doctors speculated that it might not be polio at all but beri-beri, a wasting disease caused by deficiency of the newly discovered vitamin, B_1. Lehmann had worked at the physiological institute in Lund with beri-beri in rats. Suddenly – it would always be "suddenly" – he took a particular interest in saving the life of this unfortunate woman.

He was faced with an immediate problem: was it beri-beri or not? Nobody could say because there was no method of measuring the level of vitamin B_1 in her blood (this is extremely difficult even today). Lehmann invented a new method of estimating the vitamin, using living micro-organisms. Using his technique, he confirmed that she was indeed grossly deficient in this very important vitamin. Immediately he was faced with an even greater problem. Vitamin B_1 could not be obtained. It was not commercially available. Yet time was rapidly running out for this woman, who would soon be permanently paralysed. How could he possibly save her?

Lehmann approached a local drug manufacturer, called Ferrosan, based in Copenhagen. He explained the gravity of the situation and asked if they were prepared to help. Purely on a charitable basis, Ferrosan put its chemists to work. They worked night and day to prepare a mould extract of vitamin B_1 that could be injected intramuscularly. The patient was given injections of this vitamin every day for three weeks, then every other day for three weeks and then once a week. After one week she could lift her legs and a month later she could walk with help. Just as the doctors and the pharmaceutical company were celebrating her recovery, her condition deteriorated. Suddenly, and quite mysteriously, she became extremely weak, profoundly depressed, cried all the time and had frequent diarrhoea. A striking brown pigmentation erupted over her hands, and the skin over her elbows became as thick as crocodile skin. While the doctors were racking their brains to discover what was wrong, she lapsed into a dangerous coma. The physicians looking after her realized that she now had a different disease called pellagra. She was deteriorating very rapidly and death seemed inevitable.

Lehmann had read in a medical journal from Hungary that vitamin B_1 could sometimes antagonize the action within the body of another vitamin then called pellagra factor. Maybe by giving her large doses of vitamin B_1, they had opposed the small amounts of the pellagra factor in her body and caused her to develop the disease called pellagra, in which these same skin signs were usually found. He wrote once more to the helpful pharmaceutical company, Ferrosan in Copenhagen, and asked for their very urgent help. "Can we have another vitamin preparation that contains the pellagra factor." Ferrosan once again, without financial recompense for wages or materials, worked night and day to produce another new vitamin preparation. On this treatment, the diarrhoea disappeared in a week and the skin changes began to improve. Most rewarding of all, she recovered consciousness. It would take a further three and a half months of intensive medical and nursing treatment, but after that time she walked home, completely cured.[10]

Barely a year after his return from America, this amazing doctor, Jorgen Lehmann, had acquired a reputation in Scandinavia.

ii

HE COULD SEE little prospects for further research at Aarhus, when he was approached in 1938 by a surgeon called Sved Johansson, who had invented the nail to repair fractured hips. Johansson, who was chief of surgery at the Sahlgren's Hospital, in Gothenburg, Sweden, tempted Jorgen with the post of chief of the chemical pathology laboratory at his hospital, an offer which certainly interested Lehmann, but he refused to consider it unless they agreed to enlarge the size and scope of the laboratory. What was the point of moving back to Sweden if he could not perform high quality research! The director of the hospital agreed with this but it excited a furious jealousy amongst several of the physicians already working at the hospital.

The chief physician thought that a laboratory doctor should have no say whatsoever in the ward or outpatient treatment of patients; and Odin, the Professor of Medicine, was adamantly opposed to the whole arrangement. He refused to allow Lehmann the title of professor, which he had previously enjoyed at Aarhus. Johansson was equally adamant that this potentially brilliant colleague should come and work at the Sahlgren's Hospital and he negotiated an arrangement whereby Lehmann should be made Chief of Chemical Pathology and Associate Professor, while having no formal employment with the university. Lehmann accepted the post of Chief but refused the status of Associate Professor. In a curious twist of fate much later, after his compulsory retirement at sixty-five years of age, Lehmann began a second career in pharmacology, with a research interest in mental diseases, when he was at last granted the honorary rank of professor at the same hospital. Tempests would rage between these two divergent careers.

This was a wonderful time to be in biochemical research. The latest fashion was the newly discovered vitamins. In December 1939, as soon as he had taken up his new post in Gothenburg, Lehmann read two fascinating articles, published independently of each other, which described the chemical structure of one of the new discoveries, vitamin K. One article was by Fieser, the other by a different scientist called Doisy, who, with

the Dane Henrik Dam, would subsequently be awarded the
Nobel Prize for this in 1943. Dam had gone no further than
showing that the lack of a mystery ingredient in the diets of
chickens caused them to bleed to death internally. This
bleeding tendency was not helped in the slightest if you gave
them vitamin C. What intrigued Lehmann about this newly
discovered vitamin K was the fact it had a dramatic effect on the
clotting of blood in human beings as well as chickens.

Now another Dane, Schönheyder, working in Copenhagen,
showed the bleeding that Dam had noticed in chickens was
caused by deficiency of a vital blood clotting protein, what we
now call prothrombin. In the normal process of blood clotting,
prothrombin is converted into thrombin, an essential step in
making a solid blood clot. Of course it is essential that the body
should be able to make blood clots, otherwise we would bleed
to death from every little cut or knock. What Fieser and Doisy
had shown was that the prothrombin deficiency in the
chicken's blood was in turn due to deficiency of vitamin K. In
other words, the chickens were bleeding to death because they
lacked vitamin K in their diet.

In an instant, Lehmann completed quite a different jigsaw in
his mind: he could see that this would make it possible to use
this newly discovered vitamin K to treat patients, for example in
the bleeding disorders that sometimes threatened the lives of
newborn babies.

But again there were unsolved mysteries. Before he could
assess any possible use for vitamin K in treating human
sufferers, he would need to be able to measure its effects on the
blood clotting processes. He decided he would invent a method
to do this. While he was brushing up on other known ways of
doing similar measurements, he sat down and read a paper on
the subject, which had been written by an American scientist,
called Quick. In this same paper, something quite different
caught his eye, a curious aside: cattle that ate mouldy sweet
clover suffered from a bleeding disorder called "sweet clover
disease". On a single farm, twenty-three out of twenty-four
young bulls had bled to death after the simple operation of
castration. All at once a much bigger notion occurred to him,
something quite the opposite of what he had just been

considering. In Lehmann's words: "The knowledge of this disease at once gave me the idea that a toxic substance in the mouldy sweet clover might be useful to reduce the coagulability of the blood in thrombotic conditions."[11]

What followed was typical of his single-minded eccentricity.

He knew that Roderick, a Canadian veterinary surgeon, had found that something in mouldy sweet clover was very poisonous to living cells: but Roderick had no idea what this substance was. Lehmann believed that perhaps he might succeed where the veterinary surgeon had failed – "who knows!" If he could only purify this poison, he might be able to use it as a treatment for blood clots in the leg veins that moved up into the lungs and killed many patients after childbirth or surgery.

"So I went to Professor Rennerfeldt at the botanical institute and asked him where I could find this sweet clover.

"'Well,' he declared, 'you will find it all over the refuse heap at Hisingen (an island in the river Gota, just outside Gothenburg, and on which there was a well-known farm).'

"Then I spoke to the hospital gardener and asked for a ruck wagon and some scythes and off we went, my assistant Johan Martensson and I. We collected a huge mass of sweet clover and rode back through the streets of Gothenburg to the Sahlgren's Hospital along Park Avenue. No wonder the girls at the laboratory made saucer eyes and thought this new professor must be crazy, bringing this cargo of sweet clover to the hospital."[12]

He put the clover in the cellar and sprayed it with water, thinking this was the way to make it mouldy. But the hay derived from it had not a scrap of effect on rabbits when he fed it to them.

He tried again. This time he sprayed the clover not just with water but also with moulds he obtained from the botanical institute, called *Aspergillus niger* and *fumigatus*. This time it worked perfectly. "I found a reduced coagulability of blood in the rabbits and my assistant, Elizabeth, and I started new experiments with this substance. Next I tried to extract the active principle. But I could not tell what it was."[13]

There was no question of his giving up. Off he went to discuss the problem with his brother-in-law, Gote Turesson, an expert in plant genetics, in Uppsala, in the north of Sweden.

"You do know," remarked Turesson, "that sweet clover contains a very strong aromatic substance, called coumarin, which causes cattle to avoid it – indeed botanists in Canada are trying to produce types of sweet clover which contain very little of this substance."[14]

Jorgen in fact knew nothing of the kind, no more did he know the formula for coumarin, but he decided he would look it up that same evening. When he did so he received a shock. The chemical formulae for vitamin K and coumarin were almost identical. The sixty thousand dollar question was now obvious: was coumarin the toxic agent in spoiled sweet clover?

Throughout his apprentice years with Thunberg, Lehmann had learnt a very important principle in organic chemistry: this was the principle of competitive inhibition. It was precisely this principle that Thunberg had eloquently demonstrated in experiments with malonic and succinic acid and which he claimed had laid the groundwork for Krebs' Nobel-Prize-winning discovery. The question Lehmann now asked himself was as follows:

We know that vitamin K plays an essential role in the chemical pathways in the liver which manufacture the blood clotting protein, prothrombin. What will happen now if the body is offered coumarin, which is so very similar in its structure to vitamin K? Is it not likely that the coumarin will sit in the chemical slot normally occupied by vitamin K, throwing a spanner in the normal workings of that chemical pathway?

Lehmann's understanding of this competitive principle, his growing confidence in its manipulation, would soon prove vital in a different story.

If coumarin blocked the effects of vitamin K, this would in turn reduce the level of the vital blood clotting protein, prothrombin, in the circulation. But there was more to his conjecture even than that. Not only would this explain the poisonous effect of the spoiled clover but it would also give him the exact formula for the wonder drug he was searching for. On 15 August 1940, in a mood of great expectancy, he got hold of some coumarin, dissolved it in oil and gave it intramuscularly to some experimental rabbits. He couldn't believe it when it had no effect whatsoever on the prothrombin level.

In November that same year, 1940, he received news from America that alarmed him. It seemed that Professor Karl Link, at the Agricultural Experiment Station in Madison, was already working on the anticoagulant in mouldy sweet clover. Even more devastating: they had gone so far as to extract an active ingredient which they were already purifying and analysing. This active ingredient must, he reasoned, be very close in structure to the coumarin he had been testing. Having taken his research so far, Jorgen Lehmann knew that he faced defeat. How could he compete with a major organization of chemists backed up by "American know-how".

In April 1941, his fears worsened when he read another paper from the Link group in which they went so far as to describe the chemical nature of the new active formula, a derivative of coumarin, called dicoumarol. As soon as he read it, he rushed off and contacted the Malmö office of Ferrosan, that same drug company he had previously worked with on the vitamin research. He urged the company to synthesize this drug.

At the Malmö branch of Ferrosan, the chief chemist was a man called Karl-Gustav Rosdahl. In the cautious world of drug companies, who think hard and long before they commit themselves to anything that might make losses, this contact with Rosdahl, who was an exceptional practical chemist, was crucial. In Sweden at this time there were no really large pharmaceutical companies and Ferrosan was a small family company which had to be very prudent about any large financial commitments. Now the foresight on Lehmann's part during those difficult days of controversy about his appointment at Gothenburg became important.

He could begin the animal experiments with dicoumarol because the new laboratory, which he had insisted upon as part of the bargain on his appointment at the Sahlgren's Hospital, had been built by 1 September 1940. He had everything he needed, animal operation facilities, autoclaves, animal houses, feeding facilities, perhaps some of the best research facilities connected to a hospital in all Scandinavia.

"Rosdahl helped me at very short notice. I started clinical tests on rabbits and the new substance prolonged the coagulation time as expected. After clinical tests on animals came the first tests on humans. I used myself as the guinea pig."[15]

In a radio interview many years later, he would be asked if he knew then that there was a race going on. Lehmann would reply, "No, I did not. I recall I wrote to my assistant Johan Martensson, in Kalmar at this time, telling him not to worry because the Americans didn't know how to use it."[16] In an even more extraordinary development, several years later, Link would contract tuberculosis, which caused him to be admitted to an American sanatorium, when in controversial circumstances, a discovery made by Lehmann would help to save his life.[17]

At this time, however, Lehmann could not have been more mistaken. The Americans well understood the potential usefulness of the new drug, dicoumarol. Convinced he was ahead of them, Lehmann went on conducting experiments in total secrecy, working night and day in the attic of his laboratory. He used himself as a guinea pig for the first human experiment. But how could he tell how much of the drug to give himself since it had never been given to a human being before? If he gave himself too much, he could suffer a fatal internal haemorrhage. . .

It was a gamble and a dangerous one at that. He started with a small dose, and gradually increased it. When he reached the higher doses he experienced a prolongation of his bleeding time and he knew then roughly the quantity he would need to treat human disease. He hadn't had the slightest qualms at all in exposing himself to the unknown danger of the untried drug. Now, however, it would take a good deal more courage to treat his first sick patient.

"It so happened that my old friend, the surgeon, Gustaf Pettersson, was in charge of a surgical ward. I visited him and told him about the work nurse Elizabeth and I had been carrying on in secret up in the attic of the laboratory. Maybe the time was right to treat a real patient? Pettersson reacted very enthusiastically. It could not have come at a more opportune moment. He explained to Lehmann: "I've just operated on a woman with abdominal cancer. I had to remove half the stomach and some of the colon. Now, after surgery, she has developed a big venous thrombosis in her leg." Lehmann rushed to his laboratory and brought back a supply of the new drug and treated this unfortunate woman, visiting her daily to assess her bleeding tests and to see how she was progressing. On the third day she shook his hand with delight. The pain and swelling in her leg had disappeared.[18]

Jorgen Lehmann had acquired a new reputation, much as he had earlier at Aarhus. But where his first "case" had saved the life of one young woman, this discovery might benefit millions of people worldwide. After this first case, he treated every patient with a thrombosis or embolus at the Sahlgren's Hospital, very often in the maternity department, where life-threatening thromboses were a common complication after childbirth.

This work was exhilarating and he worked very long hours, falling into bed at two or three in the morning. Over the following twelve months, he gathered enough evidence for the effectiveness of the anticoagulant treatment to present it at a scientific meeting in Stockholm, where the surgeons were very impressed with what was clearly a major medical breakthrough. But there was a secondary effect of this staggering workrate: although he denied it during the radio interview, the race with his American rivals was a vital factor which had forced Lehmann to put everything else aside. And this would overshadow another idea, even more important than the anticoagulant research.

Dicoumarol, jointly discovered by Link in America and Lehmann in Sweden, went on to become a standard drug worldwide in the treatment of life-threatening blood clots. But at the very heart of all this excitement, a letter was making its slow and tortuous way, across the war-torn Atlantic ocean. That letter would give Lehmann a new idea so potent it would eclipse every idea he had ever had before, indeed every idea this brilliant man would ever have again in his long and eventful life. It began, in Lehmann's own words:

"It was rather a strange story. One morning, in 1940, I was sitting on my couch in my office at the Central Laboratory, when I received the morning post. For the most part it was just the usual rubbish and advertisements. There was a single exception. This was a small brown envelope, from the Duke University School of Medicine, Durham, North Carolina. It came from my friend, the biochemist and pharmacologist, Frederick Bernheim. Frederick had once been described to me by another American as a man who wrote exceedingly short papers. This proved absolutely right. In this simple brown envelope I found a tiny article, printed on just one page. The title was, 'The effect of salicylate on the oxygen uptake of the tubercle bacillus'.[19] What it said was that if you added one milligram of salicylic acid to tuberculous bacteria, you could stimulate the oxygen uptake of the bacteria by more than one hundred per cent."

Suddenly, as for Dubos, Domagk, and Waksman before him, it was Lehmann's turn to experience the revelatory moment that would change his life. "That was it! Immediately I saw the significance. I remember that I sat on my couch in my study with my spine erect and read the article over and over again."[20]

iii

THERE WAS NO personal reason why Jorgen Lehmann should be interested in tuberculosis. No close member of his family, no friend, had died from it. His attitude was no different from that of any other doctor of his day: he could not be other than desperately familiar with the disease. It ravaged the world. Sweden itself, particularly in the north, was devastated by it. A century earlier, the city of Stockholm had suffered the most appalling mortality rates from tuberculosis of any major city in the entire world.[21] Whole families were wiped out by it.

In 1904 the Swedish National Association for Tuberculosis had declared war upon the disease. The Swedish Royal family had always taken a very active interest in this Association and in 1940, the Crown Prince and later King Gustav VI was President. Indeed the Prince had a deep personal interest in the struggle against tuberculosis. His beautiful first wife, Princess Margaret of Connaught, had died at a tragically young age from the disease in 1920. His second wife, Lady Louise Mountbatten, sister of Lord Louis, was just as deeply committed to the

National Association and would take up the Presidency after his retirement from it. There was no doubting the importance of the disease in everybody's consciousness. Lehmann was also well aware of the pessimism that reigned worldwide with regard to finding a cure. "One could say that the situation in 1940 was one of utter defeatism. People had given up any hope of a cure."

Tuberculosis was without doubt the ultimate challenge for any doctor at this time. It was against this background that Lehmann had read Bernheim's tiny paper.

The salicylic acid used in Bernheim's experiment was of course nothing other than aspirin. But because aspirin was so common-place – even then it had long been abused by extravagant marketing – this did not mean it was ineffective. The very success story of aspirin owed much to the fact that this drug was, and remains today, a true wonder drug, which interestingly had been first discovered by the Bayer laboratories at Elberfeld towards the end of the nineteenth century. What Bernheim was now saying was that the internal chemistry of the tuberculosis germ seemed in some way to make use of and was stimulated by the presence of aspirin.

Lehmann remarked: "I particularly noticed that this was an effect that seemed specific for the tuberculosis bacterium. This meant that we had an insight into the internal workings of the tuberculosis bacterium – something that might be significant for its very life."[22]   In a second article, published in June 1941, Bernheim and his colleague, Arthur K. Saz, described how they had tried to block this internal chemistry of the germ by making chemicals that were variations of the aspirin molecule and adding them to the culture medium.[23] Bernheim too was well aware of this guiding principle of competitive inhibition. He was looking for a chemical, derived from aspirin, that would damage the bacterium's internal chemistry.

In the 1941 paper, Bernheim reported a further dramatic discovery. He found that a chemical derived from benzoic acid, called 2,3,5, tri-iodobenzoate, did indeed cause a marked inhibition of oxygen uptake by the germ. Bernheim now took this further. If he added this chemical to tuberculous bacteria growing in bottles of broth, he showed that it dramatically inhibited the growth of the bacteria.

Something else struck Bernheim as fascinating: if he took
tuberculous bacteria that had been suppressed by the tri-
iodobenzoate and transferred them to a new culture medium
without the inhibitor, the bacteria swarmed and multiplied.
The chemical clearly had not killed them. Bernheim racked his
brains over this. What was the chemical really doing to the
bacteria? It seemed that the tri-iodobenzoate did not kill the
bacteria but froze them in a form of suspended animation, preventing them from dividing and multiplying. How important
might this be? He simply did not know – but he surmised it
might well be very important. "What," he now asked himself,
will happen if I change the chemical molecule of the tri-
iodobenzoate? I wonder what effect that will have on the
germ?" Soon he had his answer, and it was even more fascinating: the slightest change ruined the entire effect.

In May 1940, a British research scientist was attracted by the
heady excitement that was charging the air in chemical research
circles.

Dr Paul Fildes, a Fellow of The London Royal Society and
Director of the Department of Bacterial Chemistry at the British
Medical Research Council, attempted to rationalize what was
happening. He published his thoughts in the *Lancet*, under the
title, "A rational approach to research in chemotherapy."[24] This
summarized exactly what should be expected of an anti-
bacterial drug and how antibiotics might be expected to work.
Fildes concentrated his attentions onto things which he called
essential metabolites; in other words chemicals which were
vital for bacterial growth and survival. How else could anti-
bacterial drugs work except by interfering with such vital internal chemical processes?

Fildes gave as his example the way he thought sulphanilamide worked. Sulphanilamide, the active principle of Prontosil, was very similar in its structure to a molecule that bacteria
needed for life, para-aminobenzoic acid. Sulphanilamide
worked because of this very similarity, by taking up the place in
the internal chemistry of the bacteria that would normally be
taken by the para-aminobenzoic acid, while at the same time it
did not do the work done by the para-aminobenzoic acid. This
was the meaning of competitive inhibition.

A year later, reading Bernheim's second paper, Lehmann remarked at once the similarity between para-aminobenzoic acid and the tri-iodobenzoic acid Bernheim was getting excited about. And this was that same chemical which Bernheim had described as having a dramatic effect on the growth of tuberculosis germs in cultures. Lehmann already knew the answer. He had known it since the arrival of that first tiny paper – a realization that had, in his own confession, already set his imagination aflame. What else was his own discovery of the anticoagulant drug all about if not the principle of competitive inhibition? The anticoagulant he had found in spoiled sweet clover sat in the chemical pathways of the liver which were responsible for the manufacture of the blood clotting factor, prothrombin.

So it was, on that vital morning, early in 1940, that Jorgen Lehmann had sat back on his couch, in his office on the first floor of the three-storey stone building of the chemical pathology laboratory at the Sahlgren's Hospital. Over and over, with his mind in a state of bemused shock, he read that tiny communication from his friend, Frederick Bernheim, while about him winter's wind and snow buffeted the window. Suddenly, in his imagination a question whirled and turned, a question that was at once exhilarating, bewildering, even terrifying in its potential significance.

What if the humble aspirin molecule was the key to the greatest of medical mysteries? What if he could take this key and open the door to the cure for tuberculosis?

For the twinkling of an eye, a candle of hope burst into flame. But . . . "I was occupied at the time with the clinical testing of dicoumarol. I realized that I couldn't concentrate on two things at the same time."

The race with Link's group in America had proved crucial. And in that decision to put this new idea to one side, the little candle of hope was snuffed out.

10

Triumph and Tragedy

Your remedy does not treat the real seat of evil. It continually removes the traces of the enemy, but it still leaves him deep in the invaded country.

Arthur Conan Doyle: reporting Koch's invention
of a vaccine against tuberculosis.

i

THE DISCOVERY OF Prontosil had thrown the work of René Dubos and Oswald Avery into gloom and self-doubt. Avery in particular was devastated by it. Unmarried, living within easy walking distance of the Rockefeller Institute, in essence he had only one life. He would come to the laboratory in the morning, perform his work, go back home in the evening, sleep, then return to work. He had no family and hardly any friends. He never read and he never participated in public affairs. His work was all that mattered to him – and now his entire philosphy had been turned upside down. In Dubos' own words. . . "He began to experience severe difficulties in his laboratory. Nothing worked any more. Most of his effort had been focused on the production of serums and vaccines for pneumonia. But the sulphonamide drugs appeared in 1937, and overnight his approach appeared useless, out of date. He felt that he'd wasted his entire life. He had a disease that could have been considered serious, a goitre, Graves' disease (an overactive thyroid gland). Then his Graves' disease literally erupted;

he couldn't bear it any longer. He had to have an operation, and for two or three years he was a dispirited man; he thought it was the end."[1]

The endearing and eccentric Oswald Avery suffered this crisis in silence – "he, too, wanted to keep his own counsel and face his destiny alone."[2] Avery did not discuss his health with anybody except to answer the concern of friends with the refrain that he was always getting better. Even to the end of his life, Avery left no record of his personal thoughts, so that Dubos, who would subsequently write his biography[3], was left to imagine, from "very tenuous clues", some of the factors that influenced the important decisions in his life. At the heart of this very difficult period in their joint researches, in 1934, a year before Lehmann came to work in the same institution, René surprised Avery by announcing that he was about to get married.

Deeply moved by this news, the shy bachelor congratulated his young assistant, while appearing to sense just how profoundly marriage would alter the course of Dubos' life and career. "At one point in our conversation, he slowly walked to the window and looked outside, lost in thought for a few seconds. Coming back to his chair, he casually mentioned that he, too, had contemplated such a move years before, but that circumstances had stood in his way. Then he turned the conversation back to my own life, although his attitude tacitly expressed a longing for the kind of intimate relationship which he had not known."[4]

The man who had so flirted with English girls in Rome had now fallen in love with an attractive young Frenchwoman, Marie Louise Bonnet, who taught French in New York and was a gifted pianist. Her influence on Dubos' subsequent life and career would prove great yet we know very little about her. Nobody knows how they first met although Carol Moberg, who subsequently worked as Dubos' assistant, thinks they probably met at a party or social evening.[5] In his leisure time, René enjoyed the company of the ex-patriate Europeans who flitted about the margins of university life in New York and it is likely that they met at such a gathering. Perhaps the young man was lonely for his native France. She was already in her early thirties when he first met her, dark-haired, brown eyes, highly intelligent with a likeably impulsive nature. René appears to have been captivated from their first meeting. Much the same age as René, she had probably lived in America from a young age since her English was only slightly accented.[6] They were married on 23 March 1934.

Events would subseqently make René Dubos almost as secretive as Avery with regard to this period in his life and in particular with regard to the intimate details of his relationship with Marie Louise.

Although they were both of humble origins, each was unusually gifted. René was just sensing the breadth of his vision, his scientific ambitions, his gift for language, both as writer and orator; Marie Louise had struggled since childhood with the tempestuous imagination of a wildly emotional nature. The few of her writings which have survived reveal a deeply spiritual person, shy in company, so overflowing with love for the natural world as to seem woundingly vulnerable.[7] We know that she was very close to her family, who still lived in Limoges, and that she felt the separation from them poignantly.[8] A large man, powerfully built with all too profound an understanding of the raw and exciting environment of New York, René must have felt an overwhelming desire to protect her.

A year or so after their marriage, a new determination is evident in René's philosophy.

"When Avery became ill, the department broke down immediately. Each and every one of us went into something else."[9] Dubos wandered into a vague line of research on bacterial enzymes, which was getting him nowhere. By the time Avery was fit enough to return to work, it was quite obvious that the sulphonamides had made his previous line of research redundant and the work on the pneumococcus was completely abandoned.[10] Henry Dawson, a Canadian, had meanwhile pioneered an entirely new line of pneumococcal research. Dawson had noticed something that would soon shake the scientific world down to its roots. It began with a puzzling observation: that pneumococcal germs could actually parcel up hereditary material and move this parcel from one bacterium to another. How could germs move such vital information from one germ to another? Until this time, the world believed that hereditary material was contained within the nucleus of all cells and could only be passed on during cell division or in the coming together of male and female cells during reproduction. Yet Dawson's observation had nothing to do with bacterial division or reproduction. How was this possible? At first people simply refused to believe it.

For Oswald Avery, however, this sensational discovery would lead to a totally new biological concept called "transformation". A decade later, he would take this to its breathtaking conclusion, when he discovered for the first time in history that DNA was the master code of heredity and life itself.[11] This discovery would enable Crick and Watson to solve the problem of its three-dimensional structure in space, the almost mystical double-helix, for which they were awarded the Nobel Prize in 1962.

Yet at the time of Avery's illness, and with his work ended in stalemate, what was René Dubos to do? He knew he had to break free of the pneumococcal capsule experiments. He had to fall back onto the naive self-confidence that had brought him to the Rockefeller. He asked himself a brutally honest question: "Well now, am I fooling myself in thinking I can do this job – or do I really have the gift to do it?"

Like his delightful superior, René Dubos was also searching for a new scientific truth, a philosophical avenue that would lead him to the greatest scientific discovery of his life.

ii

IN THE PNEUMOCOCCAL capsule experiments, he had performed more than just a single successful experiment; he had discovered a general principle. The Cranberry Bog Bacillus did not just produce the enzyme that dissolved the pneumococcal capsule by accident. He had grown the bacillus in an environment that contained only the pneumococcal capsule as the source of sugar. It had been forced to adapt to this sole source of food and it had produced the remarkable enzyme as a result of this. He had studied the effect of the Cranberry Bog Bacillus enzyme in mice, rabbits, monkeys – if you gave them the enzyme, the deadly pneumococcus, denuded of its protective coat, was mopped up by the animals' white cells and utterly destroyed.

Dust to dust: this, the most fundamental lesson of the Bible, had been the thinking behind his innovatory experiment. If this philosophy had worked for the capsule of the pneumococcus – could it just conceivably work for a whole bacterium? It might! But how exactly should he put his new theory to work?

What if he allowed his cultures of soil micro-organisms a new sole food source – nothing other than the deadly bacterium he wanted to destroy? Not a piece of that deadly germ, not a capsule, but the whole living micro-organism?

The staphylococcus is one of the most vicious of the acute bacterial infections, the cause of boils, abscesses, wound infections, and in its worst form of all, infection within the heart itself. It causes a fatal form of blood poisoning, where it "boils up" as destructive and incurable abscesses in every internal organ of the body. Unlike the streptococcus, the staphylococcus was often resistant to treatment by Prontosil or the sulphonamides derived from it. In time it would often become resistant to penicillin too. Dubos now took this dangerous germ as enemy number one in an exciting new experiment, in which he added staphylococci to a large number of mixed soil samples.

He had no laboratory of his own, but this did not matter at all. "The climate at the Rockefeller in those days was extraordinary. I had no department then, but the ease with which I could collaborate with anybody – Hotchkiss, an organic chemist; the people in the streptococcus department; or the institute's animal pathology laboratory at Princeton – was phenomenal. I never even had to bother about a budget, though I did not spend much money anyway. All this was done with incredibly simple equipment ... essentially in enamelware designed for hotel kitchens. The fact is that I never had to worry about money. Dr Avery arranged whatever I needed."[12] So he began a new and equally wonderful voyage of discovery into territory that had never been explored in history. Just as in the pneumococcal capsule experiment, he prepared soil samples which contained the staphylococcus germ as the sole source of food. He varied the conditions so that they encouraged only a single type of microbe to grow in the soil, one that would be capable of devouring the staphylococcus in order to survive.

It took him two years to grow a new wonder germ from one of his soil samples. The bacillus, called *Bacillus brevis* had never been seen before, yet it had a voracious appetite for the staphylococcal bacteria. The very manner in which he had found the new bacillus was ample proof of his theory: he had isolated it from a soil sample to which he had been adding suspensions of staphylococci over a long period of time. But exactly what mysterious effluvium did this newly discovered bacillus produce that was so deadly to other germs? With mounting excitement, he performed experiment after experiment, testing it further.

From the soil containing the new bacillus, he extracted a very unusual chemical. His chemical looked a sticky impure mess, yet when he added it to growing cultures of deadly staphylococci, pneumococci and even the notorious streptococcus, it destroyed them all. Dubos was no chemist, but he did his best to purify the strange new chemical further. When he reduced the temperature of the solution containing the chemical to zero Centigrade, and kept it cold for a period of time, the chemical solidified out of the solution as a precipitate that resembled a sticky brownish mud. Next he tested different concentrations of this mud against standard quantities of germs. On the culture plates, in the test tubes, down the lens of his microscope, he found himself gazing at a miracle. A thousandth of a gram added to ten billion pneumococci destroyed them completely within an hour. The germs simply dissolved away until they had disappeared. Even the tougher staphylococci and streptococci could not survive against his new discovery. They too disintegrated, although more slowly.

If all he wanted was to kill the germs rather than completely dissolve them, he found that a thousandth of a gram killed a hundred billion pneumococcal germs in two hours when incubated together at body temperature.

When he took this a stage further, assessing the chemical extract against infection in experimental animals, the results were exhilarating. A single injection of two milligrams protected white mice against 10,000 to 100,000 times the fatal dose of virulent pneumococci. More exciting still, the protective effect worked even if the extract was injected several hours after the fatal dose of bacteria had been injected. Preliminary work showed a similar protection against the deadly streptococcus.

Dubos had found precisely what he and Avery had been searching for all these years. It was the first antibiotic ever to be found from a deliberate programme of screening soil microorganisms. In February 1939, he wrote a preliminary report of his findings, which was published a few months later in a medical journal.[13] Immediately, he was deluged with congratulations from excited colleagues. It occurred to him that he had no name for his new antibiotic. One of Pasteur's early collaborators named Duclaux had discovered a bacillus that was very similar to his wonderful *Bacillus brevis*. This had also been capable of killing other bacteria. Curiously, this bacillus had been known for almost a century to play a part in the fermentation of cheese. Duclaux had called his bacillus tyrothrix, "tyro" meaning cheese and "thrix" meaning a thread. "Well I thought the kind of bacillus I have discovered is very similar to tyrothrix and might as well be called by a name similar to the one Duclaux has invented. For this reason, I called the substance tyrothricin."[14]

In the first week of September 1939, in a lecture on tyrothricin given to the fateful Third International Congress for Microbiology, René Dubos gave further details of his antibiotic breakthrough[15]. Alexander Fleming and Selman Waksman were in his audience. Dubos had the opportunity of talking to Fleming, who was depressed about difficulties in producing penicillin in soluble form. Dubos encouraged him to persist. Dubos also found the opportunity of talking to Howard Florey, who only two years later, together with Ernst Chain, would revolutionize the production methods for penicillin.[16]

Dubos had entered the most exciting research of his life. Tyrothricin was the talk of medical microbiologists and was surely the beginning of something bigger, far more exciting still. Still relatively young, his marriage to Marie Louise had blossomed. Life, in every facet, was vibrant with promise. In

1938 he had become an American citizen. Soon afterwards, he was elected to the National Academy of Sciences. The Rockefeller Institute, of which he was now a fellow, provided him with a new laboratory. But already, unknown to the media currently extolling his praises, tragedy had entered his private life.

At the peak of this success, René suffered a third attack of rheumatic fever. While he was still recovering and simultaneously reporting his discovery of tyrothricin to the world, his wife, Marie Louise, fell desperately ill. To René's horror her illness was confirmed as pulmonary tuberculosis.

iii

HE COULD NOT believe the diagnosis. Surely tuberculosis was a disease of the poor, of the undernourished, of developing countries. Marie Louise lived a relatively protected life, on Villard Hill in the rural surroundings of Dobbs Ferry, a village twenty miles north of New York, on the East bank of the Hudson River. Her work was fairly comfortable, teaching French at the Master's, a fashionable girls' school locally. She was not exposed to tuberculosis. "Why," he asked himself, "did she get tuberculosis, when we live as well as we do?"[17,18]

Years later he would discover that his wife's father, who had worked as a painter of porcelain in a factory at Limoges, had suffered from silicosis, the consequence of a lifetime of inhaling silica-containing kaolin dust.[19] Silicosis is a very unpleasant disease, where thick fibrous scars spread throughout the delicate tissues of the lungs, irreversibly ruining them. It is not uncommon in this condition for tuberculosis to invade the damaged lungs, bringing about a fatal end. Marie Louise had contracted tuberculosis from her father when she was five or six years of age; but while he, in his weakened condition, had died from it, she had made an apparently good recovery with nothing more than rest and the healing powers of her own tissues.

Tuberculosis, healed by the body's own defences, is never fully cured. In the tiny calcified scars that show up on the chest X-rays, like little tombstones, the relentless germ lives on, dividing with its curious slow metabolism, ever dangerous and threatening. With the outbreak of the second world war, his wife had been cut off from all communication with her family in Limoges, which had deeply worried her. At this time Marie Louise's sister, living with them or very close by, became severely disturbed by those same worries, developing a psychotic illness, and had to be treated in a psychiatric hospital. Highly emotional and sensitive, Marie Louise fell into a profound despair so severe that she completely lost her appetite.[20] Depression, as doctors have long realized, can impair the body's defences, making the sufferer more liable to illnesses, particularly those affecting the immune system. Avery's thyroid disease was typical of such illnesses, which are often activated by shock or a period of great worry. René Dubos would in time become convinced that it had been these emotional pressures, exhausting his wife's strength and spiritual reserves, that had triggered the relapse of tuberculosis which, for thirty-five years, had lain dormant within her lungs.

The situation was extremely serious. Marie Louise was losing weight and deteriorating rapidly. The specialist they now consulted had no doubt that her life was threatened and he recommended that she should be admitted straight away to a sanitorium. In that eventful year, 1939, at the time of René's greatest triumph with his discovery of tyrothricin, Marie Louise moved north of New York, into the Adirondack Mountains, to become a patient at the Raybrook Sanitorium, between Saranac and Lake Placid.

iv

RENÉ DUBOS WAS now cruelly torn between his research, which had reached a critical stage, and caring for Marie Louise, who was struggling for her own survival, so far away from him. Weekdays he continued the exhausting research while every weekend he travelled north to be with her.

At this time, he had only completed the most preliminary studies on the new antibiotic. Now, under such circumstances, and hardly qualified as a master chemist, he was faced with the mammoth task of manufacturing much larger quantities of the drug and attempting to purify it for further testing. With his own hands, he managed to prepare several hundred grams, huge amounts in terms of a solitary laboratory worker, a work of arduous labour. Then he had a stroke of luck. At that time "a very good and young organic chemist called Rollin Hotchkiss" was working in Avery's laboratory and René frequently asked his advice on purifying the sticky mud that comprised the new antibiotic. René found himself asking Hotchkiss for more and more assistance. "Soon enough Rollin Hotchkiss asked me to give him some of my tyrothricin, and in his typical mysterious way (because he's a person who often likes to work alone) he disappeared for a few weeks or months."[21]

In Rollin Hotchkiss, Dubos had found the perfect working companion. Hotchkiss had a brilliant mind, coupled with an eccentric sense of humour, and a dedication to hard work equal to Dubos' own. The fact that Hotchkiss was already engaged in other research and had also been called up by the American Navy, following Pearl Harbor, was not allowed to get in the way. Hotchkiss' own words uniquely and vividly capture what it is like for a scientist to become caught up in this whirlwind of new discovery.[22]

"Quite on my own, in the middle of 1939, I volunteered to help Dubos purify the bacterial extract he had produced. My adventure did not have the sanction or encouragement of my administrative superiors – not until I had made some progress and we were deeper into World War Two. But I shall always be grateful to the Rockefeller Institute for permitting us to initiate our own war research project.

"We contrived to commandeer some laboratory help and some large equipment for a summer of growing gallons of the soil organism *Bacillus brevis* and preparing the raw material that Dubos had isolated. The crude brownish material was practically incompatible with water and, under organic solvents, congealed into a sticky mass as uncouth as earwax. But it was powerful wax all right. Its amber alcohol solutions could be finessed into acceptable suspensions in water, and at great dilutions it would powerfully block bacterial growths, both in the test tube and in the peritoneal cavity of an infected mouse.

Starting with some half a pound of the material, I set out that fall to find the nature of its powers.

"Needing to manipulate a good many litres of different hot organic solvents, including ether, I soon attracted the attention of other colleagues. I was banished to the power house roof for fears I would set fire to our hospital patients, rather than simply reduce their fevers."

The results proved more and more exciting – so much so that the experiment was now officially adopted by the Institute. Hotchkiss was excused his previous duties and given proper laboratory space and assistance. "Soon I was granted my first technical assistant, and we were given keys to unlock and work in the lavish mouse dormitory and surgery which Alexis Carrel had built and abandoned when he moved to Europe. There I was enabled to set up some explosion-proof, safe electrical equipment and bring in other supplies."[23]

Hotchkiss now performed a myriad of chemical tests and manipulations on tyrothricin. Gradually it became clear that the antibiotic was not one substance at all but two totally different compounds. "Arriving at the laboratory each day a good hour before I did, René would absorb the information the night had brought. From my end, I could usually tell him whether the mice had looked feverish or nonchalant – noncalorific – at midnight. With all night to think about it, my cautious evaluations had usually caught up to his instant insights of the next day, so we quickly made our conclusions."[24] One day Hotchkiss, who had gone away to work on his own, came back to Dubos and asked him to look at something down the microscope.

René had his first sight of beautiful crystals, elegant, needle-shaped, as pure as ice. He knew he was gazing down on a pure chemical that had been extracted from the mishmash that had comprised his original brown sticky mud. Those first needle-shaped crystals, which Hotchkiss had purified and which they now called tyrocidine, were capable of killing bacteria in test tubes but not in animals. Hotchkiss soon christened it a "roughneck" lysin: it seemed to destroy everything equally, bacterial cells, red blood cells, tadpoles – indeed it was useless as an antibiotic substance because it was so poisonous. On 4 November 1939, their fortunes improved dramatically with the discovery of the second substance present, in Hotchkiss' expression, a "gentle protector", which, because it killed Gram-positive bacteria (in other words, bacteria that stained with a dye invented by a man called Gram: these include many of the common bacteria such as staphylococci, streptococci and pneumococci), they christened gramicidin. Gramicidin emerged in its pure form as beautiful boat-shaped crystals.

Great excitement now followed each new step in the chain of discoveries. In December 1939, Dubos and Hotchkiss each presented papers at a bacteriology meeting in New Haven, where René Dubos reported that a single microgram of gramicidin would protect mice from a thousand times the fatal dose of the pneumococcus.

In a very short space of time, they had taken the discovery so far, yet a vast amount of further research was still necessary. It would need to be tested in more animal experiments before anybody would even think of trying it out in human volunteers. It would need to be assessed for the massive commercial production essential before any new antibiotic could be marketed and thereby made available to doctors and chemists worldwide. Before the year was out, they freely doled out cultures of *Bacillus brevis* to any drug company that was interested. They even added complete instructions for making the new antibiotic substances.

In fact neither man was remotely interested in the commercial applications – money being regarded as an evil notion in academic circles – but they needed to ensure that there were no restrictions placed by avaricious entrepreneurs on the drug's production and availability. Rollin Hotchkiss had fond memories of their joint application for a patent. "When Dubos and I were officially assigning these patent revelations over to the Institute, we pointed optimistically to the clause 'in consideration of the sum of one dollar' – what we understood to be the legal minimum to bid one forever hold his peace. At this the Institute's kindly business manager, the towering E. B. Smith, disappeared and then returned, bringing into the room two shiny half dollars, with which he crossed our respective palms – one for each! That has kept me 'halfway peaceful'."[25]

v

STILL JUST THIRTY-NINE years old, René Dubos was now famous. On 22 March 1940, the *New York Times* carried a detailed report of the gramicidin discovery, brimming with congratulation and praise. Another newspaper hailed the discovery as a medical miracle. Antibiotics were headline material – the cure of Roosevelt Jnr with Prontosil had guaranteed that. On 25 April 1940, the *New York Times* carried a second and even more complimentary article:

"Ever since Pasteur's time it has been known that bacteria keep the soil fit for the growth of trees and plants. It is somewhat like the blood, this soil on which we depend. Were deadly hosts of unseen organisms to take possession of it there would be no animal life on this earth." The article, which moved on to discuss a new and related development at Rutgers conducted by Selman Waksman, went on to conclude: "What we have in the work of Drs Dubos, Avery, Waksman and Woodruff, is something more than an extension of the traditional way of fighting bacterial diseases, something more than the discovery that the soil is both the giver and the preserver of animal life. . . We have, then, the beginning of a new kind of chemotherapy."

Eminent scientists wanted samples of the new antibiotic for their own researches. Florey and Chain, of penicillin fame, were already planning research into the properties of tyrothricin.

Dubos and Hotchkiss had every reason to hope that they had the most important anti-bacterial agent since Prontosil in their hands. Over just a few months there was an intense interest in gramicidin from pharmaceutical companies worldwide, including Germany and France. In the United States major drug companies such as Parke Davis & Co., Squibb, Lederle and Lilly, had gone into a crash programme of chemical investigation of gramicidin, reporting their results and sending back samples of their analysis to Hotchkiss for testing. One such company, which took a very active interest, was George Merck & Co., of Rahway, New Jersey, an early interest that would subsequently prove important.

While the chemical analyses were being performed by the big companies, the two drugs, gramicidin and tyrocidine, were tested exhaustively in a wide range of experimental animals. It was at this late stage that Dubos and Hotchkiss suffered their most bitter disappointment. Not only was tyrocidine, as they already knew, extremely poisonous, but gramicidin was too, if to a lesser degree. When given by mouth or by injection, it combined with the membrane lining the red cells and caused them to rupture, a condition known as haemolysis. Soon afterwards, it was also shown to cause kidney damage when it was injected intravenously.

Further research showed that all was far from lost. Even if the drug could not be given my mouth or by injection, it could be used in local powders and creams to treat skin infections, in nasal sprays for nose and sinus infections, and as a wash in the treatment of infections of the mouth and throat. In animals, it could be used for more serious infections and Elsie, the Borden cow at the 1939 World Fair, was one of the first to benefit from its use in mastitis. It would find an important role in the treatment of war wounds, when it was applied as a cream or incorporated into the wound packs and dressings. Howard Florey, who shared the Nobel Prize with Fleming and Chain, gave credit to Dubos and his discovery of gramicidin for the resurrection of interest in the largely forgotten penicillin. When Florey visited New York, at the time of the 1939 World Congress, Dubos introduced him to the people at the Merck Pharmaceutical Company. This contact would lead to the mass production of penicillin, which, having little toxicity and a very similar spectrum of action to gramicidin, would make gramicidin largely redundant.

Perhaps this proved a little disappointing for René Dubos. Yet there was an inference to be drawn from the discovery itself. It was an inference of such colossal importance that it must surely have suggested itself to René as he travelled north to the Raybrook sanitorium every weekend to visit Marie Louise.

vi

THERE ARE FEW records of Marie Louise's experiences during her three years at Raybrook but we can be certain that she suffered a great deal, mentally as well as physically. She would have spent her first six months or more bed bound, being fed by a nurse and putting up with the indignities of the bed bath and bedpans. Once allowed out of bed, she would have been permitted only a very gentle exercise, gradually increasing until at last she was permitted out of doors. Photographs taken at the time show her wrapped in furs outside buildings covered in deep snow on one of the occasions when, much later on, she was allowed to take a gentle walk with René.

Three years is a long time to spend in a sanitorium and it emphasizes the gravity of her illness. How many nights did she spend tossing and turning in high fever, her bedclothes saturated with sweat? Did her tuberculosis spill over, as it so often did, from the infected lungs into her throat, then into the intestines and throughout the abdomen? Did it spread to involve the long bones of her legs, her spine, her kidneys, bladder, skin, eyes? Or come out through the chest wall, as it so often did as a complication of pus eating its way out of the delicate pleural spaces round the lungs, to discharge in never ending livid purple abscesses through the wall of her chest? We do not know the answers to such questions – only that she must have suffered along some of these lines. How often did she make young friends amongst the other patients, only to suffer the shock of their deaths later on from the disease? This was the common lot of sanitorium life. Yet nobody can endure this protracted mental and physical torment without its having a profound effect on his or her soul.

In the archives of the Rockefeller Foundation, set in the beautiful Pocantico Hills, twenty miles north of New York, there is a typescript written by her at this time. Written in French, it may be part fact and part fiction, but it is written in an impassioned language, imbued with a love of God and His universe, and a haunting nostalgia for the harmony of nature. The archives also contain snatches of her diary and a poem or two, deeply emotional, sensitive to the feelings of the young people who shared the long years in the sanitorium with her.

The following is a part quote from her poem, *En Bateau*,

which ends with what is almost certainly the presentiment of
her own fate:

> Les herons bleus, rapides et discrets,
> Traversent, pattes rapides, cou tendu,
> La très miroitante surface!
>
> Et le lac, immobile, parfait,
> glauque, impassible,
> Ou les blancs nénuphars mirent
>
> Avec une langoureuse coquetterie
> Leurs virginales graces,
> L'allonge au pied des montagnes infinies!
> Va mon joli bateau, va vers l'eau perfide
> Cruelle et savamment enchanteresse!
> Le temps s'évanouit, plus de regrets!
>
> Plus d'effrois, plus de doutes!
> Va mon joli bateau vers ton rêve
> et ta suprème illusion! Va ...
> Coule ... mon joli bateau.[26]

vii

T H E *New York Times* article of 22 March had drawn attention to a
new and extraordinary possibility under the subheading:
TUBERCULOSIS HOPE SEEN, when it continued ... "Since
the bacillus of tuberculosis belongs to the Gram-positive group
of microbes, it is hoped that the road has at last been opened up
for a chemical attack on the white plague."

As long ago as 1932, a fascinating experiment had been performed in Waksman's laboratory, regarded at the time as
routine. The American Tuberculosis Society asked Waksman to
test the ability of tuberculosis germs to survive in normal soil.
Waksman handed the task to Chester Rhines, one of his assistants, who published his findings in 1934.[27] What was this
strange experiment about?

Rhines wanted to know if tuberculosis germs died when they

were put into soil. He began with a bizarre, almost sinister, hypothesis: that tuberculosis germs must get into soil from contamination with infected animals and human bodies – clearly if such germs survived for a long period in the soil, this might lead to spread of the disease. He cultured avian tuberculosis for up to ninety-seven days in soil samples that contained various other bacteria and fungi. He repeated the experiments with these same competing organisms but this time used soil to which fresh manure had been added. Then he counted the numbers of tuberculosis germs which had survived for periods of seventeen, sixty-seven and ninety-seven days.

What he found was very curious. Tuberculosis often did survive extremely well in soil, perhaps confirming its own origins in the earth. But there was a secondary finding that was truly startling. When bacteria that needed the presence of oxygen, called aerobic bacteria, were added to the soil sample, the tuberculosis germs increased and multiplied to vast numbers. Exactly the same thing happened if bacteria that preferred to live without oxygen, called anaerobic bacteria, were added to the soil samples. But if Rhines added fungi instead of the aerobic or anaerobic bacteria, the numbers of tuberculosis germs appeared to die off within just seventeen days. This was particularly so if he used manured soil. Why did this happen?

If it is true, as Waksman must surely have suspected, that tuberculosis began its evolution in the primitive soil of the earth, if it had indeed fought out its wars for survival against other living organisms in that primeval mud, then the experiment must have exactly replicated that desperate struggle. Something else in soil had successfully fought back against it. Some other living organism, either the fungus, or another living creature in the manure, had triumphed over tuberculosis. What was this mysterious life form that was killing the tuberculosis germs?

The results were duly recorded. And that was it. Nobody took the slightest notice. Bewilderingly, even Waksman did not take the study further. Why on earth did the Tuberculosis Society themselves not follow it up? If they weren't interested, why request the study in the first place? But there was a more far-reaching omission. Dubos had left Waksman's department some five years before this study was started but he had always kept in touch with his former teacher. Dubos must surely have known the results of this experiment. No man in the world was more armed with the necessary knowledge to discover an antibiotic that would cure tuberculosis than René Dubos at this moment in time. The *New York Times* article had underlined this vital message when it had quoted Dubos' own words:

"It may be reasoned that, since a soil bacillus, when fed on Gram-positive bacilli, develops chemicals that counteract Gram-positive bacteria, other soil bacilli may be found that would develop potent bactericidal substances ..."

Gramicidin was routinely tested against tuberculosis but it had no more effect against the germ than penicillin. Why not begin again, seeding his soil sample not with the staphylococcus, but with the most deadly germ of all, the germ that caused the most virulent form of human tuberculosis?

vii

IN 1908 A LONDON physician, reacting to a lecture given by Robert Koch to the Royal Society of Medicine, boasted he could cure tuberculosis in anyone, given fresh air, good food, and isolation. After three long years in the sanitorium, in the winter of 1942, a frail Marie Louise came back home. While she was in Raybrook, René had moved from the rural surroundings of Rosalind Gardens, Dobbs Ferry, to York Avenue, New York City, so it was to the streets of Manhattan that she now returned, hoping for the opportunity of a normal married life and to play a part once again in supporting René in his pioneering scientific researches. Although fragile and weak, she felt much improved. She had gained a marvellous amount of weight. They both believed she had defeated the disease at last.[28]

Fearful that the stresses of living in New York City might threaten this fragile improvement in her health, René resigned from the Rockefeller, applying for a position as Professor of Comparative Pathology at Harvard. He was prepared to sacrifice everything for her. He would give up the entire line of antibiotic research and start something entirely new. Before leaving New York, there was a little time in which they could walk the streets together, see the familiar places, perhaps visit the theatre and see their many friends. In late winter, on a day gentle with the promise of spring, they walked arm in arm through the streets of Manhattan, in the vicinity of Carnegie Hall. Close to where Marie Louise herself used to play her music, they overheard a professional concert pianist at practice. The beauty of the music touched Marie Louise very deeply. She could not help but feel a poignant longing for the ability she so recently had in her own fingers and which she realized was no longer within her physical capabilities. At the end of three years of suffering, this was the last straw. She simply could not bear it. Shattered by this experience, her tuberculosis went into a fulminating relapse and she had to be rushed into the New York Hospital.[29]

Rollin Hotchkiss, who was working very closely with René at this time, could not fail to notice René's distress. Although he spoke little during their working hours about his wife, he was clearly very worried about her. Yet even now, as Marie Louise lay gravely ill in the New York Hospital, which was very close to the Rockefeller Institute, René tried to carry on with his work, taking time off each day to sit by her bedside. On 23 April 1942, a month or so after she had been been admitted to the giant hospital, with its famous gleaming tower, René had left the laboratory as usual to visit her. It was early in the evening. Hours went by and Rollin Hotchkiss realized that something was seriously wrong. Pearl Harbor had been attacked the December previously and Hotchkiss, a volunteer, was wearing his naval uniform, in preparation for an evening meeting. On impulse, he decided instead to go and meet René at the hospital, where he found him pacing the hallway of a ward that was many storeys high in the skyscraper building, directly in front of some large uncurtained windows. He asked René how Marie Louise was feeling.

"Marie Louise," René spoke softly, "has just died."

Rollin gazed in sympathy towards René, who was standing in front of the window, looking out over the lights of Manhattan.

"Thank you for coming!" René spoke again, placing his hand

on Rollin's arm. "But you can't do anything for me now. I have many things that require settling."

Rollin could say nothing. It was a very touching moment when speech was redundant.[30]

ix

RENÉ WAS INCONSOLABLE. That September he abandoned the Rockefeller Institute, where he had known such success and happiness, and now such grief. In a letter to Dr Gasser, head of the Institute, dated just six days before her death, he had given a brief and clearly pained explanation for this emotionally-laden move.

> "I have tried to express to Dr Rivers the factors which have influenced me, none of which concern in any way my relation to the Institute. May I assure you again, as I have in the past, that I have been perfectly happy here, that I never hope to live and work under such ideal conditions as you have given me. If I have not tried to communicate with you at the time of taking this decision, it is because I believed you could not help me at this time, and any discussion would have rendered this experience even more painful to me."[31]

From this moment onwards, his life would veer radically away from the research that had made him famous. Refusing to work any further on antibiotic research yet determined to fight on against the disease which had killed his wife, in his letter of acceptance to Harvard he indicated his desire to study the physiology and immunology of the tubercle bacillus. But this proved impossible. The critical wartime need for tropical medicine research led him to work on the problem of bacillary dysentery. Lonely, restless, still bewildered in his continuing grief over Marie Louise, when Thomas Rivers and Herbert Gasser asked him to return to the Rockefeller in 1944, inviting him to continue with his new interest in tuberculosis and offering him a laboratory specifically devoted to tuberculosis research, he agreed to return to his true home.

"I came back primarily for two things. They told me I could do what I wanted and I said I wanted to work on tuberculosis. I also came back because the avenue of trees as you enter the institute here is one of the most important elements of my life."[32] He would never leave the Rockefeller again.

From now on he would look to the social causes, to the environmental factors that had allowed the disease to plague whole countries and even continents. That vision, which had first come to him in the Palatine Gardens, would once again inspire him into extraordinary creativity. His colleague, Lewis Thomas, would subsequently comment that "although Dubos was not a doctor, he learned more about medicine than most physicians. He knew the power of scientific medicine to reverse mortal infections. But he also knew that mankind's changing of his own environment has much more to do with susceptibility or resistance to infection than anything in the modern pharmacopoeia."[33]

In the words of Carol Moberg, he was no longer concerned with treating individual sufferers, but . . . "Working and thinking ecologically, Dubos' revisions in the germ theory implicated the total environment as a determinant of disease. He showed that a microbe is necessary but not sufficient to cause disease. He reasoned that men coexist with microbes, both good and bad. He found disease-producing microbes are not inherently destructive and can persist in a quiescent state in the body for long periods. His new theme became: 'if we want to improve our physical and spiritual wellbeing, we must first understand and then control our impact on our surroundings.'"[34] For these contributions, the editor of the *American Review of Tuberculosis*, Walsh McDermott, referred to Dubos as "the conscience" of modern medicine.

With the assistance of Dr Bernard Davis, René would discover a culture medium that produced rapid, luxuriant growth of tuberculosis in the test tube, which greatly helped doctors to develop a safe BCG vaccine for global use. He would search for environmental and human explanations for the way in which the disease had plagued mankind for millenia, for example the influence of poor diet and malnutrition. He would write a book on this aspect, *The White Plague*, brilliant in its comprehensive and global analysis of the social causes behind the epidemic nature of tuberculosis.[35] During this research, his assistants Bernard Davis and Jean Porter, would contract tuberculosis from their contact with the bacillus as part of their work and their lives would only be saved by the intervention of the cure.[36] In time the innovatory young scientist who had destroyed the capsule that surrounded the pneumococcus would find new and even greater fame as a pioneer in our modern concern for the polluted atmosphere that envelops our small and all too vulnerable planet. In 1968 he would present his warning on the health of the earth in *So Human an Animal*, for which he was awarded the Pulitzer Prize. Lauded with many other prestigious prizes and eulogies from the great centres of learning worldwide, he would write in excess of two dozen deeply caring and brilliantly evocative books for both scientist and layman, earning the virtually unheard of distinction of a second Pulitzer Prize.[37] In many lectures, articles and books, he would develop his philosophy of caring about humanity and the human environment, using earthy terms and experiences of daily life to show that humans can act to shape their own destiny through manipulations of the environment. *Only One Earth*, written in association with political scientist Barbara Ward in 1972, served as the unofficial scientific and social guideline for the First United Nations Conference on the Human Environment.

Such famous environmental slogans as "Think globally, act locally", were coined by René Dubos. He would be the recipient of more than forty honorary degrees. But he would never perform any more work to further the search for the antibiotic cure for tuberculosis.

In the vast and prolific outpouring of his written words, his lectures and interviews, this "despairing optimist", so skilled at communication and so open in the expression of his views, would remain curiously reticent in describing even the smallest detail of Marie Louise and their life together. The pain of loss, the anguish, was too deep. On 28 April 1943, on the first anniversary of her death, he wrote eight handwritten pages in her memory, in French with the title, *Le Passé Vivant*.[38] In its simple eloquence, its immense sadness and the evocation of great loss, this unpublished elegy speaks for itself. These are a few illustrative lines:

> Marie Louise left us on a mild April evening. The spring air was misty, semi-lucent. For an anxious spirit, spring promises the coming of new life. One senses the vastness of the world, so much greater than the narrow horizon which chokes our own lives. The early spring brings blustery winds which seem to echo the confused voice of the universe, felt without being perceived. Nevertheless, these strong winds die out, leaving just a few sweet remains of the anticipated treasures, a few flowers, birdsong, some fruit for our small lives. . .
>
> Marie Louise wished to know nothing else of life than this spring. Although she came from a humble family in provincial France, she loved the universe and listened to its voice every day of her life.

PART III

THE GREAT
CURE

11

New Beginnings

Now I have touched the bottom of the sea – now I can go no deeper, one goes deeper. I do not want to die without a record of my belief that suffering can be overcome. Everything that we really accept undergoes a change. Suffering becomes love.

Katherine Mansfield

i

FROM THE BEGINNING of the first world war, the death rate from tuberculosis in Western Europe increased steadily until by the end of the war, four years later, it had doubled. The threat of the disease was so great that in 1920 delegates from thirty-one nations gathered in the Sorbonne in Paris and swore, one by one, in an impressive procession, to unite in the fight against it. The International Union Against Tuberculosis was born, which would, by 1992, have affiliated members in no less than 118 nations. However, with the outbreak of the second world war and in spite of such good intentions and all of the lessons learnt from the first, this same pattern had begun to repeat itself. The *blitzkrieg* bombing of cities such as London caused the mass evacuation of civilians, including half the entire nation's school children, to the countryside. A million and a quarter children and adults were evacuated from areas of danger, such evacuees often ending up in overcrowded houses or temporary billets.[1] Tuberculous children from the poorer wards of the cities were thrown into

173

contact with healthy households, greatly increasing the risk of
spread. No matter how prepared the authorities were, and in
spite of the precaution of compulsory medical examination,
many cases remained undiscovered. At the peak period of the
evacuation, no health measures could cope with the sheer
volume of numbers, a problem which was at its greatest in the
first and second years of the war.

There were many instances where infected children transmitted the disease to the entire family of their host.[2] In one
unfortunate example a girl suffering from acute tuberculosis
infected eight out of thirty-nine classmates in her new school
before her disease was recognized.[3] Adults too saw a marked
increase in the numbers suffering from the disease. The bombing caused an acute shortage of housing. Long factory hours,
the blacking out of windows, food rationing, all weakened the
resistance of the population. Most of the sanitoria were redesig-
nated for military pupuses and the patients were discharged
into the community, even though they were still sick with the
disease. "Some of them even had open cavities of the lungs and
their sputum contained millions of tuberculosis germs."[4] Dr
Marc Daniels, who visited many European countries soon after
peace, called tuberculosis "the major health disaster of the
second world war".[5]

In the first two years of the war the death rate from tuberculosis in Britain increased by fifteen per cent, two thirds of this
from pulmonary tuberculosis and the remaining third from
tuberculosis of bones, intestine, throat and the dreaded meningitis. Where, throughout 1939, the death rate from British war
casualties amounted to 2,000, just the *increase* alone in deaths
from tuberculosis over the two years 1939 to 1940 amounted to a
staggering 11,000 lives, all the more tragic for the fact that this
increase was mainly in children and young women.[6] It was a
pattern repeated in almost every country involved in the conflict. In Poland the death rate would rise progressively until it
equalled the worst epidemic figures in the country's history. At
the same time the researches of the disparate handful of doctors
and scientists, scattered in their different hospitals and
laboratories throughout the world, appeared to have ended in
stalemate.

Yet, in gramicidin, Dubos had discovered more than an antibiotic: he had discovered a general principle. Soil microbes were creators of antibiotics. No man in the world knew more about soil microbes than Waksman. In 1932, Chester Rhines, working with Waksman, had, after an exhaustive study, shown that if tuberculosis germs were added to certain types of soil, they died. Why had that vital research ended so prematurely?

These are Waksman's own words of explanation: "On the completion of this study, in 1935, I was not yet prepared to take advantage of these findings and did not attempt to determine the exact mechanisms involved in the process of destruction of the mycobacterium."[7]

Even more extraordinary: "Neither was I prepared to undertake such a study a year or so later when a test tube culture of the avian form of the tuberculosis organism, apparently killed by a contaminating mould, was brought to me by a colleague from the Poultry Department of my university."[8]

Why was Waksman so reluctant to study tuberculosis further? In fact the truth is perfectly simple. Waksman was not medically qualified. In his small laboratory, within the grounds of Rutgers Agricultural College, he was divorced from the mainstream of medical research at that time. Unlike Dubos, in daily contact with the medically qualified Avery, Selman Waksman had no contact whatsoever with doctors. He knew nothing about the pathology of diseases.

Selman Waksman was interested in bacteria not as the causes of diseases but as life forms in their minuscule selves. He candidly admitted that not only did he know, by 1935, that tuberculosis germs survived in sterile soil, that they died out slowly in soil contaminated by other organisms, but he even knew that it was certain fungi in the soil that seemed to kill the tuberculosis germs off. As far as he was concerned, this was all very interesting but it was leading him nowhere.

ii

ON THE OTHER HAND, Waksman was very interested indeed in the effects one microbe had on another when they lived together in the soil. There was something very curious – even beautiful – to the harmonious way in which different life forms lived cheek by jowl with their neighbours.

"Only one type (of microbe) is capable of causing typhoid fever, another is responsible for gas gangrene, still another for influenza, or polio, or scarlet fever, or diphtheria . . . In the soil, in the manure pile, and in the sea – those natural substrates for microbial development which I have studied most of my life – microbes do not live alone, or as pure cultures, but as *mixed populations*. Every particle of soil contains many millions of microbes, representing many thousands of kinds or groups. The microbes that live in the soil exist there side by side, without destroying one another completely and without one kind becoming predominant in suppressing all the others.

"I often raised the question, as no doubt many others have done . . . how are all these microbes able to get along together? Do they fight one another occasionally, or do they help one another as good neighbours? Do they compete for food or do they live upon one another?"[9]

To a soil microbiologist, these questions were fundamental. They fascinated Waksman. Why did some microbes come out on top in the struggle for survival and not others? As he peered down his microscope at their wriggling forms, the mysteries disturbed him. At first sight, there seemed to be no reason why, in a certain type of soil, one should do any better than another. What he was observing down the microscope seemed little better than anarchy. But slowly, in experiment after experiment, he began to untangle the skein of this complex mystery. One thing he did know: if a microbe lost its food supply, it died. Even the way it died was curious. It didn't just shrivel up, as might be imagined. It seemed to melt away to nothingness. Sometimes, he noticed too, this ghostly dissolution happened when one microbe was put too near another. So sometimes they really did fight. But when they did so, lacking tooth and claw, they fought it out with chemical weapons. One microbe produced a chemical which killed and dissolved another.

What were these killer chemicals? Why were they produced? Even more vitally – was Dubos' gramicidin exactly such a chemical weapon? The growing racial menace in Europe and

Asia made him wonder if there might even be a similarity here to the conflicts of mankind, to the great migrations of people down the ages, maybe even to the very appearance and disappearance of whole races of people? Was it really a practical notion to think he might find a beneficial use for these chemicals that one microbe produced to kill and devour another?

At the end of 1936, he wrote a series of papers, in which he summarized all he knew of how microbes affect one another's lives. But he was thinking still in terms of soil microbiology and not using his knowledge to fight diseases. His perceptions would soon undergo a dramatic change. "The opportune time came about two years later when Dubos succeeded, in 1939, in demonstrating that by systematic study of the soil microbes, it is relatively easy to isolate microbes which are able to kill disease-producing germs."[10]

Throughout 1938 and 1939, Waksman and Dubos had been in constant touch, writing to each other, meeting, endlessly discussing the possibilities of Dubos' new line of research. Could something extraordinary result from Dubos' pioneering ideas? Waksman was not as yet committed. However, it was a man already primed by Dubos' ideas and by the practical success of gramicidin who attended the Third International Congress of Microbiology in New York, where he heard Fleming say that penicillin was at last about to benefit mankind.

iii

IN 1939, H. BOYD WOODRUFF graduated at Rutgers with a BSc in which he had majored in soil chemistry. A farmer's son from Bridgeton, New Jersey, this young man had been impressed by the teaching of soil microbiology at Rutgers. Rather like Dubos before him, Woodruff found Waksman a truly inspirational teacher. "For the first time I realized the unity of biology and chemistry, that each biological observation has an underlying chemical cause, that in unravelling the latter, one could understand the other."[11]

Woodruff was thinking about a career in chemistry. Not for a moment did he anticipate an offer from Dr Waksman to join him on a university fellowship, which would allow him to do full-time research on a relatively generous stipend of $900 a year. No mention at all was made of antibiotics. Woodruff joined several other postgraduate students with origins as diverse as mainland China, India, South America and Europe, in addition to various corners of the United States, all engaged in a multitude of research studies on such processes as soil erosion, decomposition of cyanide in soil, the nature of marine micro-organisms, even to the composting of human excrement. He had already begun to research how sulphur was oxidized in compost at various temperatures, when suddenly everything changed. This was the day that a highly agitated Waksman burst through the doors of the laboratory and exclaimed, "Drop everything!"

Woodruff was left in no doubt as to the future: from now on every effort of Waksman's laboratory would be devoted to the search for anti-bacterial substances produced by soil micro-organisms.

But how should they go about testing for such substances? The soil was a harbour for billions of micro-organisms. How, from these billions, could they select the very organisms they wanted? Bacteria and fungi for example grew very differently on different growth media: while some, most notably tuberculosis germs, grew very reluctantly indeed, others would swarm across the surface of a culture plate, engulfing everything in their path. They already knew there were many micro-organisms in soil with anti-bacterial potential, from the commonest of everyday bacteria, to spore bearing bacteria, such as the *Bacillus brevis* discovered by René Dubos, from the actinomyces, which Waksman had studied so closely all his life and which had earned him his early reputation, to the ubiquitous fungi that floated about in the laboratory air, contaminating all manner of rotting food, an example of which produced Fleming's penicillin. Any of these might contain the wonder germs they were looking for.

They had to start right from the beginning. Two thousand years of advance had brought the medical world to its present understanding of infectious diseases; yet neither man, working in this small agricultural college laboratory, had the slightest knowledge of this other than what they could read for themselves in books. Neither had attended a single medical lecture and their only contact with hospitals had been to visit an occasional sick relative. Incredible as it might seem in retrospect, Waksman and Woodruff actually sat round a table and discussed which of the many bacterial infections in humans they should try to cure. From what they knew about the sulphonamides, penicillin and gramicidin, it was clear that a certain large group of disease-causing bacteria were resistant to all of these recently discovered drugs. These, called the Gram-negatives because they failed to stain with a dye invented by Gram, were commonly found as the normal flora of the bowel. They caused bladder and kidney infections. They killed thousands, maybe even millions of people globally, when they infected gall bladders and bile ducts. They were a nightmare to the abdominal surgeons, when they infected surgical wounds or swarmed throughout the delicate tissues and organs of the abdomen, causing huge abscesses and destruction. Everybody knew of one of their most common effects, the deadly peritonitis. What better challenge than to search for an antibiotic that would kill these Gram-negative germs!

The first step therefore was to think of some way in which they could detect the presence of a microbe capable of killing such bacteria. A marvellously simple test system was the "plate method". The technique was as follows.

A sample of soil was diluted in tap water and a tiny quantity evenly dispersed over the bottom of a culture plate. A second layer of soft agar, seeded with a disease-causing germ, was then poured over this same plate and allowed to set like jelly before the plate was incubated at body temperature overnight. Normally the disease-causing germ would proliferate in the soft agar, visible the next day as a diffuse cloudiness – as if milk had been added to a jelly mix. The presence of even a single antibacterial microbe in the soil wash under the agar layer showed up as a clear circle in the cloud, where the dangerous bacteria had been completely destroyed.

Almost as soon as they had started this testing, Waksman

and Woodruff discovered two distinct micro-organisms from soil that killed Gram-negative bacteria. The first, and less effective of the two, was a bacterium of the *Pseudomonas aeruginosa* group, and the second, and by far the most promising, was an actinomyces.

For Selman Waksman the actinomyces was a wonderful portent. These were the tiny life forms which had fascinated him all of his life. His very first scientific paper had been devoted to them. The first lecture he had ever given in his scientific career, back in 1915, had described their distribution in soil. In his textbook, the chapter that would most inspire an entire generation of students focused on these delightful micro-organisms.

After testing nearly 500 different strains of actinomyces, only a single species was promising enough for further testing. They found that it produced a chemical which was soluble in ether and that the extract, even in very great dilution, completely inhibited the growth of several harmful germs. Within just a year, they had discovered their first anti-bacterial drug. They called it actinomycin.

When they purified the new drug to its active form, it was found, like Prontosil, to comprise beautiful red crystals. It was easy to produce and extract, was sufficiently stable to be analysed chemically, and was so highly active that, in the words of Woodruff, "we could dream of practical applications."[12]. Sadly it would never be tested in human infection: it was much too poisonous. Even small amounts, when administered to mice, killed them within twenty-four to forty-eight hours. Years later, those very poisonous effects would make it an important drug in the suppression of the rejection of organ transplants. But for Waksman and Woodruff, unaware of its future potential, it brought heartbreak. "All our dreams were defeated by toxicity."[13]

They had of course learnt a great deal in terms of technique and application. Most important of all, with the discovery of actinomycin, the pharmaceutical company, Merck & Co., only a single station down the line on the New York run from New Brunswick, was interested in the antibiotic research now taking shape in Waksman's laboratory.

iv

MERCK WAS WELL-KNOWN for its success in the purification of natural products for clinical use, particularly the vitamins. This company had also taken an interest in Dubos' gramicidin. It was inevitable that this budding relationship should now extend to the search for antibiotics. Just how important this would prove to be, Waksman subsequently made clear.

> When I started my search for a new antibiotic in 1939, I had merely a theory, two and a half decades of stored knowledge of the interrelationships of soil bacteria, a systematic method of investigation and plenty of enthusiasm. All these put together, plus persistent, painstaking labour and more than any man's share of good luck would probably not have brought me much closer to my goal than another demonstration, like Fleming's, in a glass dish.
>
> Any promising substance would have to be isolated and purified by chemists. It would have to be manufactured in quantity and tested by pharmacologists in thousands of animals. If exhaustive animal tests showed it to be both safe and effective, it would have to be mass-produced for clinical trials in man, and, finally, for worldwide distribution. How was a soil microbiologist in a small laboratory going to do all this?
>
> Fortunately, I did not have to answer this question. It was answered for me by Dr Randolph T. Major, then head of the Merck research laboratories. He and his colleagues, intrigued by Dubos' experiments, had started to make tyrothricin and came to me for advice. When Dr Major learned that I had already launched my own search for an antibiotic, he asked me if I needed help. I needed all the help I could get, I told him.[14]

Merck took the patent on actinomycin and arranged the facilities for large-scale production. The hundreds of flasks incubated at Merck were inoculated by Waksman himself. The Merck chemist, Dr Max Tishler, later to become president of Merck Sharpe & Dohme Research Laboratories, joined forces with Waksman in bringing actinomycin to a final state of purity and in investigating its chemical structure. Meanwhile, helped by funding from Merck, the antibiotic research in Waksman's laboratory expanded.

Incoming graduate students were now specifically assigned to the antibiotic research. Many spent all of their time just screening actinomyces cultures to see if they had any antibiotic potential. Hardly had they recovered from their disappointment over actinomycin, when an assistant called Walter Kocholaty found an actinomyces, with wonderful properties, which grew in beautiful lavender-coloured colonies. This new microbe was called *Streptomyces lavendulae*. It was passed on to Woodruff for further testing.

From *Streptomyces lavendulae*, Woodruff isolated a new antibacterial drug, streptothricin, which was more exciting than anything they had ever found before. Unlike actinomycin, it was soluble in water – a factor which lent it great promise.

In experiment after experiment, streptothricin swept everything before it. In bacterial cultures, it killed not only Gram-positive bacteria, such as were killed by penicillin and the sulphonamides, but it also showed great promise against the previously resistant Gram-negatives. Although they had not yet tested it against tuberculosis, this could only be a matter of time.[15]

As with actinomycin, the next step was to test it for safety and effectiveness against infection in experimental animals. Here, however, they ran into difficulty. Although it was easy enough to test streptothricin against bacterial infections in mice, they simply did not have the facilities for more comprehensive testing in animals. A colleague, Dr Metzger, in the dairy department at Rutgers, helped them out. Metzger had for some time been studying contagious abortion in cattle, caused by infection with a bacterium called *Brucellus abortus*. At this time, there was no treatment available to cure this infection. Metzeger agreed to test streptothricin in his infected cattle. The results were dramatically effective. Streptothricin completely cured the animals of their unpleasant infections.

In Woodruff's own words: "The excitement in our group was intense. From that time on . . . the advantage of variety in research experience was lost to its students. We talked of antibacterial substances, nothing else."[16]

The new drug caused just as much excitement at Merck's drug company as it did in Waksman's laboratory. Waksman kept the Merck research directors informed of progress. He also suggested that Woodruff should spend the last six months of his PhD programme in residence at Merck's research laboratories. Here, Woodruff shared the same laboratory bench with Norman Heatley, who had only recently arrived in America to help Merck produce penicillin in large quantity.

At Merck, the research had reached a very advanced stage. They had invented techniques for measuring streptothricin in blood and body tissues. A factory for the production of streptothricin was designed and in preparation. At last, in early 1943, they were ready for the first clinical trials in human volunteers. But such trials were instantly terminated. Nobody had the slightest warning that there would be a mysterious delayed toxicity. Mice that had been given the drug died many days later, from a poisonous effect on the kidneys. This effect was all the more dramatically poisonous in larger animals, such as monkeys. There was no question of human application. For Woodruff it was the greatest disappointment of his life.[17]

For Waksman it was just as great a blow. Streptothricin seemed to embody all that he was searching for in an antibiotic. The fact they had been so close to success made the disappointment all the harder to bear. If only they could find something similar to streptothricin, an antibiotic that had all of its wonderful activity against harmful bacteria and yet none of its poisonous effects!

v

IN SPITE OF such disappointments, a thrill of excitement never left the laboratory and those working in it. Everybody involved in the new research were now part of an "enchanted circle".[18] No disappointment could stop the progress of this spectacular new field of science. People wanted to know what to call these new discoveries. In 1941, at the request of a journal editor, Waksman redefined a term, *antibiosis*, which had been in circulation since the days of Pasteur, hailing the new discoveries by the name the world would instantly accept and recognize from then on – *antibiotics*. "In doing this, I made use of an old adjective, which was at one time used to designate the injurious effect of one organism upon another."[19]   New side avenues opened before the scientist with incredible rapidity. In Waksman's own words: "Here were the miraculous substances that would do away with infections and epidemics! No wonder the public gasped in amazement at these compounds and at once designated them as 'miracle drugs'. The horizons were now unlimited. New fields were opened. Was it not time to attack the most difficult of all infectious diseases, tuber-culosis?"[20]

Waksman himself drew attention to a sparkling sunny morning. "I shall never forget the bright morning of 1 June 1943, a small group of people met in one of the rooms of the Pennsylvania Hotel in New York to discuss possible approaches to the problem of the chemotherapy of tuber-culosis."[21] Those present included Leroy U. Gardner, a bac-teriologist from the Saranac Sanitorium, Dr William C. White, two or three others from university laboratories and several representatives from interested pharmaceutical companies, including his close collaborators, George Merck & Co. There was no programme for discussion. The very atmosphere seemed imbued with a profound pessimism. Not surprisingly, they failed to reach any common conclusion from the discus-sions.

The topic of conversation was of course the new antibiotics. Dr White's presence guaranteed that they would discuss tuberculosis. During the course of the day, Waksman would remember discussing Domagk's sulphonamides, which had proved disappointing against tuberculosis. Penicillin also was discussed only to be dismissed in this particular role. They moved on to consider the new group of drugs which were still being assessed for an anti-tuberculous role by Hinshaw and Feldman at the Mayo Clinic, the sulphones, which had ultimately derived from the sulphonamides. The sulphones seemed more promising than anything that had been tested before but already there had been side-effects. Nobody in the room regarded sulphones as the answer.

What was to be done? Conversation drifted to new ideas. Could anybody suggest the way forward?

White spoke about the possibility of extracting digestive enzymes from earthworms. To Waksman, this seemed utterly ludicrous. Yet it was being taken seriously by no less authorities than the National Tuberculosis Association, the Research Corporation and Merck's drug company. A study was taking place right now in Washington. White spoke enthusiastically on what he thought might be the explanation for Rhines' earlier findings. The disappearance of tuberculosis germs from soil was almost certainly due to their being devoured by earthworms. White was as obsessed with finding an enzyme to dissolve the waxy capsule of the tuberculosis germ as Avery had been with that of the pneumococcus.

Hadn't Dubos, who was after all Waksman's protégé, successfully extracted an enzyme capable of destroying the pneumococcus capsule from soil? And now White gave some scientific credibilty to his argument. Earthworms, it seemed, had actually been studied. They really were very interesting in a number of respects. For example, did his colleagues realize that earthworms could digest tuberculosis bacteria and remain uninfected? The common earthworm must contain an enzyme that would strip the tuberculosis bacterium of its protective coat . . .

Waksman's scepticism annoyed White. It seemed to him that in the unlikely event that such an enzyme could be extracted from earthworms – and furthermore if it would digest the almost indestructible capsule of mycobacteria – it would more than likely digest the internal organs of any human being to whom it was administered. White reacted angrily.

"How do you propose to go about this problem?"

Waksman's answer was simple. "The cure for tuberculosis must come not from enzymes but from antibiotics. The antibiotics will do it. Just give us time."[22]

Waksman was all too well aware that his argument had carried no weight with his colleagues. Yet, with the help of his assistants at Rutgers, he had already discovered two new antibiotics, no matter that they had been spoiled by toxicity. What was needed now was not some far-fetched enzyme derived from the humble earthworm but a renewed search along the lines he was already taking.

In May 1942, in an astonishing development, Waksman's son, Byron, then a medical student at the University of Pennsylvania, wrote a letter to him. "In reading the reprints you sent me, I was struck again with the urge to do some work in the direction of finding an effective antagonist to the tubercle bacillus. I was particularly impressed with the relative simplicity of the method you used in isolating fungi capable of producing antibiotic substances, and I wondered if exactly the same method could not be used with equal ease to isolate a number of strains of fungi or actinomycetes which would act against M. tuberculosis . . . "[23]

Later, rereading the letter from his son, Waksman was struck with regret. Byron was described by a fellow student as one of the brightest in his university. There is no doubt that had Waksman followed his son's suggestion, Byron's career would have been transformed. Waksman replied to his son with the following words:

"The time has not come yet. We are not quite prepared to undertake this problem. But we are rapidly approaching it."[24]

12

A Phoenix from the Ashes of Elberfeld

*I am on the verge of mysteries and the veil is getting thinner and
thinner.*

Louis Pasteur

i

FOR GERHARD DOMAGK, the nightmare did not end
with that terse letter, in which, under duress, he had been
forced to refuse the Nobel Prize. Those experiences
would cast a long dark shadow which blighted his life and work
for many years afterwards, when the indomitable spirit that
had seen him through the bitter years of hunger and loss following the first world war seemed lost to him. Even a year later,
in 1940, he found it impossible to concentrate. Yet, in the darkest moments of his depression, he struggled bravely to shake
himself free of this debilitating melancholy. Never, since the
end of the first war, had humanity so needed his courage and
intellect. With the new war, thousands of soldiers and civilians
were once again dying from the appalling wound infections
that he had witnessed in the field hospitals of the Eastern Front
in the first world war.

In the summer of 1940, seeking comfort through the pleas-
ures of family life, Domagk took Gertrud and their four children
to the little resort of Dammeshöved on the Baltic. En route, they
spent a night in the hotel, Stadt Hamburg, in Lübek, where
they were forced to shelter in the cellars from a heavy bombing

attack. After just a few days at the resort, he was compelled to return to Elberfeld . . . "because I was still very much run down. I had not recovered normal health since the shock of my imprisonment."[1] It seemed that no matter how hard he fought back against it, the long dark shadow would not leave him. "The new continuing working day had catastrophic consequences for somebody like me, who relied completely on creative mental effort. My mind was always full of thoughts and ideas that would not turn off in the evening and all through the night. Under such pressures, the quality of my research was drastically reduced."[2]

His nervous state was not helped by the effect the war was having on his children. They were already experiencing difficulties with obtaining such basic items as shoes. At least they did not as yet have to worry about decent supplies of food. When, at the end of July 1940, he was awarded a prize from Berlin for experimental therapy, he passed the money on to the German Red Cross. Day after day, in spite of the support of his colleagues, Gerhard Domagk faced a hard and protracted inner battle for his former determination and self-confidence. He was well aware that terrible as the war would prove in terms of death and destruction, the social consequences would usher in a familiar and even more apocalyptic danger. Tuberculosis would soon return in epidemic proportion to the towns and cities of Germany.

Gerhard Domagk regarded this fearsome disease as the greatest challenge of his life. Although the Bayer researchers were no nearer to finding the cure than they had been two years earlier, intermittently during these last two years of debilitating nervousness, Gerhard Domagk had felt that extraordinary challenge rise again: the exhilaration of pitting every fibre of his being against impossible odds. Nothing could be more vital to his work, to his imagination and efforts, than this single disease. But how could he possibly rediscover his former spirit of adamantine determination? In his diary of February 1941, Domagk found it necessary to remind himself where his sense of purpose had first begun.

"The real birth of chemotherapy as far as I am concerned took place in the great war of 1914–18, when I swore an allegiance with my fallen comrades. Those were my first principles and they are still valid. They stand over my work like a shining star. Man must want more than he is able to achieve. No matter that the borders may be drawn in harsh reality very early and very soon. If we do not reach for the impossible, we shall never reach far enough to discover the possible. Our wishes have to be boundless. Yet this need to reach for the stars, the desire to do more than one is physically able to achieve, to want to do more than is humanly possible – all this is often the first step that will lead to modest success."[3]

No man was more dedicated to discovering the cure for tuberculosis. But before he could once more apply himself to that almighty struggle, a struggle in which he would have to pit himself totally, body and soul, he must first keep his vow made under the appalling conditions of the field hospitals before Verdun. Gas gangrene had to be defeated.

In July 1940 the first edition of his book, *The Chemotherapy of Bacterial Infections*, was published by Hirzel in Leipzig. He fondly hoped that the information it contained would give the army surgeons a vital message for the treatment of the wounded. However, it soon became evident that the army doctors were taking no notice. Domagk wrote to Professor Waldmann, Director General of the Army, with details of the Bayer team's new discovery, Marfanil, synthesized by the brilliant Klarer, and which was the first ever drug to be effective in the treatment of gas gangrene. Still the army surgeons ignored him. On 9 November 1940, he wrote a letter to the Bayer directorate, suggesting that they increase their efforts to discover even better drugs for the treatment of gas gangrene. Importantly, in that same letter, he suggested that they should restart the tuberculosis research, which had been abandoned with the outbreak of war.

On 15 May he was invited to give a series of lectures in Rome. Following his return, he found his suggestions for the treatment of gas gangrene enmeshed in even greater controversy. While some of the army surgeons welcomed his ideas, Kirschner, the surgical director, was downright insulting in the manner in which he threw Domagk's ideas aside. He enlisted the help of eminent medical colleagues, such as Bauer at Breslau and Frey at Düsseldorf. Meanwhile, the Bayer factory at Leverkusen was bombed and a large quantity of mesodine was destroyed. Münster and Cologne were under heavy air raids. Domagk's colleague, Schürmann, was killed in a huge tank battle involving the Panzers near Beresina in the Ukraine. Nevertheless, the vital work continued, if with agonizing slowness.

Early on 1 June 1942, his wife, Gertrud, called him at work to say there was an urgent phone call. Could he return home immediately to take it. "On my arrival, Hildegard came tripping towards me in her impetuous way and declared, 'Pappy, Pappy, Berlin wants you!' " This call was not the one he had hoped for. It was merely an invitation to travel to Oslo to give a talk to the German/Norwegian Association. No sooner had he agreed and returned to work than his busy little secretary, Miss Sauer, came towards him... "Quick, Professor – a call from Brussels!" Maybe this was another routine call? He found himself speaking to Dr Wachsmuth, the leader of the field surgeons group. Would Domagk be prepared to travel to Brussels to talk about the treatment of wound infections? Domagk could hardly believe what he was hearing. Wachsmuth was known to be utterly sceptical about the Bayer drugs and had made derisive comments about them to a colleague very recently in Bonn. Domagk donned his army uniform and reported for duty on the 16th.

Arriving in Brussels between 10 and 11 p.m., he was given a room at the Hotel Metropol by the quartermaster. The following morning, at eight o'clock, he reported to Professor Wachsmuth for a short briefing. In the casino he met Professor Pfeissler from Hamburg, a foremost bacteriologist. Apart from the two professors, their audience consisted solely of army surgeons. Nothing suited Domagk better. Pfeissler had brought some growth media and some earth containing spores of the bacteria that caused gas gangrene. It was his intention to reproduce the very conditions of gas gangrene infection before the eyes of the surgeons.

Pfeissler began his first experiment by demonstrating exactly how gas gangrene developed in a wound. Although the bacteria that caused this had been known for over fifty years, many of the surgeons in his audience doubted that it was due to a bacterial infection at all, convinced it was the result of some obscure poisonous process which could not be cured except by removal of the infected tissue, even if this meant disarticulating the entire arm at the shoulder or the leg at the hip joint. Now Pfeissler and Domagk performed a devastatingly simple experiment. They infected wounds in rats with earth containing the spores, leaving half the animals untreated while sprinkling Marfanil into the wounds of the other half. No form of surgical treatment whatsoever was attempted... "On the following day we went to Bruges, to admire the architecture of the old town, and in the evening we returned to the army hospital, where the experiments had been carried out. All of the untreated rats had died while all those treated with Marfanil were still alive."[5]

It was an experiment that could hardly miss its mark. By Christmas 1942, the fourth of the war, a new inspiration had delivered Gerhard Domagk from the black maw of depression. He had kept his word to his fallen colleagues on the first world war battlefield. The army was at last taking the chemotherapy of gas gangrene seriously. "Packed in convenient small sifter-top containers, it was to be found not only in every soldier's kitbag but also in the medicine chests of many homes ... when it saved the lives of thousands of wounded soldiers and civilians."[6] Resting from his exhausting labours with his family over the holiday period, he felt sufficiently bolstered by the recent success to engage himself once more in the most important challenge of his life.

ii

"FOR MONTHS I HAVE been suggesting to Hörlein that we should extend the researches of the chemotherapy department to tuberculosis. So far there has been no reaction. No new ideas are coming through from the chemists. Not even from Klarer, who used to be the most productive of all. All initiative appears to have been killed off."[7] There was good reason for their reluctance. The war was worsening from day to day.

Tuberculosis research was extremely time-consuming. To devote any substantial effort to a radical new programme of research would mean putting aside the productive research they were already engaged in, work that was an integral part of the war effort. How could Hörlein possibly convince the company's management, itself under pressure for increased production in other directions from the Reich government, that precious time and a substantial allocation of their rapidly dwindling manpower should be diverted to something that had no benefit at all to the troops on the front line, indeed a line of research, which to judge from their previous efforts would inevitably prove a wild goose chase. Everybody was convinced that the cure for tuberculosis was a pipe dream.

Between 1937 and 1940, Domagk had tested more than two thousand permutations of the sulphonamide molecule against tuberculosis – and what had he proven? A slowing down of bacterial growth in test tube cultures and a lessening of the disease in guinea pigs at doses that would have been fatal, projected to a human scale. That small initial promise had ended in vapid disappointment.

In the turmoil of destruction and death that surrounded Elberfeld and Leverkusen, there were many cogent reasons why Bayer should not become embroiled in a major new effort against tuberculosis. The majority of the Bayer workers, chemists and management, could think of little other than the havoc the war was causing. Each day brought heartbreaking news of friends and loved ones.

The youngest son of one of Domagk's dear old colleagues, Dr Bearendez, had fallen in the east at the age of nineteen. His parents had been expecting him home for Christmas. Gerhard Domagk had met him at a school performance of '*Young Mozart*' when he had come home on holiday the previous year. What a strapping young fellow he had seemed. "How many," Domagk reflected, "will wait in vain this Christmas?"

On his way home from a meeting in Hungary, where Domagk was appalled by the fact that one in two newborn babies were dying from an umbilical infection that could have been prevented by the simple measure of sprinkling the skin with a sulphonamide powder, the air raid alarm was raised on the train. Through the window he could see the town of Dortmund in flames. Eight days later it was the turn of his home town, Wuppertal, where his friend Professor Klee, at present suffering his own by persecution under the Nazi regime, had performed the first clinical trials of Prontosil.

Domagk was still lecturing away from home when he heard the news. "When I returned to the hotel, after giving a lecture to the association on how to prevent the infant deaths, I found a telegram from my wife. 'Nothing has been destroyed here.'" A few minutes later it was announced over the radio that Wuppertal had suffered heavily from bomb attacks. In fifty minutes one hundred thousand people lost their homes. For weeks, every day, there were up to one hundred obituaries in the newspapers. Shattering tragedies – whole families destroyed. A medical colleague newly arrived home to his family was killed with his wife and four children. Many were burned to death in the streets as they were running for safety. It was a tragic night for Wuppertal, even for Koenigsberg. Fortunately the damage to the factory was repairable and they were able to put out the incendiary bombs. I asked that a prize of 10,000 Marks, which had been awarded to me at Koenisberg, should be donated to the Red Cross to help the injured of the war. But how little one can help those maimed victims of air attacks. Our pitiful efforts just can't keep pace with the raging destruction."[8]

A few days later it was the turn of Düsseldorf to burn. "When we opened the shutters in the morning, the sunlight was dimmed with yellow, red, white thick fog and everywhere was soot and ash covering an area of fifteen square kilometres." Unexpectedly, in the eye of the storm, he was to find support for his tuberculosis proposals.

He was taken by surprise when an article he had written, *Ten Years of Sulphonamide Therapy*, caused a storm of controversy within the Bayer research laboratories. He had offended Klarer and Mietzsch with his opening sentence, which, in their opinions, underrated their contribution to the Prontosil discovery. To be fair to the chemists, their contribution to the sulphonamides had been largely ignored by the outside world. Hörlein, who sympathized with the hurt felt by Klarer in particular, was equally upset by the closing sentence of the paper, which he judged less than fair to the company. The matter blew up into a heated row, where resentments that had been smouldering for years erupted into the open. These differences emerged at a time of great personal duress, with the omnipresent ravages of the war. In their frank exchange of views, Professor Hörlein threatened he would not renew Domagk's contract. And in the heat of the moment, Domagk retorted he did not care. He would don his uniform and go out to serve his country in the army.

But in fact, behind the volcanic release of pent-up anger and emotions, it had never been Domagk's intention to belittle the contribution of the chemists or the Bayer company. With Hörlein's guidance, the controversies in the paper were ironed out and an amicable agreement was reached. But the internecine exchange had an unexpected outcome. During their argument, Domagk had stressed once again his contention that Bayer would not support his tuberculosis research. When tempers had cooled down, Hörlein reflected upon those arguments. There was never any question of his not taking the suggestions seriously. Yet the logic against restarting the tuberculosis research was as persuasive as ever. Indeed, with the worsening conditions of war, the arguments against it were all the more overwhelming. Somehow Hörlein persuaded the management to support the idea, no matter how crazy it seemed at that highly charged moment, no matter what his own reservations or those of so many others. This decision was to be the watershed.

In Domagk's diary, soon after Christmas 1942, a new tone of optimism is apparent. "Our tuberculosis work has progressed so far that I am convinced we can do something with it. I have concrete proof that we are on the right track and I have put forward suggestions for further work to the chemists. At last, they are beginning to listen. How extraordinary it is that this major objective has been achieved as a result of a storm in a teacup. The chemists are really getting down to it and now it is full steam ahead in our battle against tuberculosis."[9]

iii

IN SPITE OF DOMAGK'S enthusiasm, the reason for Hörlein's

initial reluctance was immediately apparent. Working conditions in the research laboratory at Elberfeld were not such as to permit a new and great leap into the unknown. They were desperately cramped for space. Experiments that could be decided within days in the case of acute bacterial infections took weeks and even months when it came to tuberculosis. The mycobacteria that caused the disease took weeks to grow on the jade-coloured Lowenstein-Jensen slopes, the culture media that contained a strikingly beautiful and highly poisonous dye called malachite green that was added to kill all bacteria other than the tuberculosis germ. When they inoculated tuberculosis germs into experimental guinea pigs and rabbits, it took weeks and even months before the outcome became apparent. More worrying still, tuberculosis was a much more dangerous organism to work with than anything they had tested previously. It was notoriously prone to kill the researchers who worked with it. If one of his laboratory assistants contracted the disease from the virulent germs they were testing, nobody could do a thing to cure him. Domagk began to worry about those cramped conditions, and the impact of the chaos of war on the quality of the work. The perils his technicians were exposed to, his memories of what tuberculosis did to people on those hopeless wards during his years as a younger doctor, were a constant source of alarm. He wrote letters to the directorate, warning of the dangers. In reply, the directorate could only assure him that they would do everything in their power to improve safety for the staff. Domagk lay in his sleepless bed praying that . . . "the English Tommies do not spoil everything by destroying the modest facilities that remain functioning – our laboratories. Everything in our power should be tried to make this contribution to humanity."

As early as 1938, Domagk was convinced that only two in particular of the thousands of sulphonamides tested – sulphathiazole, which had made its reputation in the treatment of gonorrhoea, and sulphathiodiazole – showed any worthwhile effect against experimental tuberculosis in guinea pigs and rabbits. When they had carried out tests in test tubes, where the drugs were added in very diluted amounts to the egg culture media, dilutions of one in 25,000 of these drugs had shown a promising effect against the germs. At this time, in 1941, a thirty-two year old chemist called Robert Behnisch, the youngest of the chemists working at Bayer, volunteered to take part in the project. Behnisch had a personal reason for his strong faith in Gerhard Domagk.

In 1933, his mother, then sixty-years-old, had had a fall and broken a metacarpal bone in her hand. A large wooden splinter that had penetrated deeply into the flesh had been overlooked and amputation was required to save her life from blood poisoning. With a tremendous fever and in a semi-comatose state, she was too sick to sign for the operation and the surgeon was forced to make an urgent phone call to her son, Robert, to obtain his permission... "Immediately I got in touch with Domagk who directly contacted the head of the Breslau pharma office. The latter set out for the clinic with a hospital pack of Prontosil. Doctors there had not yet had occasion to test the drug which had only recently been launched. With great hesitation they agreed to try chemotherapy since they felt the patient had little chance of surviving the amputation because of her poor general condition. Intensive treatment cured the blood poisoning, the splinter could be removed and the fracture treated. She went on to make a good recovery and was discharged from hospital after five weeks."[10] Little wonder that the young man should relish the opportunity to join forces with Domagk in the tuberculosis research.

In examining their very limited past success, Behnisch at once realized something crucial. If only two of the thousands of sulphonamide drugs had shown any useful effect against tuberculosis, it was obvious that ... "the sulphonamide chemical group could not be the part of the molecule that mattered."[11] By chance Klarer and Mietzsch had added some other cluster of atoms to the basic sulphanilamide molecule – and it was this entirely unrelated chemical substance that was responsible for the anti-tuberculous effect. But what atoms were responsible? "Perhaps," Behnisch wondered, "it was the order of the atoms of sulphur and nitrogen in the molecule which was responsible for the effect?"[12]

Now Behnisch, the inspired newcomer, asked himself a second question, a very daring question indeed, that seemed to contradict all that had been learnt from the research to date. Was part of the molecule of sulphathiazole, an atomic structure called the thiazole ring, as sacred as everybody believed? This chemical ring was nothing so substantial as to be visible even under the most powerful microscope. In fact it wasn't a ring at all, but one of the most basic structures in the chemical universe, a mysterious pentagon, with its corners made up of five conjoined atoms. Two of these were nitrogen atoms, two were carbon atoms, with the remaining and perhaps the most interesting atom of all, sulphur. Behnisch now commited a cardinal sin. Using chemical means, he cut open the thiazole ring, laying bare a tiny chain in which those five atoms of sulphur, carbon and nitrogen were the jewels. Since there were five bonds that held the ring together, he was able to cut the ring at five different places, giving him five different chains of atoms.

They all seemed unprepossessing substances. Next he experimented a little further, adding different chemical side chains. Some of these new inventions were very poisonous and had to be handled with extreme caution. Nevertheless he passed on some examples of his ingenious new chemical groupings to Domagk for testing. The first of these, chemical substances called thiosemicarbazides, had no activity against tuberculosis. Then, on 25 November 1941, their luck changed. Behnisch created a new compound, based on the cloven thiazole ring, a chemical with the tongue twisting title of benzaldehye-thiosemicarbazone. It was the breakthrough they had been looking for.

When this strange new chemical was added to the jade green test tube slopes, the tuberculosis germs stopped growing. When guinea pigs infected with tuberculosis were given injections of the new substances they lived longer. In larger doses the guinea pigs showed a dramatic recovery from an otherwise fatal tuberculosis.

An incandescent excitement gave a much-needed uplift to the little group of researchers. In his tiny chain of atoms that formed the nucleus of the thiosemicarbazones, Behnisch had discovered a theme of atomic structure which, like the mystical four notes of Beethoven's fifth symphony, seemed capable of almost infinite variation. That primary discovery was soon

followed by hundreds of new substances, chemically simpler
than the sulphonamides, and all moulded about the progeni-
tive theme of the five atoms. After a long and arduous series of
experiments, involving a myriad of different chemical permutations, it was confirmed that the anti-tuberculous properties of
these new compounds were attributable to just one chemical
grouping, a grouping that all of the successful compounds had
in common. This was the wonderful theme of thiosemicarbazone.

For Gerhard Domagk, intensely aware of the human importance of this discovery, the exhilaration must have been unbearable. But every instinct boded caution. There had been
wonder cures for tuberculosis before and every single one of
them had ended in disappointment. Would this prove to be just
another such example? They would need to be certain that the
cure really worked since . . . "even a hint of it would be hotly
denied by most other experts if we begin to publicize our results
now. So let us wait and see." He was all too aware that they
were leagues away as yet from a formulation that could be
tested against the disease in human sufferers. They would need
to find even more powerful molecular derivatives, more overwhelming evidence.

Still the production of sulphonamides for the war effort demanded the lion's share of the company's energies and the
tuberculosis research was not progressing as quickly as Domagk and Behnisch would have liked it to. To evaluate the new
drug in test tube experiments involved many hours of examination down the microscope. There simply wasn't the manpower to be thorough enough. Domagk tried to press Hörlein
further but there was nothing the director could do about it.
Professor Heinrich Hörlein had more pressing worries.

The horrific dangers in which Domagk, Behnisch and the
other scientists were continuing to work may be judged from an
entry in Domagk's diary, dated 26 June 1943:

"I am sitting here at my work and since hardly anybody else
has turned up I shall use this time to put pen to paper to describe the last eventful days and nights here. Of sixty-five
employees here in my laboratory, there are hardly ten left.
Many are dead. Others have been made homeless and are now

desperately searching for a roof over their heads. Some are having difficulty in getting to work because of lack of transport – there are still a great many fires burning and many roads are not passable. Tramcars and railways are not running at the moment. Fortunately our lives have been spared yet again. I didn't even hear the fire alarm – I had gone to bed late and utterly exhausted, but when I woke in the morning the whole town was ablaze. Above us roared the all too familiar concatenation of attack, the bombs and the anti-aircraft guns and a deafening noise. Minutes later the whole sky over us, from Elberfeld to Cronenberg and Remscheid, was a burning red. As soon as the shooting stopped, I went to where help was most needed.

"The factory had escaped serious damage. It had been hit by a few incendiary devices which were soon put out, so I decided to go to the hospital to see if I could help. But the road was already closed. Together with my laboratory assistant, I tried to get there by an alternative route, behind the power station across Schiller Square. Behind the power station we crept along the rubble-covered streets, under the large chimney which was still standing. Most of the fires had been put out. The houses in Schiller Square were still burning; in front of them sat the people who lived in them, with the few belongings they had been able to save. People were throwing mattresses, blankets and clothes out of the windows of burning houses.

"My laboratory assistant and I made our way through the smoke and sparks and between burning falling wooden beams. The hospital itself was ablaze. Block 1, where Dr Gehrt had his children's clinic had quickly been cleared, as had Block 2, the surgical clinic. In Block 3, the roof rafters were ablaze. Some of the buildings were preserved. All the sick people had been successfully evacuated. Professor Klee had been able to save some of the medical records and books. I came back through the subway under the rail track to the tarmac road – that was the only way through. In the subway people were sitting about with beds and clothes in front of them. Outside they were surrounded by flaming buildings and debris. I am taking a family with two children into my house – the mother couldn't move any further.

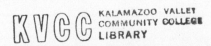

"The area of Steinbeck around the station was decimated, as was the main railway station. Many of my colleagues are completely destitute. Klarer's flat was badly damaged. On Friday morning we effected some essential repair work on the factory and then went to the hospital to help with the injured. All the shrapnel wounds were treated with Marfanil-Prontalbin. In this attack the English started up at exactly the same spot where they left off last time. Elberfeld as you know it, no longer exists. Our house is full to the brim with the family and two children. Our air raid shelter is home to two men who were bombed out completely at Barmen for the first time and now again for the second time at Elberfeld. We opened a casualty ward to bomb injuries. Many had damage to the eyes from phosphorous vapour. In the course of the day many were evacuated, mainly by lorry and bus. In the evening two trains left for Bavaria – trying to get out, not caring if they can save any of their belongings. All they want is to avoid a second night of this. For many it was the second time round. Slowly the biting smell of smoke is shifting away from the town. . . I estimate the number of dead in Wuppertal between 5,000 and 6,000. Accurate numbers are not known since there may be some people under the rubble. The death rate may be as high as 20,000 in Barmen and the same number in Elberfeld. I am very glad that Gertrud and the children are not here."[13]

iv

IT IS SCARCELY believable that in this Dante's inferno, with Elberfeld, Cologne, Düsseldorf, Leverkusen, Münster, all reduced to piles of rubble, the universities were determined to carry on with academic life. In mid 1943, Domagk received the following telegram: "The Chancellor and the Senate of the University of Greifswald have bestowed upon you the title of honorary senator. For this occasion, the medical association would like you to give a talk here next Wednesday or Friday."

Domagk, who shared that same heroic spirit, did not know how to tell them he would be arriving. There was no telephone. The local post offices no longer existed. He walked through two small towns only to find he could not obtain an envelope in which to place a letter. Somehow he found a way to send on his message. He had already decided that he would stop at Greifswald and give them their talk, and then carry on to Dammeshöved for his summer holiday. He arranged to pick up his son, Wolfgang, along the way, but first he must return to his laboratory for his postmortem examination of the animals infected with experimental tuberculosis. Nothing would be allowed to interfere with the great experiment. No matter that test after test was showing little change, today might be that momentous day when there might be something new to see, the slightest change that would herald a new breakthrough.

Behnisch, who worked very closely with Domagk at this time, described exactly how Domagk still worked on the tuberculosis researches. "In his studies he observed and followed up even the slightest deviation from the norm. He would do his own postmortem dissections and microscopic examinations of animal organ sections. When carrying out his weekly postmortem examinations he was accessible to no-one, took no telephone calls and received no visitors. He would dissect until he could no longer stand on his feet and gaze down through the microscope until he could no longer see. This was his normal habit until his last working day."[14] That Monday, his work at the laboratory finished so late in the day it was ten o'clock at night before he could set out, accompanied by Gertrud, Götz, Hildegard, and Heinz, the young friend of Götz', whose family had lost their home during the bombing. It was eleven o'clock by the time they arrived at the station, a pile of rubble, indistinguishable from its surroundings. The train was so full of fleeing people, he could hardly get through the door with his three suitcases. They alighted at Eisenach, to pick up an exhausted Wolfgang, who had travelled to meet them on the train from Streufdorf. After delivering his lecture in the main hall at the Institute of Pathology, where some nineteen years previously he had qualified as a university lecturer, Domagk took the family on a long and roundabout route to their old family room in the summer resort of Dammeshöved on the Baltic, where they enjoyed a brief interval of fine weather before it ended with thunderstorms.

It would be the last family holiday for some time. On 9 August, he had to return home with Götz, who was expected to report for duty as an anti-aircraft assistant.

Domagk pitted himself once more against the colossal and slow-grinding wheel of the tuberculosis research. More formulations of thiosemicarbazone were tested but the results showed nothing better than they had already. Since the first discovery of the thiosemicarbazones in November 1941, many hundreds of new compounds had been synthesized and tested, resulting in thousands of test tube and animal experiments, a gargantuan labour that was even more exhausting than the five years that had first led to the discovery of Prontosil. Nobody knew how much longer the factory would be be able to keep going. Many of the workforce were dead. Most of the survivors were homeless. Few of these had returned to work after the mass bombing of Leverkusen and Elberfeld. The fact that the work was continuing at all was a miracle under such circumstances, yet Domagk's determination appeared undiminished.

"Eventually I will succeed in broadening the basis for experiments and that in spite of the Tommies who provided us with a lively night again last night." Hörlein had just given Behnisch permission to spend all of his hours on the tuberculosis research.

Mietzsch now added his great experience to the struggle, as did a third chemist, Hans Schmidt. By degrees, with the addition of yet more chemical groups to the basic chain structure, more new substances were created which were put into the test system. Some were more effective, some less so. By now they were certain that it was the sulphur atom that played an essential role. With a courage and endurance that can scarcely be imagined, the dwindling numbers of chemists and technicians still working, rose out of their temporary shelters after the bombing raids of the previous nights, and walked through the rubble of Elberfeld to the factory, where they worked on, by degrees finding better thiosemicarbazones, gradually improving their effectiveness in test tubes and experimental animals.

Week by week, fewer workers arrived in the laboratory. Domagk continued to lead them, searching for every small way

to direct the increasingly precious resources towards the tuberculosis research ... "But there are many problems to solve:
shortage of space, animals, limited resources for animal and
animal feed. For a long time we have had no gas to work with
and even now it is closely rationed so that intensive work is
made very difficult. We are running out of glycerine and this
and that. A few hours of relaxation in the evenings, after work
and before the bomb alarms start. The boys spend these hours
reading from a book which Götz had received from his grandfather on 17 August, his seventeenth birthday. The speeches
and letters of Frederick the Great, Bismark, and others.
Speeches for and against the Monarchy. Stories about the anti-
quities of Egypt, the Sumarians ..."

Götz still lived at home but now they had to find somewhere
in the country where they could send the younger children.
Götz' friend Heinz, who lived with them, was now old
enough to join him in anti-aircraft training, but he was still able
to come home every evening. Hildegard aged fourteen and
Jörg aged twelve had been taken to safety in Brandenstein
where Baroness von Breitenbuch agreed to look after them.

The social fabric of family life was disintegrating. Clothing
ration cards were meaningless because there was no clothing to
be bought. Only the barest essentials in food were available.

They attempted to sign on new technicians to enable the
work to continue but more and more of the technicians, both
new and old, had lost all incentive to work. Women whose
homes had been bombed and whose husbands were fighting
on the front could no longer face the long hours, let alone the
necessary overtime. At home, Gertrud was rushing about,
sewing and mending old clothes for the children. Domagk was
asked if he could take in another homeless family, who hadn't a
stick of furniture left. He had barely agreed to accommodate the
family when he was approached by another woman from his
laboratory, in just as desperate a situation.

On 22 August 1943 they received the news that their nephew,
Fritz Robra, had fallen near Bjelgorod, seven weeks before the
birth of his first child. Another nephew, Klaus Umbelang,
ejected from his plane at a height of 3,000 metres and was saved
by a miracle.

The Baroness had a few words of comforting news of the younger children, which she sent by letter to Domagk's sister, Charlotte, still living in Brandenburg with his mother. "At last you are able to hear from me again and I can let you have news about my children (Domagk's children). They are both very well brought up and sweet little darlings and I love having them with me. Hille is working very hard in school. Jörg is not so good, but I think he is spending a lot of time growing and hasn't got the energy."[15]

How ironic it was that at this desperate hour, the tuberculosis research was proving more and more promising. Domagk would have liked to intensify his researches but it was insane to continue to work under such appalling conditions with such a deadly bacterium, using a greatly reduced number of sufficiently trained assistants, people whose lives were constantly disturbed by bomb alarms and who were overtired and hardly as attentive as they should be.

On 9 December 1943, he travelled to Hamburg, in an attempt to complete the third edition of his book, *The Chemotherapy of Bacterial Infections*. Professor Hegler, who had been cooperating with him on the typescript, had died from dysentery, but his son had taken notes from the Professor on his deathbed. Domagk looked through the draft papers before making his way to the publisher, Hirzel in Leipzig. He only got as far as Halle because bombing had disrupted the trains. The next day he found a train to Wahren and made his way from there to the badly damaged Leipzig. When he reached the publishers, all that was left was a pile of smouldering rubble.

Christmas 1943 was a modest affair, with Wolfgang unable to join the family because of diphtheria. At two o'clock in the afternoon, there was a bomb alert. It was the harbinger of even more desperate days.

The new year saw a marked escalation with bombers appearing in vast numbers – many hundred planes at a time. The neighbouring cities of Düsseldorf and Cologne were completely destroyed. People did not talk about Barmen and Elberfeld any more. A former school friend of Gertrud wrote to her from Berlin following a raid in which ten firebombs were found in her home and had to be defused. "About five o'clock we lay

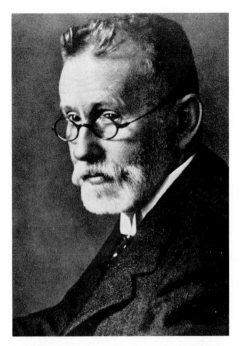

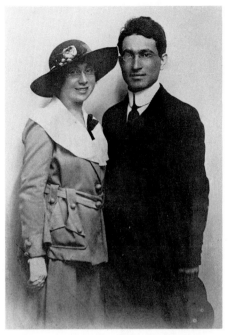

Paul Ehrlich, who first invented the idea of treating infections with drugs. (*Bayer Archives*)

Selman Waksman and his wife, Bobili, on their wedding day. (*Special Collections and Archives, Rutgers University Libraries*)

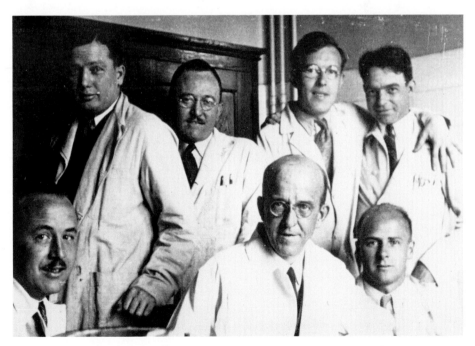

The research group in Oswald Avery's laboratory at the Rockefeller Institute in the early 1930s. Avery, center foreground. René Dubos, back row, second from right. (*The Rockefeller Archive Center*)

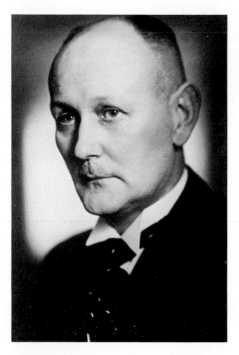

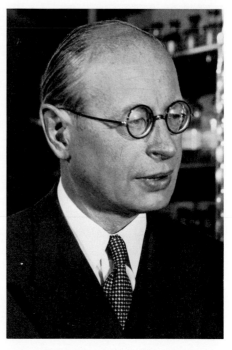

Gerhard Domagk at the time of the Prontosil discovery. (*Bayer Archives*)

Fritz Mietzsch, the chemist who helped discover Prontosil and thiosemicarbazone. (*Bayer Archives*)

Josef Klarer, the chemist who first synthesized Prontosil rubrum. (*Bayer Archives*)

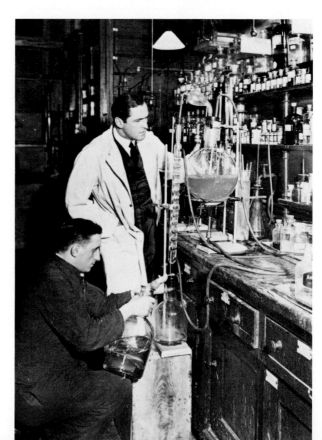

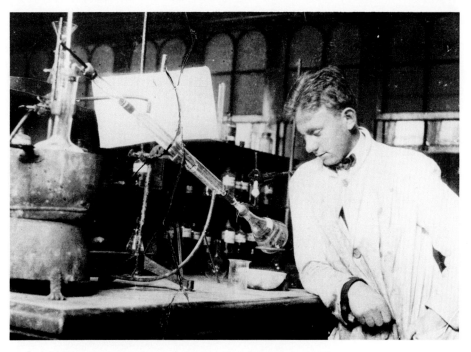

Jorgen Lehmann, as a young doctor in Lund. (*Ferrosan Archives*)

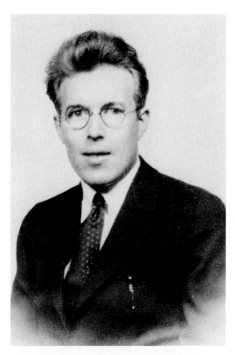

René Dubos c. 1930. (*The Rockefeller Archive Center*)

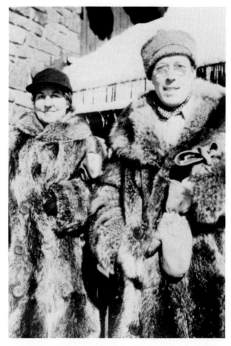

René Dubos and his wife, Marie Louise, at the Raybrook Sanitorium during her illness. (*The Rockefeller Archive Center*)

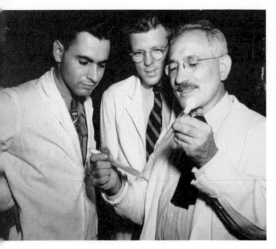

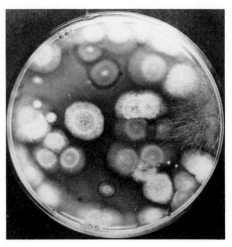

Albert Schatz (left) and Selman Waksman (right) looking at cultures of *Streptomyces griseus* in the laboratory at Rutgers Agricultural College, New Jersey. (*Courtesy Albert Schatz and Doris Jones*)

Culture plate showing the wonderful diversity of different Actinomyces growing on agar. (*Courtesy Albert Schatz, from his PhD thesis on streptomycin*)

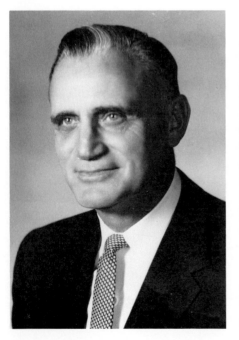

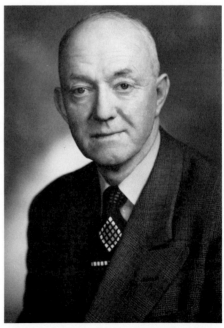

H. Corwin Hinshaw, who, in association with William Feldman, first tested streptomycin in human tuberculosis. (*Courtesy Professor H. Corwin Hinshaw*)

William Feldman, who, in association with Hinshaw, carried out the first experimental animal trials of streptomycin. (*Courtesy Professor H. Corwin Hinshaw*)

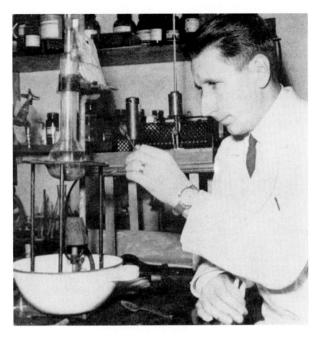

Karl-Gustav Rosdahl, the chemist who first synthesized PAS. (*Courtesy Mr K-G Rosdahl*)

Patients marching through the grounds of the Kronoborgs Sanitorium. Their banners read: *We want more PAS! Long live Lehmann!* (*Ferrosan Archives*)

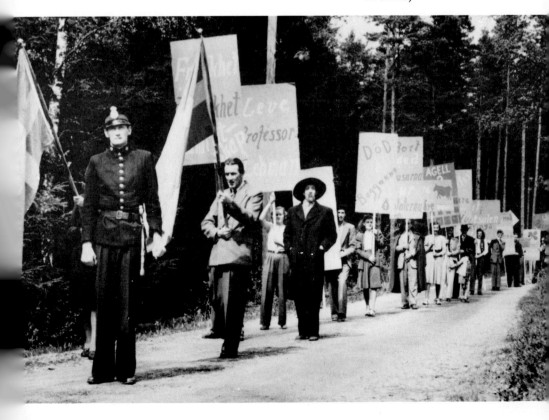

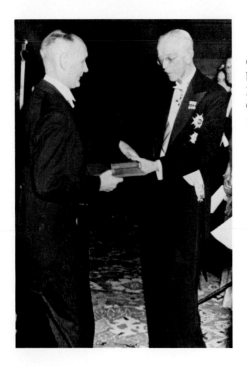

Gerhard Domagk (left) belatedly received his Nobel Prize from King Gustav V of Sweden in 1947. (*Bayer Archives*)

The bomb-damaged entrance to the Bayer factory in 1944 when Domagk, Robert Behnisch and their assistants continued to work on thiosemicarbazone. (*Bayer Archives*)

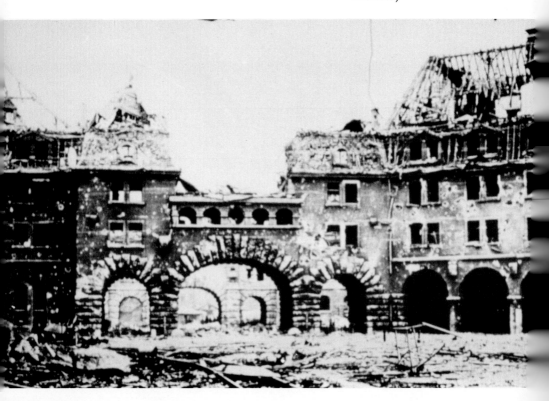

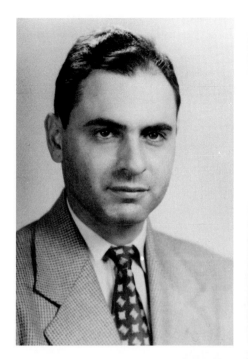

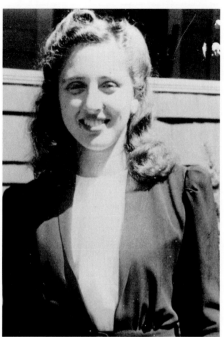

Above: Albert Schatz, co-discoverer of streptomy-cin, at the time of his marriage to Vivian Rosen-feld. (*Courtesy Albert and Vivian Schatz*)

Above right: Vivian Rosenfeld, at the time she was courting Albert Schatz. (*Courtesy Albert and Vivian Schatz*)

Right: Selman Waksman (left) before one of the 15,000 gallon fermentors for mass production of streptomycin at the George Merck factory at Elkton, Virginia, December 1945. (*Merck Sharpe & Dohme Archives*)

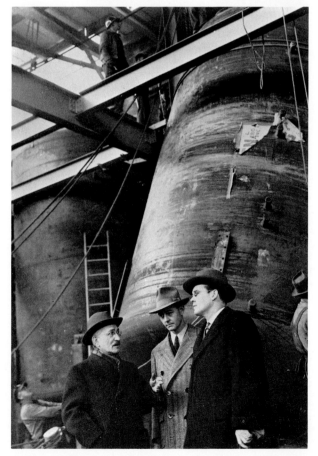

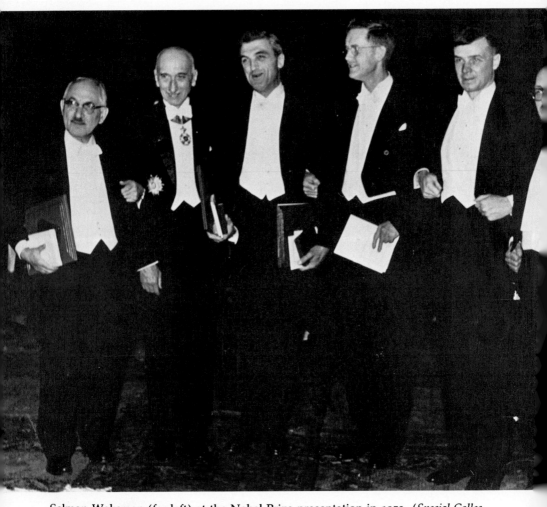

Selman Waksman (far left) at the Nobel Prize presentation in 1952. (*Special Collections and Archives, Rutgers University Libraries*)

down, the smoke was coming in from the broken windows – all the time one could hear the cracking and breaking of masonry, the sirens of the fire engines and the pumps of the motor hoses. The following night I couldn't help shaking all over when the sirens started all over again."[16]

Still the great labour struggled onwards, in fits and starts, hopelessly understaffed, on the tormented backs of a dwindling band of men and women, every one of them hungry, desperate and demoralized by the bombing. It had become almost impossible to obtain animal supplies. "On Tuesday, I had an adventurous journey to the office which usually takes about fifteen minutes, but now I had to do it largely on foot through an area littered with debris. Even in my liveliest imagination I could never have thought of anything like this. The following day I found a lady colleague in the ruins of her burnt out home and we dragged her and some lost children to the home of her friend in a cart made for street cleaning. She used to live in the Hansa district – all one can say now is that it does not exist any more. Our office is the only one left standing in the area, badly damaged, without windows and doors and the library is burned out, but still repairable. On the way, one had to wade through glass, water and thick yellow smoke. Lower down the street, only the outer walls of houses remained standing."

Yet, by February 1944, Behnisch, assisted by Mietzsch and Schmidt, had found a new thiosemicarbazone which could stop tuberculosis growing in test tubes at a dilution of one in forty thousand. That same week, Domagk received a letter from the Rector of Münster University, telling him he had been nominated by the university for the *Ritterkreuz*, the equivalent of the George Cross. It was the first time in history this medal had been awarded for purely scientific merit.

While pleased with the award, Domagk made no pretence of supporting the Nazi party, as he now made abundantly clear from a diary entry. "The National Socialist system started with lies and suffocated in cruelty and blood. It was easy for Hitler to get to power with six million people out of work. He was the only one who gave the masses what they asked for."[17]

Domagk's close friend and colleague, Professor Philipp Klee, was fighting a desperate struggle to protect his Jewish wife, Flora. But he was made to suffer for his obstinacy. From as early as 1933, at the very time he was treating the first patients in history with Prontosil, this courageous man had been subjected to intimidation and insults. Although they could not prevent such a highly respected doctor from carrying on with his work at the Wuppertal-Elberfeld Hospital, they made this work as difficult as they could. He found it impossible to obtain funds to buy equipment. The more prejudiced of his patients discharged themselves from his care. Others were intimidated from going to see him. He was prevented from supplementing his modest salary by seeing private patients. For five years, from 1939 to 1944, armed with nothing more than his reputation and unlimited courage, he had blocked every attempt by the SS to arrest Flora. Just how extraordinary an achievement this was can be judged by the fact that not another Jewish woman in Wuppertal survived. But now, in the gathering nightmare of November 1944, even his heroic efforts were not able to save her. Flora, the gifted artist, was torn from his embrace and taken away to Theresienstadt concentration camp, a thousand kilometres away, in Czechoslovakia.[18]

In the face of such brutality, the obsequiousness with which certain people still supported Hitler was a source of amazement to Domagk. "Our baker was strutting along like an Italian cockerel in his brown gala uniform when he arranged for the victims of the next night of bombings to be taken by lorries to an undecided destination. They were even grateful for the fact that they, burned out paupers, without a scrap of luggage, had been able to escape this hell. The spies of the party were crawling round the houses. Every Sunday they had collections and they were sticking their noses into things. The man who was looking after the central heating in our district was wearing a thin elegant summer uniform – never mind the weather and the fact that he was bow-legged. Trousers made of finest black cloth, brown coat and brown raincoat. Every time I saw him he appeared more magnificent. When I didn't react to his loud 'Heil Hitler' he stopped it and just walked by quietly when we met."[19]

Work had already stopped in the Bayer research laboratories.

It had simply petered out during the first half of 1944. They had run out of materials, animals, but most important of all they had run out of technical assistants, most of whom were wounded, homeless, indeed many of whom were now dead.

As east and west Prussia, Pomerania and Silesia were taken by the Allies, Domagk became increasingly worried about his mother and sister, who still lived in the east. News filtered through to Elberfeld of endless lines of refugees attempting to flee from their farms and homes, to face attack by tanks and low flying aircraft. When in the first days of May the last motor and fishing boats tried to escape from Pommern and Mecklenburg across the Baltic, they were sunk. For six months there was no news at all. Then, in November, Domagk received the first intimation that they were still alive. When their home town was taken by the Russians, they had been moved out. But now that the front had moved onwards, they were allowed back into the villages and his mother had been allowed to go into an old people's home. A little later they were ordered out of the town, which had now been incorporated within the borders of the newly defined Poland.

"Mother couldn't walk very far on foot. At last she was seated onto a cart. When they got as far as the river, her coat was ripped off her and all her gold and jewellery stolen. They were put into a refugee camp on the other side of the river, where mother died of hunger. Of hundreds who were camping there only a few survived. Of 153 inmates placed in the camp there were only 50 still alive by 25 October. By 11 November only 25 were still alive."[20]

For Philipp Klee, news of the Allied victories brought the first small ray of hope. As Germany was collapsing, he threw personal safety aside and rushed across the war stricken country into Czechoslovakia, determined to get Flora out of the concentration camp while she was still alive. But the thousand kilometres journey was painfully slow and when he arrived at the camp, he found it had already been liberated by the Americans. Flora was nowhere to be found. Fearing the worst, Klee made his sad progress homewards. But in fact she had fled the camp, where she had been forced to do shameful work under the constant threat of death, and now, heavily disguised, she travelled as part of a liberated gipsy group along the slow and dangerous road to Wuppertal, where she was waiting for Philipp when he finally arrived home.[21]

After the harrowing death of her mother, Domagk's sister, Charlotte, survived "dreadful living conditions in a refugee camp where typhoid, TB and lice are the order of the day," to reach her brother in Elberfeld. She was taken in by a neighbour because the Domagk home was serving as a billet for allied soldiers. Gertrud was now safe in Dammeshöved with the younger children and meanwhile Domagk slept in the factory. In January, 1945, when their house became vacant again, Charlotte was accommodated in the attic together with Götz. "Then every evening after work we started the long task of cleaning the house, beginning with the simple furnishing of a single room. Then came the painter and decorator and the joiner and we were content to have things repaired in the most basic way."

For the moment Gerhard Domagk was concerned only with recreating a home to which his wife and youngest children could return. All work had stopped at the Bayer laboratories in Elberfeld, although the factory at Leverkusen was still largely intact. The town of Elberfeld no longer existed, apart from piles of rubble. Yet, in testimony to those two years of heroic struggle on the part of a small group of one doctor, several chemists and seventy technical assistants, an important advance had been made in the search for the cure for tuberculosis. One day a phoenix with the unlikely name of thiosemicarbazone would rise again from the ashes of Elberfeld.

13

Streptomycin

Eva ... did everything she could to conceal from Picasso the fact that she was suffering not from a passing bout of bronchitis but from tuberculosis. She hid the blood-stained handkerchiefs and applied thicker and thicker layers of rouge to disguise the pallor of her cheeks. She was terrified that if he knew, he would leave her.[1]

Arianna Stassinopoulos Huffington: *Picasso, Creator
and Destroyer*

i

IN JUNE 1943, in the more tranquil setting of Rutgers Agricultural College, New Jersey, Selman Waksman was approached by a young man called Albert Schatz, who wanted to return to the college to study for his doctorate. Albert was a very welcome applicant. Highly intelligent, he had impressed Waksman as a student at Rutgers, where he had graduated top of his year with a bachelors degree in May of the previous year. Woodruff had now moved to George Merck's pharmaceutical firm and, with virtually every able-bodied graduate involved in the war effort, Waksman was eager for exactly such a bright young man to continue the research for new antibiotics. There was however an immediate problem. Schatz did not want to work in antibiotics.

In Schatz' own words: "When I originally thought of working for a PhD, I wanted to work in soil microbiology. What I had in mind was combining my knowledge of soil microbiology with pedology (soil science)."[2]

Waksman told him that he was welcome to work in soil microbiology as such, but there were no funds available to support him. Schatz, only recently discharged from the armed forces because of a back complaint, was penniless so there was no question of his being able to support himself. However he had another option. It would have been very easy for him, as a discharged soldier, to get a part-time job. But this very bright young man had no ambition to spend his life working in a service laboratory. In antibiotics, Professor Waksman was prepared to offer him the stipend of forty dollars a month, only half what he had offered Woodruff. Although initially somewhat reluctant, Albert Schatz soon agreed to divert his interests to antibiotic research. There were interesting reasons why he should do so.

He had begun his schooling in a two-roomed schoolhouse in Connecticut before the family moved to Passaic, a small town close to Patterson, New Jersey. "I lived through the depression. I saw people fighting on garbage dumps when the garbage came in to get the scraps of food. Some of these people used to live in shacks on the garbage dumps which they built out of wood from fruit and vegetable crates. I remember during the depression that my mother bought eggs four at a time and an eighth of a pound of butter. I remember people hanging around outside restaurants on trash days and going through the trash to get something to eat from whatever was discarded from the plates."[3] An intelligent and sensitive boy, growing up in humble surroundings, Albert had known friends contract pneumonia or diphtheria – what the ordinary folk called blood poisoning – and with an alarmingly high frequency the friend would never turn up for school again. Most terrifying of all, as a boy he had seen people suffering from tuberculosis. He remembered the more fortunate going to a sanitorium at Lake Placid. But most of the people he knew could not afford that. Albert's father, Julius, when not working on the farm, was a house painter, who certainly would not have been able to afford any such treatment. "Poorer people, such as we were, could afford little treatment at all – they just wasted away."[4] The opportunity of working on these two problems overrode any misgivings Albert had felt in working with antibiotics.

The salary was miserable but he arranged to sleep in a side room in the plant physiology greenhouse, where he earned his keep by maintaining the temperature, watering the plants and sweeping up. In such penurious circumstances, the young man took up the hands-on aspects of the antibiotic research at the point where Woodruff had left it only months earlier.

Under Waksman's direction, Albert Schatz now addressed himself to the Graduate Faculty of Rutgers University, setting out the purpose and scope of his thesis for the degree of doctor of philosophy. The few introductory paragraphs, in their terse scientific prose, evoke in retrospect the spell of prophecy. The thesis would address itself to two very important problems; namely, "(1) a search for an antibiotic agent possessing a broader range of activity, especially against Gram-negative bacteria, than that offered by streptothricin; and (2) a search for a specific antimycobacterial agent."[5] By "antimycobacterial agent" was meant the search for an antibiotic cure for tuberculosis.

ii

ALBERT SCHATZ WAS an unusual young man in other respects. Born in Norwich, Connecticut, on 2 February 1920, like Selman Waksman, he was Jewish, his family having fled the Minsk area of Czarist Russia when his father was just nine years old. When they arrived in America, his grandparents had to make an immediate choice. They could either go into a small business in a large city such as New York or settle down on a farm. His grandfather chose farming, buying one hundred and forty acres of land in Connecticut, a farm which, in Schatz' own words "was not marginal land but sub-marginal". It was a wonderful farm for Christmas trees but that was about all, guaranteeing that life for Albert's father and subsequently Albert himself would be unflinchingly hard. Even so, Albert Schatz would remember his early years on the farm as a very positive experience. It was the reason why he majored in soil chemistry as an undergraduate and in soil microbiology for his PhD at Rutgers University.

There was an additional very important furnace that drove him. For this young man, just twenty-three years old, the opportunity of studying for his doctorate was more than just the chance for a higher education. It was his dream. He wanted it desperately, not merely for himself but for the pride of his family, to whom he was very close. All of their lives, from their first steps onto American soil, Albert's family had known little other than grinding poverty. "My uncle worked in a mattress factory and a meat market to put himself through dental school. My mother never went to high school. She went to work in a bakery and sat on a stool with rats running around her feet. The opportunity for me to get a PhD – it validated their lives."[6] This single-minded young man, toughened by his childhood years in the depression, supplemented his meagre salary by picking up cheap fruit and vegetables from colleagues undertaking research in agronomy in the college fields and free ice cream from the dairy department.

At the time he joined it, the department of soil microbiology was a small, closely-knit group of students and assistants, with two professors, Selman Waksman and Robert Starkey. Doris Jones, who was a contemporary of Schatz', furnishes a sparkling description of the others who formed the team. "Dark-eyed Viola is the secretary; Clara a laboratory assistant. Portly Mr Adams makes media and washes glassware. Cooper, a conscientious and friendly black man, is a laboratory helper. Then there is a collection of graduate students. If they are not working on iron or sulphur metabolism with Starkey, they are involved with antibiotics. There is Betty Bugie and Chris Reilly, Sam Green, Monti Reynolds – who dubs me 'Moose' because I bellow so loudly – and others (many from Merck & Co). Every Friday there is a brown bag lunch in the third floor laboratory and a journal discussion around a big table. Next to it is a walk-in incubator with a rather newish shaking machine, and just outside a large still, perpetually recovering ether. No one seems to worry about it leaking or blowing up. Materials are always in short supply. The odour of bag lunches mixes with scents of mould and actinomycetes. We all adore Dr Starkey; and Dr Waksman is our great white father. He is wise, demanding yet understanding. He doesn't seem pretentious. His clothing is worn, and his vest always seems to carry traces of his last few meals, maybe a moth hole or two. He wants us to work hard, not waste lots of time studying extraneous things in books. I worship him."[7]

Selman Waksman's office, together with his personal laboratory with walk-in incubator, was on the third floor of the small detached building within the grounds of the agricultural college, that housed soil microbiology. Albert Schatz was to begin work two floors below, in the basement laboratory, which he shared with Kent White, another graduate student who was working for his PhD under the supervision of Dr Starkey. Doris Jones occupied an adjoining laboratory in the basement, where she worked under the tutelage of Dr F.R. Beaudette, "a red-haired, flaring-tempered pathologist, who I'm told hates women, but who is helping me in my struggles to look for antiviral agents."[8] The basement laboratory, being larger than that on Waksman's top floor, was also used for classes when they had students. "At one end is a sink, always full of dirty glassware, which we all must wash. At the other end an antiquated autoclave which has to be manually filled with water to make the steam. If you forget it, it overheats, and ker-plow! Here in this lab with its stacks and stacks of plates and flasks and tubes is Al Schatz' scientific nest, and he seems to be testing everything . . ."[9]

This was the research environment in which Albert Schatz began the work for his thesis in June 1943. The laboratory was just eighteen feet square. It had two windows but part of it was below ground level. After an initial period in which Waksman explained the basic techniques and brought Schatz up to date with the discoveries of actinomycin and streptothricin, Schatz worked on his own in the basement laboratory, although Waksman would come and check progress from time to time. If there was a problem to be overcome, or if there was anything interesting to report, Albert would take it up to Waksman's office on the third floor.

The arrangement implies an unusually close relationship between Waksman and Schatz. Waksman regarded Schatz as one of the brightest of all his pupils. He trusted Schatz to the extent that he allowed him very much a free rein as to how he designed and performed the experiments. "I worked, I probably worked, I undoubtedly worked, more independently than any other graduate student."[10]

Albert Schatz was inspired by a sense not only of mission but of curious certainty. "I was pretty confident I would find something. I had an intuitive feeling about the work I did – and an intuitive feeling about the way to set up the experiments. I also had an intuitive feeling about the results I would get."[11] He would have similar deeply spiritual perceptions about work he would do throughout his life and in his experience, such prescience always proved true.

Schatz was small, of much the same stature as Waksman himself, dark-haired, ruggedly handsome, with the pugnacious determination of a bantamweight fighter. In photographs taken at the time, he would demonstrate his physical fitness by gripping a vertical pole and powering his tensed body into a perfect horizontal and then hold it there for as long as he wanted. There was only one way in which he would approach something this important to him: this was in a spirit of blood and guts commitment.

iii

THERE WAS SOMETHING in soil that killed the germs that caused tuberculosis. Waksman was certain of this because Rhines' experiment in 1932 had proved it. That something was most markedly demonstrable in soils that had been heavily manured, soils indeed which would contain millions of different micro-organisms. At first Schatz looked at a range of microbes, much as Woodruff had tested before him, but he very quickly gravitated to the actinomyces. Streptothricin pointed to these as the most likely to produce new antibiotic substances. These fascinating life forms were instantly recognizable even as colonies on a culture plate. Although halfway in evolution between the bacteria and fungi, they were much more delicate than fungi. The diameter of one of the filamentous threads of an actinomyces was as minuscule as that of a bacterium. "You could look at colonies and pick out ninety-nine per cent of the actinomyces."[12]

Mostly Schatz just grew them on agar plates, where the production of millions of microscopic spores gave the actinomyces colonies a delicate powdery appearance. Often they were exquisitely beautiful, displaying every shade of white, red, brown, green, blue or black, growing to a maximum of five to six or seven millimetres or so, with a pastel surface sheen that was unmistakable. He soon became expert enough to spot an actinomyces colony at a glance.

For Albert Schatz, the quest for the wonder microbe in this chaos of nature owed more to intuition than any systematic scientific search. "If you ask me why I picked one colony of actinomyces over another, I cannot tell you. There was no rationale for picking one colony of an actinomyces over another. Naturally if a plate had five colonies which morphologically and grossly looked alike, I would not pick all five."[13]

The screening test for antibiotic potential had evolved into a very simple technique, called the "streak test". For example, if Schatz had a colony of actinomyces he wanted to test for antibiotic activity – say against the streptococcus germ – he brushed a wire loop which had been dipped in the actinomyces down the middle of the plate, so that he eventually got a growth of actinomyces that took the form of a thick diagonal band bisecting the plate. Next he dipped a clean and sterile wire into a culture of the dangerous streptococcus, streaking this microbe across the plate at right angles to the line of actinomyces, so they crossed at right angles in the middle. This second streak could be done either on the same day as the actinomyces streak, or several days later, when the actinomyces was already well established and secreting any potential antibiotic into the growing medium. In practice, he would screen a new actinomyces against several different disease-causing bacteria at once, repeating this same experiment over and over until he found a strain of actinomyces that looked interesting. Hunting for these new strains of actinomyces in soil, in manure heaps, in drains, even from the culture plates that were being thrown away by colleagues working on other unrelated projects, indeed anywhere in the world that his imagination would take him – this was Albert's entire life.

He would never know or remember just how many actinomyces he eventually tested since he made no attempt to tabulate them all in his thesis. It might have been hundreds, perhaps even thousands. By this stage he had realized that it made no difference if he tested a hundred or a hundred thousand. "If I got something effective, I could stop. If I didn't get anything effective, I wouldn't get a PhD dissertation simply because I had found that a quarter of a million organisms didn't produce anything. So that after a while, I stopped recording the number of organisms I had tested." He did however keep a culture of every actinomyces he tested on agar slants, because he never knew when he began if this one of the myriads he had tested would eventually prove to be what he was searching for. After he had cross-streaked, he would wait one or two days to give the test organisms time to develop. Different bacteria grew at different rates and it was vital that each different germ was given plenty of opportunity to grow as near to the actinomyces streak as possible. If those cross-streaks of dangerous bacteria refused to grow when they came near to the diagonal streak containing the test actinomyces, he knew he had something interesting. Even then he didn't know whether it was active simply because it had depleted the medium of a lot of nutrients needed by a bacterium or if it changed the pH sufficiently to prevent growth, or whether the effect was caused by an antibiotic produced by the actinomyces.

From the very beginning, the research had become an obsession for Albert Schatz. While other graduate students found time to relax, to have parties in the evenings, time even for romance, Albert was conspicuously absent from such occasions. In his own words: "I generally began my work in the laboratory between five and six in the morning, and continued until midnight or even later. I also often prepared my own meals and ate in the laboratory. I worked this intensively for several reasons. First I was fascinated by what I was doing; it intrigued me no end. Secondly, I fully realized how important it would be to find antibiotics effective in treating diseases caused by Gram-negative bacteria and even more so tuberculosis. Finally, with an income of only US $40.00 per month, I simply could not afford to buy an automobile or have much social life.

Most girls had little or no interest in dating anyone in my very limited financial circumstances.

"I, therefore, worked literally day and night in the laboratory. Many times I even slept there because I was too tired to get to the room which I rented in a private home in the city or because it was already so late that I could get only one or two hours of sleep at the most."[14]

With little money, living in cheap digs, he could not afford to take girls to dances or nightclubs. And the girls took little interest in the young scientist who hardly knew or cared about the Glen Miller sound, whose prospects appeared so uncertain and whose notion of an evening's entertainment was a solitary stroll. One morning, at 2.00 a.m., the night watchman found Albert lying unconscious in the snow outside the laboratory and had him transferred to hospital by emergency ambulance where he was found to be suffering from pneumonia. Within a week or two he was back at his usual work, searching for new actinomyces.

Barely a month or two of starting work on his thesis, the combination of frenetic labour and mysterious instinct was already showing dividends. He was finding actinomyces that had an inhibiting effect on disease-causing germs.

He could afford to dismiss the very slight inhibition that was shown by very many actinomyces. But if the disease-causing germ refused to grow within two millimetres of the actinomyces streak, then he would take a closer look. These were now grown in much larger quantity in a liquid culture medium after which he would test it all over again, this time with a modification of the original plate test. He would inoculate warm soft agar with a disease-causing germ, such as the staphylococcus, then pour this over the whole surface of a plate. When the agar hardened, he would insert a tiny cylinder of glass containing the actinomyces into the centre of the plate. After overnight incubation, growth of the staphylococcus germ in the agar would turn the plate cloudy throughout. If the actinomyces was still promising, it would produce a zone of translucency around where the little glass cylinder was inserted. "Depending on the size of the zone of inhibition, I would or would not follow it up. If I got a significant zone of inhibiton, lets say five or ten millimetres away from the glass cylinder, I would then produce a large volume, maybe four or five litres, of culture medium and from there the testing would start all over again, but in many different ways."[15]

In the words of Doris Jones, this was "the salt mine, where, in order to pull a practical antibiotic producer out of Mother Nature, we literally have to work our asses off. The failure rate is about 99.99 per cent."[16]

This Herculean labour would soon be rewarded with success. Albert Schatz would remember the day and time exactly, 19 October 1943, just three and a half months after he had begun his searches, at about 2.00 p.m., when, in the words of Doris Jones, "Despite all the odds, Al hit paydirt!"[17]

Albert Schatz had found not one but two separate colonies of actinomyces which had properties unlike any other that had ever been seen before. On the plates they had a greenish grey pastel shade that pointed to their being very similar to an organism found some twenty-eight years earlier by Waksman and Curtis, which, because of their colour had been called *Actinomyces griseus*. One of the colonies had come from Doris Jones herself, from one of her discarded agar plates, which she had been passing through the window between the two laboratories.

The plate passed to Schatz by Doris Jones had come from a throat swab taken from a sick chicken. Most fascinating, in the light of Rhines' earlier experiment with the survival of tuberculosis germs in soil, the second colony, and subsequently the more productive of the two, had come from a sample of heavily manured soil. Barely six months earlier, Waksman, together with a colleague, Henrici, had changed the name of the species of *Actinomyces* to the new name which would soon become world famous, *Streptomyces*. In Schatz' words: "That organism produced something we subsequently called streptomycin."[18]

iv

ON THAT GREY AFTERNOON in the autumn of 1943, Albert Schatz found himself gazing down upon a streak test of the new actinomyces for the first time. Running diagonally across the plate, unmistakable in its pastel grey-green shade, was the thick line of primary growth of *Actinomyces griseus*, while running across the plate at right angles were five or six lines of test culture, where he had drawn the inoculum loop right across and through the line of actinomyces. Now, to his amazement, wide zones of inhibition were dramatically clear of every single bacterial growth, extending for many millimetres and even centimetres away from that central grey-green line. These were the most dramatic results ever witnessed in the laboratory. Albert Schatz had found his antibiotic, just as his curious prescience had suggested he would. In Schatz's words: "I was too thoroughly exhausted to feel elated. I had worked day and night. But nevertheless I had a good feeling about it."[19]

When Schatz took that first dramatic plate up to Selman Waksman in his third-floor office, the results were so striking that Waksman couldn't believe it. Was it possible that his young assistant, after only a few months of effort, had found the miracle Waksman had been searching for since 1939? He told Schatz to repeat the experiment.

It did not take Schatz long to convince Waksman that he had indeed discovered an antibiotic that looked more interesting than actinomycin or streptothricin. Schatz continued to experiment, testing the new substance further, discussing each step with his jubilant superior, working out the methodology of each new experiment between them. "I reported frequently to him, whenever I had something new to report. I knew now I had my thesis dissertation. I also knew this finding was potentially important. However, I had no idea of what the purity was and I had no idea of the toxicity or lack of toxicity in people. Nor did I have any idea, if it proved to be non-toxic to people, whether it would be effective in treating people suffering from infections. So there were a lot of unanswered questions."[20]

With the help of Betty Bugie and Waksman, he found out what this fascinating micro-organism needed as an ideal source of food. This allowed them to move on to much larger scale production of the actinomyces and its subsequent delivery of the antibiotic. Repeated testing, in gradually more refined and exacting cirumstances, confirmed that the new antibiotic would annihilate very many of the germs that caused common and deadly diseases, including that most resistant germ, the staphylococcus. More exciting still, it had dramatic killing effects on the Gram-negatives, those very bacteria that were untouched by penicillin.

Exhilarating results crowned every experiment. But Waksman himself remained wary. He remembered only too well the heartbreak with streptothricin when it came to that most difficult hurdle of all, the potential for poisonous side-effects that would only show up when they tested streptomycin in animals, and finally, in human beings. Within just weeks of its first discovery, Waksman arranged for its first testing against infections in living animals. Doris Jones was asked to study its effects in chick embryos.

Using a dental drill, she drilled holes in fertile eggs, infecting them with the bacteria that caused fowl typhoid. Half the infected eggs were treated with tiny doses of streptomycin and half were left untreated to act as controls. Within a day or two, all the untreated embryos were dead while most of the treated eggs went on to hatch. "I am so new at this business, I have never watched them peck their way out. Fluffy little chicks and I am told to autopsy them for *Salmonella gallinarum*."[21] With tears rolling down her cheeks, Doris sacrificed the chicks only to confirm the reason why they had survived the salmonella injection. There were no bacteria to be found in their blood or internal organs. The streptomycin had cured them of their infection.

Hardly noticed, at the very heart of this pandemonium of success, Albert Schatz moved on to the next stage of his research. It had been a fundamental aim of his thesis to search for an antibiotic that would cure tuberculosis. From the beginning, he had felt that same prescience with regard to tuberculosis that he had felt generally with regard to the success of his quest, a curious confidence born out of an almost religious sense of faith. Many of his colleagues, realizing what he was now undertaking, repeatedly warned him that he was wasting his time looking for a cure for tuberculosis. "They told me that the tubercle bacilli were covered with a heavy waxy capsule and nothing could get in. And that's why the drugs were not effective. My feeling was that if nothing got in we wouldn't have tuberculosis, because nutrients would have to get in and waste products would have to get out. If food and waste products could get through, so could an antibiotic. So that argument did not hold water with me. I therefore kept on working."[22]

So, calmly and methodically, Albert Schatz, barely twenty-three years old, now performed an experiment that would ultimately prove one of the most important in the history of medicine. He tested streptomycin against tuberculosis. Although the strain of germ he used in the very early experiments was said to be relatively safe, he took sensible precautions. For example, he minimized his risk of inhaling the germ by growing it in Lowenstein Jenson medium that had been poured into tall narrow tubes, called agar slants, which exposed much less of the growing bacterial cultures to the open air when the caps were lifted. Streptomycin was added to the green medium in various dilutions before the germs were brushed onto the surface. Now, instead of being able to read the results the following morning, as was usual, he had to sit it out for several weeks, to give this, the slowest germ of all, time to become visible. He knew exactly what to expect. Nothing else would grow in the medium made poisonous by the addition of malachite green. Soon he would be gazing at the strange crusty arabesques, like miniature versions of the thick brown fungi that sprouted from the rotting stumps of trees, which were the typical slow-growing colonies of the tuberculosis germ. By seven or eight days, Albert thought he could spot the first pale brown specks. Within three weeks he was absolutely certain. In the slants to which he had added streptomycin, even in very dilute amounts, the sloping green surface was a perfect mirror, devoid of growth. In the control slants, the waxy arabesques were densely sprouting. The new antibiotic was dramatically effective in inhibiting the growth of tuberculosis germs.

v

IN *The Ascent of Man*, Bronowski attempted to convey in words the essential nature of scientific discovery using the analogy of the grain in stone. From a time lost in antiquity humanity made tools by working stone. Sometimes the stone had a natural grain, sometimes the tool-maker created the lines of cleavage by learning how to strike the stone. From such a simple beginning, mankind discovered how to prise open the nature of things to reveal the magic and the wonder of creation.

The chain of discovery which would eventually lead to streptomycin had begun with Waksman himself in his very earliest researches with the actinomyces. Dubos and Shatz had begun their scientific careers as students of Waksman. They would subsequently admit to being inspired by him. Dubos had taken this inspiration and, guided by Avery, had made the original breakthrough, which would become the template for all that was to follow, when he discovered gramicidin. Dubos had, in Bronowski's analogy, first split the stone, exploring its very heart and discovering there the *secret law of nature* itself. But this was as far as he had taken it. From Dubos the baton had passed back to Waksman again and it was finally Waksman, encouraged by the earlier discoveries of Woodruff, and now at last, with the assistance of his brightest student, Albert Schatz, who had brought it to the state of practical fruition. That Albert Schatz had brought his own unique talent to the search was undoubtable. For many years, researcher after researcher would use the "Rutgers" techniques to discover more than thirty new antibiotics. The unassuming Hubert Lechevalier, who would one day succeed Waksman in streptomyces research, discovered the very important antibiotic, Neomycin. But in all of this research, extending over twenty years, nobody at Rutgers would ever discover anything that killed tuberculosis germs like streptomycin.[23]

These are Schatz' own words to describe the way he felt when he saw for the first time that the new antibiotic, streptomycin, had a promising effect against the germs that cause tuberculosis.

I was fortunate in many ways in my research. I was fortunate in isolating not one but two strains of *Streptomyces griseus*. I was fortunate too that the one antibiotic was the solution to both of my doctoral problems. I did not mind the long hours of solitary labour. Because I wanted to do this. This was my life at the time.

It wasn't merely a research project for a PhD degree. This tied in with the loss of people in my early grade school and with what I had seen in the army with recalcitrant infections. Now I was hopeful this would not be the end of it.[24]

Meanwhile the research on streptomycin intensified from day to day. There were various ways of extracting, purifying and concentrating a new organic chemical, such as streptomycin. Schatz performed all of these chemical techniques himself. He tried shaking the medium up with ether, then distilling the ether, and rechecking with the bacterial inhibition tests to see if he had an ether soluble fraction. He performed exactly the same experiment with chloroform. In other experiments, he shook it up with added charcoal, then eluted back from the charcoal and retested to see if he had absorbed anything on charcoal. It was another prolonged and laborious series of experiments, testing one extraction technique after another. "I was left with a brown or tan or buff sticky substance which I would then dry in a dessicator. I tested this and found to my satisfaction that it was water soluble. I therefore redissolved it in water after this, perhaps with the addition of minimal alcohol. Then I tested what I had purified. There was no doubt about it. It had still retained all of its remarkable anti-bacterial activity, even at a relatively high dilution."[25]

For Albert Schatz, it seemed that his labours were now over. "At that point, I didn't do much more work."

vi

ON 16 NOVEMBER 1943, exactly four weeks after Schatz had isolated the two strains of actinomyces, subsequently renamed *Streptomyces griseus*, Selman Waksman received an important visitor in his office on the third floor of the soil microbiology building. The name of the visitor was Dr William H. Feldman and he was very interested indeed in tuberculosis.

14

First Cures

When I identified myself as one whose work had to do with microbes, the presiding senator remarked that I must no doubt hate them all. My reply was that I dealt primarily with good microbes. To this the senator exclaimed: "I did not know there were any good microbes; if that is true, only the bad ones come my way."

Selman Waksman: *My Life with the Microbes.*

i

CURIOUSLY ENOUGH, William Feldman was not a doctor of medicine at all but a doctor of veterinary medicine; and it was an unlikely route with many a twist and turn that had led to this conversation with Selman Waksman.

Born in Glasgow, as William Gunn, his father had died when he was just two years old and he was taken by his mother to the United States. Here she had married again, taking the name Feldman and William had subsequently adopted his stepfather's surname. Chance now determined that he spent his childhood in Paonia, western Colorado, where the dry climate was thought to benefit sufferers from tuberculosis. He was impressed by the caring attitude of his mother, who, remembering the suffering caused by the disease in her native Glasgow, took pity on these unfortunate people. He was even more impressed by the fact that she did something practical to help them. One of the small ways in which she made their lives a little easier was to allow them to lie out on an open air bed on

her front porch. Many years later, when a colleague called
Myers asked him why he had devoted his life to tuberculosis,
William Feldman recalled how deeply he had been moved by
one of these unfortunate people who had died in that bed on
the front porch of his mother's home.[1]

During the work for his doctorate, Feldman had played a part
in the nationwide eradication of tuberculosis in cattle, a cause of
fatal tuberculosis in children.[2] Rumour has it that, in 1927, following his graduation from the Colorado Agricultural College,
he was head-hunted by the famous Charles ("Charlie") Mayo,
an amateur farmer, who was alarmed by an outbreak of tuberculosis in his own chickens. William Feldman soon established
a reputation for animal research at one of the most famous –
and the most unlikely – medical institutions in the world.

Three generations of the Mayo family had built the Mayo
Clinic from nothing in the tiny city of Rochester, Minnesota, on
the site of a camping ground for wagon trains. Charlie Mayo,
was the youngest son of William Worrall Mayo, who had
founded the Clinic, after emigrating to Minnesota from Manchester, England. Charlie was a surgical genius and, with his
brother and the Clinic administrator, William James, he had
helped build the Clinic's reputation until, despite the town's
population of barely 20,000, it had become one of the most
sought after medical referral centres in all of America. Here,
another chance encounter brought Feldman together with an
equally gifted colleague.

Five years before Feldman had ever heard of Waksman, in
the winter of 1938, he was travelling back to Rochester from a
tuberculosis meeting in St. Paul. Sitting next to him on the back
seat of the car was a consultant physician, who also worked at
the Mayo Clinic, H. Corwin Hinshaw.[3] The setting was hardly
one that would have suggested an historic outcome. Both men
were already on the tuberculosis committee of the State Medical
Association of Minnesota. The meeting in St. Paul had been
routine – these meetings were held several times a year. The
weather conditions were arctic, and over the ninety mile journey, as the two doctors huddled against the freezing cold in the
back of an old Ford with canvas top and sides, they talked about
tuberculosis. The Rich and Follis experiment at Johns Hopkins

Medical School had just been published, and it was exciting a
great deal of interest. Rich and Follis were, of course, the first
doctors to treat experimental tuberculosis in animals with a
sulphonamide drug called sulphanilamide. Feldman, who was
already a world authority on tuberculosis in animals, was fascinated. The sulphonamides, derived from Prontosil, were still
relatively new to America and Feldman wanted to hear more
about them. Hinshaw remarked that he had heard of a newer
sulphonamide, sulphapyridine, which had just appeared on
the market. Perhaps this might be even more promising than
sulphanilamide? During the two-hour journey, with wind and
snow battering the windows, they decided that they would do
this experiment for themselves.

ii

EVERY NOW AND then, whether in the sciences or the arts, a
partnership emerges that, because it draws its energy from the
inter-reaction of two exceptionally creative and mutually sympathetic human beings, is charged with a wonderful new dynamic force. The working relationship between William Feldman,
the veterinarian, and H. Corwin Hinshaw, would become exactly such a symbiosis.

Hinshaw had never worked on tuberculosis before but he
had a considerable experience of human research into chest
infections. Well over six feet tall, with a powerful athletic frame,
this genial man had retained the deep western accent of his
childhood, spent in the far West, near Idaho, where he was just
one of six who graduated from a tiny Quaker academy. Blessed
with the physique and strength of a line backer, he had diverted
his boundless energy and enthusiasm into medical research.
After taking his bachelors degree at Idaho, he had moved to
Berkeley, California, where he took a PhD in the field of microbiology, before spending three years teaching in the American
University of Beirut in the Lebanon. He had come back to
America to complete his doctorate in medicine before being
appointed a consultant physician on the permanent staff at the
Mayo Clinic. Corwin Hinshaw's special research interest lay in

pulmonary diseases. To Feldman's wide experience of tuberculosis in animals, Hinshaw now added his experience in humans.

Feldman and Hinshaw had the use of a first-class experimental institute several miles out of town in the surrounding countryside. This was where, in 1939, they performed that first small experiment, testing how useful sulphapyridine might be in treating experimental tuberculosis in guinea pigs. As with sulphanilamide, this only showed a limited usefulness. But the results were interesting enough for the two doctors to embark upon a further series of experiments, which multiplied and expanded, until they occupied all of their attentions over the next five years or more. They subsequently tested hundreds of other sulphonamides – and many other derivatives that never otherwise saw the commercial light of day – only to conclude that the results were really no better. Perhaps the most vital lesson learnt from these years of effort, and a lesson all the more vital for the fact that few if any of their colleagues had learnt it, was the realization that tuberculosis was not invincible. This was the turning point of their lives.

From now on, every ounce of their energies would be devoted to the search for the cure for tuberculosis. In 1940 Hinshaw heard of a totally new anti-bacterial drug, called Promin, which had been created by manipulation of the sulphonamide molecule. He persuaded Dr Elwood A. Sharp, Director of Clinical Investigation of Parke, Davis and Company, to supply him with some of the new drug for testing against tuberculosis.

The experiment began in May 1940 and was complete within five months.[4] Promin was shown to be a much more promising treatment than sulphapyridine. By early 1942, after much further research, they presented their findings to the thirty- eighth annual meeting of the American National Tuberculosis Association, which was held in Philadelphia. Sadly, "they received no encouragement from the audience, and, in fact, the report was received with cynicism,"[5] a short-sighted reaction that would become all too familiar to many of the pioneers in the tuberculosis struggle over the next few years.

But Feldman and Hinshaw were not discouraged by this. In

May 1942, in a major step forwards, they reported the first trial
of Promin in the treatment of human tuberculosis. They had
treated thirty-six people suffering from severe pulmonary
tuberculosis with the drug.[6] Eight showed marked improvement after treatment, while a further six showed a less marked
but nevertheless beneficial effect. This trial, which would never
be given its due credit in retrospect, was the first in history in
which a drug had been shown favourably to influence the
course of the disease in human beings. The trial was extended
so that by December 1943, they had amassed a great deal of
further information on Promin's potential. But while confirming the wonderful response they had reported earlier, the trial
ended in disappointment.[7] They had to conclude that the treatment had significant side-effects, the most serious of which
was a tendency for the red blood cells to rupture, causing a
"haemolytic anaemia", which made human treatment imprac-
tical.

In an astonishing development, Dr G. H. Faget, of Carville,
Louisiana, who had read Feldman and Hinshaw's paper on
human tuberculosis, tested Promin against leprosy, to discover
the first successful treatment of the most loathsome disease on
earth. Meanwhile, Hinshaw and Feldman had found an even
more promising sulphone called Promizole. This appeared to
cause fewer side-effects than Promin and they made plans for
testing it in much larger numbers of human sufferers.[8]

At this time tuberculosis was a scourge in the state mental
hospitals of Minnesota. In these large institutions for the
criminally insane, many people would spend the bulk of their
tragic lives, incarcerated together in cramped wards with scant
regard to hygiene. Not surprisingly, tuberculosis was a
fearsome problem and the commonest cause of death. Dr
Hinshaw had no difficulty obtaining permission from the
patients and their relatives in order to try out this new
treatment. They began selecting large numbers of patients to
include in a carefully controlled scientific trial, matching those
with advancing and potentially fatal disease with a balancing
control group of people with that same seriousness of disease.
The intention was to gather a hundred or so patients, fifty in
each of the treatment and control groups, who would be

decided by the toss of a coin. From this very exercise, the labyrinthine complexity of tuberculosis, in all of its protean manifestations, staggered Hinshaw. He realized that if they were to perform a study with any accuracy, it would be essential to enlist the help of some experienced sanitorium doctors.

Every county in Minnesota had its sanitorium and Hinshaw now recruited the assistance of Karl H. Pfuetze, director of the Mineral Springs Sanitorium, Cannon Falls, Minnesota, together with his assistant, Dr Marjorie M. Pyle. Corwin Hinshaw began the huge task of visiting the institutions and picking out patients who would not only be suitable from the point of view of their illness but who could be safely taken from the confines of the mental institution into the normal ward surroundings of the Rochester State Hospital.

It was at this stage, with seventy-five patients already selected and brought back to Rochester for testing, that William Feldman, tall and spare, climbed the two flights of stairs of the small building that housed soil microbiology, in the agricultural college of Rutgers, New Jersey, then walked down a corridor which smelled of moulds and actinomycetes, to be met at the office door by a much shorter but distinguished looking man, who ushered him into his office.

iii

THE DARK-HAIRED AND intense young Waksman from the Washington market days had been transformed over the years into a handsome fatherly figure, with white hair, a thick Russian moustache, and an old world courtesy of manner. During their conversation in Waksman's office, Feldman described his and Corwin Hinshaw's experiences with the sulphonamides and particularly the sulphones, Promin and Promizole. The reason he was here today was perfectly simple. He was interested in a single disease: tuberculosis. He had read of the new antibiotics that were being discovered here by Waksman and his team. He offered the expertise of the Mayo Clinic in assessing any new and promising antibiotics against tuberculosis.

The meeting went well, if cautiously. It would seem that there was the usual circumspection of scientists working in related fields, who as yet did not know one another too well. Waksman told Feldman nothing about streptomycin, in spite of the fact that the drug was at that very moment under intensive assessment by Albert Schatz. Instead he listened with interest as Feldman, unaware that tuberculosis was already included in the aims of Schatz' thesis, urged him to include tuberculosis bacteria in his line-up for testing. Feldman now made a point which Waksman had not previously considered. He explained how absolutely vital it was that any new antibiotic should be tested not against the worn-out harmless variety of tuberculosis germ, such as were usually employed for day to day teaching purposes in colleges, but against a virulent strain from human tuberculosis. Waksman, while feeling wary of importing such a dangerous bacterium into the laboratory, was impressed enough to ask Feldman to send on some cultures of this dangerous strain of tuberculosis for testing.

Feldman came away from the meeting sure that he had succeeded in his prime aim. He had impressed Waksman with the enthusiasm he and Hinshaw felt about becoming involved should anything worthwhile turn up. He had also established that collaboration would suit Waksman, who lacked the facilities for detailed animal study and who had no access at all to testing in human sufferers.

Soon after his visit, Feldman did indeed send on supplies of the virulent tuberculosis germs, which were passed on to Albert Schatz for further testing. Schatz would subsequently recall the circumstances. "Waksman agreed to work with the Mayo Clinic people because I agreed to work with the pathogenic strain of tubercle bacillus. The strain I used for most of my work from then on was the H37–Rv strain, which was the most virulent strain in existence. Nobody else in the department wanted to work with it because they were terrified they would pick up tuberculosis."[9]

Only a month or two after Feldman's visit to Rutgers, in January 1944, the discovery of streptomycin was announced to the world in a paper entitled, *Streptomycin, a substance exhibiting antibiotic activity against Gram-positive and Gram-negative bacteria*.

The authors in name order were Albert Schatz, Betty Bugie and Selman Waksman.[10] The title of the paper made no mention of tuberculosis. Indeed the paper was so focused on the Gram-negative bacteria, that the writer, Julius H. Comroe Jr, marvelled at this in retrospect: "The word 'streptomycin' is in the table, the words *M. tuberculosis* are also there, and the tenth line shows that streptomycin was an effective antibiotic against the tubercle bacillus. But nowhere else in the article (title, introduction, discussion, or summary) are the words *tubercle bacillus* or 'tuberculosis' mentioned again."[11] If streptomycin were to prove the cure for tuberculosis, it had arrived into the world unannounced.

But that tiny mention, in just a single column of one table, of streptomycin's activity against the tuberculosis germ was more than enough to galvanize Feldman and Hinshaw. While they were in the act of drafting a request to Waksman, a letter arrived from Rutgers inviting them to participate in a cooperative study of the drug's potential. For Albert Schatz, working alone in the basement laboratory, the treadmill was back in business:

"After discovering streptomycin, I thought I could relax a little. But circumstances did not permit this. Once again I found myself in the laboratory working night and day. One of the things I had to do was concentrate the antibiotic. I did this in two small stills in the basement laboratory where I worked. Because the total capacity of these stills was small, I kept them running continuously, twenty-four hours a day. I even slept in the laboratory. At night or in the early hours of the morning, when I was so exhausted that I could no longer keep my eyes open, the night watchman would come in and help me. He was curious about what was going on and it gave him the opportunity to talk to somebody through the night. I would place a red mark on each flask in the two distillation units, and then go to sleep with two old, torn blankets on the floor in the corner of the laboratory. If I was asleep and the solution was down below that red mark, he would wake me up and I would add more chloroform or whatever I was working with. Since I worked, ate and slept in the laboratory, I often did not leave the building in which the laboratory was located for several days at a time. Once I stayed in that building for an entire week. This is how I prepared the streptomycin for the earliest animal experiments at the Mayo Clinic."[12]

That first supply, a precious ten grams of streptomycin, produced as a result of such stoical endurance on the part of Schatz, arrived at the Mayo Clinic in early April 1944. By 27 April Feldman and Hinshaw had begun its testing in tuberculosis-infected guinea pigs. Guessing that they had barely enough drug for four animals, they divided the ten grams into four lots, treating just four animals already infected with tuberculosis, while eight similarly infected animals acted as controls. The supply of streptomycin ran out on 20 June, fifty-five days after the animals had been infected.

The animals were painlessly sacrificed and examined for whatever effect the drug had had on their tuberculosis. There was of course a very sound reason for choosing guinea pigs. As Koch had first discovered some three quarters of a century earlier, these delightful little creatures have no resistance whatsoever to tuberculosis. Without an effective treatment, every animal inoculated with the disease would develop an overwhelming infection and die from it. Feldman now performed the postmortem examinations, reading out his results to Hinshaw. The moment was charged with an expectancy they had never known in any previous experiment. They were not disappointed. Those meagre ten grams of very impure streptomycin, cultured, harvested and purified by Albert Schatz in the basement laboratory, had cured the tuberculosis in all four animals.

It was a Saturday so neither doctor needed to turn up for work in the Clinic. In a daze of excitement, they drove over to Hinshaw's house to talk about the possible implications. Sitting out of the late June sun in the shade of an apple tree in the back garden, they talked and talked into the afternoon. Bill Feldman had brought a bottle of his home-made gin, concocted from 200 per cent proof laboratory alcohol, to celebrate with. Five years after that freezing journey from St. Paul, in this wonderful moment of effervescent excitement, they sat back in two little canvas garden chairs, bathed in the dappled shade of the apple tree, and drank a toast to success and the new wonder drug – to streptomycin![13]

iv

ALTHOUGH THEY HAD tested the new drug in just four animals, the results were so striking that they sent an urgent telegram to Waksman, informing him of the exciting nature of their results. Then, without asking permission from the Mayo Clinic, they arranged some two weeks later to take the train for New Jersey. Arriving in New Brunswick on a Sunday evening in early July, they arranged to meet up with Waksman first thing on the Monday morning.

Little realizing just what superhuman effort was involved on Schatz' part in the production of streptomycin, Feldman and Hinshaw had taken quite a gamble. On 28 June, before setting out for New Jersey, they had already infected a large group of guinea pigs with tuberculosis, in the expectation that further larger supplies of streptomycin would be forthcoming. This sense of urgency could hardly fail to impress Waksman. "In retrospect," Feldman would later admit, "we could properly have been considered somewhat impetuous." But timing would prove vital in what was now a global race for priority in finding the cure for tuberculosis, a race in which national pride could be predicted to play its part.

The amount of streptomycin that the Mayo scientists were requesting was far more than Schatz could produce in the basement laboratory. Waksman, who had already interested Merck & Co., of Rahway, New Jersey, in the commercial possibility of streptothricin, put an urgent call through to the drug company, arranging for them to meet up the following day. This meeting, which was held in a boardroom at Rahway, took place on 10 July 1944. It was attended by a dozen or so of the company's senior administrators and chemists.

Streptomycin had been tested in just four guinea pigs. No more important meeting in the history of medicine could have been based upon such a shaky foundation. If Merck had not already had a close relationship with Waksman, the outcome of this meeting would have been only too predictable. Waksman, Feldman and Hinshaw sat with the large group round a table and used the most powerful lever they had: the vast human importance of tuberculosis. In Hinshaw's recollection: "We discussed the possibility, indeed the probability, that an effective drug suitable for the treatment of human tuberculosis might be developed – a drug that would have enormous, truly worldwide, importance. But the Merck staff told us it would be impossible for them to cooperate in such a study because they were deeply involved in producing penicillin and some other preparations for the troops in the war zone."[14]

Waksman did his utmost to persuade them. He would come over from his laboratory and plant the cultures at Merck for them. He even offered to prepare enough streptomycin to enable the larger trials, already begun in guinea pigs, to be completed. The Merck staff were courteous and interested but still they were concerned solely with penicillin. Penicillin had military significance. Hinshaw insisted that after the first world war, more people had died from tuberculosis than had been killed in action. This visibly impressed them. The Merck staff asked the company director and owner to come and join them and it was George Merck himself who finally made the decision: "Go ahead with it!"[15]

In fact all parties eventually agreed to a compromise. Merck would take a chance on streptomycin if Feldman and Hinshaw would agree to test the clinical usefulness of streptothricin at the same time. Feldman realized at once the importance of this commercial bargaining. "The prompt development of streptomycin was assured. Had Merck & Co. not consented to do this at this time, the clinical evaluations of streptomycin would in all probability have been long delayed."[16]

Now that George Merck himself was committed – even obsessed as it would soon transpire – he ordered no less than fifty scientists to begin work on streptomycin, including the inspired organic chemists, Karl Folkers and Max Tishler. Back at the Mayo Clinic, Feldman and Hinshaw could now return to the most crucial experiment of their lives.

v

WITH SOME MORE streptomycin supplied by Waksman, and the promise of much larger supplies from Merck, Feldman and

Hinshaw continued with the large batch of guinea pigs, which had been inoculated with virulent tuberculosis germs on 29 June. With its agonisingly slow but deadly progress, full blood stream spread of the disease would be detectable in every animal forty-nine days later. Biopsies of the livers of a few animals confirmed that the disease had reached this life-threatening stage. The test animals, all suffering from blood-borne spread of tuberculosis, were now started on streptomycin.

Throughout this exhaustive research effort, both doctors were expected by the Clinic to carry on with their normal duties. They took it in turns to travel out to the animal laboratories, many miles out of Rochester, and give the animals their overnight injections. The large scale experiment was complete on 29 January 1945. If there had been some uncertainty following the first four test animals, there could be no doubt at all now. The results could only be described as sensational. Not only had a fatal blood borne tuberculosis been reversed: the treated guinea pigs appeared to have suffered little if any side-effects from the streptomycin.

These results were so dramatic they immediately cabled Waksman to tell him so. Feldman and Hinshaw were very eager to tell the world. But Waksman asked them not to do so.[17] He now confessed that the germ that had been labelled "tuberculosis" in his first paper was a harmless strain, which had been supplied to him by Dr Florence Sabin of the Phipps Institute in Philadelphia.[18] Waksman asked Feldman and Hinshaw to delay the publication of the guinea pig trials until he had confirmed the efficacy of streptomycin against the much more dangerous tuberculosis germs supplied by Feldman. As with all previous work on streptomycin, the practical experiment, using solely the virulent H37–Rv strain, was performed by Albert Schatz.[19]

A little later that same year, Schatz and Waksman published their results in a second streptomycin paper, which concentrated solely on tuberculosis. Their conclusion was astonishing: they had found streptomycin fifty times more powerful than streptothricin in killing this deadly strain of human tuberculosis germ.[20] Feldman and Hinshaw immediately followed with their results in the guinea pig experiment.[21] Two very important papers, their early publication would establish the priority worldwide for streptomycin as the first antibiotic in history that promised a new hope in the fight against tuberculosis.

Hinshaw, meanwhile, was convinced that streptomycin was a much better drug than Promin or Promizole. Although the large scale trial of Promizole had started in July of that year, he decided they should suspend this in favour of streptomycin. Already he knew that Merck & Co were making rapid advances in purifying the drug. Merck had so gained in confidence that they were planning to build a new factory at Elkton, Virginia, to produce streptomycin in much larger quantities. Still there remained a single all important uncertainty. Every previous drug that had shown promise in the animal experiments had soon been thrown into the dustbin because of poisonous side-effects. With his partner and colleague, William Feldman, Corwin Hinshaw was ready to test streptomycin in its most important trial of all: human sufferers.

vi

IT SEEMS LIKELY that the first human being ever to receive streptomycin received a little of the batch that had been prepared in that final exhaustive burst by Albert Schatz. The patient was an elderly man, suffering from tuberculous meningitis in the Colonial Hospital in Rochester.[22]

Tuberculous meningitis was a death sentence so there was nothing to lose. Though he only had enough of this highly impure drug to treat the man for a few weeks, and though he had no idea whatsoever what dosage to give, Hinshaw administered streptomycin in guesswork doses by regular intramuscular injection. The man's disease was very advanced and he eventually died from it. But during those two weeks or so of this extremely tentative treatment, they had noticed some fall in the man's high temperature and some slight clinical improvement. Hinshaw felt confident enough to take a cautious step further.

At about the same time, a patient was brought to his attention with blood-borne tuberculosis, which was just as fatal as the meningitis. This man was suffering from tuberculosis of the kidneys and bladder, an agonizing condition in which the bladder wall becomes progressively thickened and contracted down, until it becomes a daylong torment. A urological surgeon had ruptured the badly diseased bladder when trying to look into it using a metal instrument, as a result of which, tuberculosis germs had escaped into the abdominal cavity and from there had got into the blood stream. The chest X-ray confirmed this, with the dramatic picture of widespread tiny shadows resembling a hailstorm that was typical of blood-borne tuberculosis. Hinshaw had enough of the drug to treat this man for two or three months.

Within days of starting streptomycin, the man's high fever fell back to normal. After a prolonged course of treatment, there was every hope that he had been cured. Unfortunately he too died, but at postmortem the pathologist confirmed that he had not died from tuberculosis but from a blood clot that had moved from his legs to his lungs, that well known complication of prolonged bed rest, childbirth and surgery. At the postmortem, the pathologist was amazed to find no evidence of active tuberculosis anywhere in his body. Even those tissues in his bladder and kidneys, which had previously been heavily infected, showed definite signs of healing.

Despite the unfortunate man's death, these results were considered promising enough to take the clinical testing still further. Hinshaw and Feldman, together with their colleagues Pfuetze and Pyle, gathered enough courage to face the most devious disease of all, the dreaded form in which it had been known throughout the ages as consumption: pulmonary tuberculosis.

In July 1943, Patricia, a 21-year-old woman, was admitted to the Mineral Springs Sanitorium, from her home town of Austin, with advanced tuberculosis affecting the upper lobe of her right lung. For a year she was treated with the conventional sanitorium regime of enforced bed rest. At first, she showed some slight improvement. However, by the summer of 1944, she was deteriorating, with chills, high fever, night sweats and an increasing cough. By October, her chest X-ray showed a dangerous worsening of the disease in the right lung. This so alarmed the doctor looking after her that she was transferred to the Mayo Clinic, where a surgeon, Dr Clagett performed an emergency thoracoplasty, in which he removed several ribs from the right upper part of her chest. The aim of this operation, carried out on 1 November, was to stop the diseased part of the lung expanding during the act of breathing. Two weeks later her chest X-ray showed an even more alarming spread of the disease to the left lung. Hinshaw was asked by Pfuetze and Clagett to come and see her.

Wearing the necessary face mask, to avoid contracting the disease himself, and accompanied by Pfuetze, Pyle and Feldman, he gazed down on a pretty dark-haired farmer's daughter, racked by persistent coughing, emaciated from consumption, and bathed in a feverish sweat. Like Pfuetze, he was in no doubt that her disease would soon prove fatal. At this time, the large scale guinea pig experiment had still not been completed, but they knew that in a subgroup of nine animals, streptomycin had caused a dramatic healing of the inoculated tuberculosis. They discussed her situation with Patricia herself, and she agreed to become the first human guinea pig. Her condition was so desperate, there was nothing to lose.

The correct treatment dose for humans was still completely unknown so that the drug was given very cautiously. The total daily dose was a mere tenth of a gram divided into eight equal doses, given by deep and very painful injections into the emaciated flesh of this sick girl. It is possible that the streptomycin used to treat her was initially from the supply manufactured by Schatz, soon to be supplanted by the first batches arriving from the Merck laboratories. It was still very impure and the injections caused her to suffer headaches, facial flushes, generalized muscular aching, pains in the joints, feelings of exhaustion and even chills and fevers.

Between 20 November 1944 and 7 April 1945, Patricia received five courses of streptomycin injections, each of which lasted ten to eighteen days. The treatment was constantly interrupted because they kept running out of supplies of the drug. At first the tiny doses of streptomycin had no real effect on her disease but with bigger doses and better purity of the supplies coming from the pharmaceutical firm, it was obvious that she was improving. Her temperature fell and the new infection that had previously appeared in her left lung melted away, implying that her tuberculosis had at least been partially cured. But this had proved no easy victory. Even in this first case in history treated with streptomycin, tuberculosis had sounded a warning. It did not behave like any other bacterial infection. It was only too clear from the protracted course of her treatment and from the fact that even months later the doctors were still locked in a desperate struggle to save her, that the treatment of tuberculosis with antibiotics would be far from a simple solution.

How mystifying it was that at the end of the streptomycin treatment her sputum still grew tuberculosis germs! Nobody knew the explanation for this. Nevertheless, Patricia was so much improved that the surgeons could now operate on the residual disease, an option that would have been out of the question prior to the streptomycin treatment. Most important of all, the streptomycin had reduced the severity of her infection for her body's own defences to bring the remaining disease under control.[23]

In the words of Pfuetze, "It was a story book ending. The patient made a remarkable recovery. She led a very active life. After leaving the sanitorium, she married and became the mother of three fine children, born in 1950, 1952 and 1954."[24] The streptomycin miracle had begun.

Of all the ways in which tuberculosis infects humans, one particular form of the disease is the most pitiable. This is the way in which the disease frequently attacks very young children, then viewed as hopeless and inevitably fatal: tuberculous meningitis. That first elderly man, treated with minute doses of the impure drug, had not survived – but this was hardly surprising, given his circumstances. Soon streptomycin would be given a fairer trial in this awesome condition.

On 12 May 1945, a one-year-old Irish-American girl was admitted to the New Haven Hospital with convulsions. After her admission, she ran a high temperature and continued to suffer convulsions, which had to be suppressed by intravenous injections of anaesthetic drugs. The doctors found abnormal signs on the left side of her chest, that would suggest a pneumonia. When she was still worsening some six days later, a lumbar puncture was performed, permitting the medical staff to study the cerebrospinal fluid which bathes and nourishes the brain and spinal cord. Tuberculous bacteria were seen in the fluid, confirming the diagnosis of tuberculous meningitis. Her situation was hopeless.

Examination of the family revealed that her father had pulmonary tuberculosis, so they knew the source of her disease. This little girl, dying from tuberculous meningitis, became the first child in the world to be treated with streptomycin.

The drug was given by intramuscular injection every two hours and once daily by direct injection through a hole in her skull into the fluid filled spaces at the centre of the brain. Such drastic measures were necessary because the pus that surrounds the brain in tuberculous meningitis is very thick and cheesy, making it very difficult for any drug given by mouth or through a venous line to penetrate deeply enough to kill the bacteria. Slowly but surely, week by week and month by month, she made a gradual recovery, until finally – and this would be after at least a year – she could at last be pronounced cured. For the doctors from far and wide who would come to the hospital to see her, for the nurses who painstakingly cared for her day after day, most of all for her parents, who had suffered the appalling trauma this disease brings to all it touches, it seemed a miracle. She was the first of the "streptomycin babies".[25]

In October 1944, while the guinea pig experiments were still under way and at a time when the first one or two patients were receiving the first cautious injections that had been prepared by Schatz in the basement laboratory, Waksman was invited to talk about streptomycin before the members and staff of the Mayo Clinic. At an informal dinner before the main meeting, the president of the Mayo Foundation, Dr D.C. Balfour, introduced him to a gathering of senior staff:

"We have with us today a representative from an agricultural institution, one who has no medical degree and has never even received any training in medicine. He is going to address us tonight on a subject that is at the moment of great importance to medical science and clinical practice. The fact that you, Dr Waksman, have been invited to deliver an address before a great medical organization, such as ours, suggests that you are bringing to us a very important message."[26]

As far as the world was concerned, no medical discovery had ever been more vital. Selman Waksman stood before the doctors at this famous medical institution and summarized the work of thirty years which had led him from his lifelong interest in the microbes that inhabited common soil to the discovery of streptomycin. As far as this distinguished gathering were concerned, streptomycin, already begun on its clinical testing in human patients, held centre stage in the world. They were unaware that competition had arisen from an unexpected source.

15

Hearing God Thinking

Einstein was a man who could ask immensely simple questions. And what his life showed, and his work, is that when the answers are simple too, then you hear God thinking.

Bronowski: *The Ascent of Man*

i

O N 3 MARCH 1943, in neutral Sweden, hemmed in by warring armies and cut off from the exciting developments in Germany and the United States, Jorgen Lehmann wrote an amazing letter to the pharmaceutical company, Ferrosan, in Malmö. In essence, though the words were couched in a more scientific language, the letter made an extraordinary prophecy: if Ferrosan could manufacture the para-amino salt of aspirin, it would have anti-tuberculous properties.[1]

Without a stroke of experiment, Lehmann had given the Swedish drug manufacturer the formula for a discovery that would change history. It was a deduction so brilliant that his fellow doctors and scientists would refuse to believe it. How could Lehmann have possibly picked out this single chemical derivative of aspirin as the one to test before a single experiment had been performed? Such vision was simply unbelievable when applied to the ordinary research worker, proceeding along conventional lines. But Lehmann was neither ordinary nor conventional.

As an old man, Jorgen Lehmann would shake his head at his own youthful temerity. "Now I sit here, eighty-three-years-old, I have to ask myself a truthful question. Should I say that my researches followed the general rules, bacteriology, animal experiments, toxicology, human work? Certainly this would have been the normal pattern. But no – that was not how it happened at all. In fact it all came about in quite a different way, a way I can only describe as personal. From the very beginning I had conceived of PAS as a unique and powerful idea. From then on, all of my labour was based upon the unshakable belief that it would be a success. This faith would take me over cliffs and into the most dangerous situations, all of which would prove perilous for the project."[2]

ii

FROM THAT VERY special moment, when, sitting on his couch in his office at the Sahlgren's Hospital, he had first read Bernheim's paper, he had realized its vital importance. Bernheim had shown that if you added aspirin to a culture of tuberculosis germs, the oxygen uptake by the germs doubled. Aspirin must therefore play a vital role in the life chemistry of the tuberculosis germ. What Lehmann had immediately realized was that if you now changed the structure of aspirin very slightly, for example by adding a small chemical subgroup to some part of the molecule, the altered aspirin molecule would be taken up by the germs in just the same way. But this new molecule would not work like aspirin. Instead, it would block the delicate internal chemistry of the germ's respiration. It was the very meaning of competitive inhibition, the principle Lehmann had been familiar with since his student days in Lund. It had been this same principle that had enabled him to invent the clot breaking drug, dicoumarol.

In 1940, when that flash of inspiration had first come to him, he was in the middle of the clinical experiments on dicoumarol, with daily anticoagulant rounds at the gynaecology clinic. But he had never forgotten the tuberculosis idea. Now, with the anticoagulant research behind him, he could concentrate all of his efforts upon this new and tantalizing challenge.

The aspirin molecule had a very striking chemical skeleton,

which, rather like the thiazole ring, took the form of a ring of six carbon atoms, held to each other by chemical bonds. This so-called benzol ring was not a ring at all but a hexagon. The carbon at the apex had an acidic chemical group attached to it. To alter the structure slightly, Lehmann would have to attach another chemical group to one of the other carbons. He now asked himself two simple questions: which chemical grouping should I add to the aspirin ring – and to which carbon about the ring should I add it?

In his own words: "In fact, it was very simple. In the sulpho-namide there was an amino group in the para position and if you changed the amino group for another group or put it into the ortho or meta position, then the bacteriostatic effect diminished or disappeared."[3] The "para" carbon was simply the carbon at the bottom of the hexagon, three atoms away from, and directly opposite, the acid-bearing carbon at the apex. Lehmann suggested therefore that Ferrosan should attach an amino group to the carbon in the para position, so the new creation was called para-aminosalicylic acid.

Chance therefore had nothing to do with it. PAS did not come from the screening of many chemical manipulations of the aspirin molecule. Like a real-life Sherlock Holmes, he had solved the puzzle logically from the facts which were available to him. And given the insight into his thoughts, we are almost tempted to play Watson: of course, in retrospect and given Lehmann's explanation, it seems *elementary*. But so elementary that not a single scientist worldwide had performed that same feat in all of the three years since Bernheim's tiny paper had first been published in *Nature*.

In his historic letter to Ferrosan, Lehmann drew attention to a curious puzzle. He had discovered that the other derivatives of aspirin, the "ortho" and "meta" amino salts, had been described in two German journals in the early 1900s.[4] Yet there was no record of those same German chemists having created the additional "para-amino" salt. Karl-Gustav Rosdahl, the senior chemist at Ferrosan, and the man who had played such a vital role in the dicoumarol research, was just as puzzled about this. He knew that a technique for synthesizing the para-aminosalicylic acid had long since been published in the book every chemist regarded as his Bible, Beilstein. How strange it was that he too could find no record of anybody ever having made it.

After sending his letter, Lehmann waited for several months: nothing at all seemed to be happening. In August he contacted Ferrosan to ask how the synthesis was going. But still he received no reply. It was all the more unusual since Ferrosan had so enthusiastically supported his earlier ideas, from the woman dying from beri-beri in Aarhus to the globally important discovery of dicoumarol. On 9 September he contacted them again only to encounter that same baffling silence. What on earth was happening?

In order to understand this – and it would continue to be an obstacle to the later development of PAS – one has to recall what had happened a generation earlier. When the sodium salt of gold was recommended as an effective treatment for tuberculosis by Professor Mollgaard, in Denmark, Ferrosan had committed itself to a major research and manufacturing involvement. It took fifteen years before gold was subjected to a controlled clinical trial, when it proved to be worthless. The Danish owners lost a million crowns, a fortune in those days. Ferrosan was a small company, employing just seventy-five employees, and another such catastrophe would bankrupt them.[5] Pinning one's hopes on the cure for tuberculosis was as perilous to the survival of a small pharmaceutical company as the disease itself was to the suffering millions. Yet the company was reluctant to dismiss any suggestion of Lehmann's, no matter how wildly improbable it might appear.

On 2 June 1943, and unknown to Lehmann, the thirty-three-year-old chief chemist, Rosdahl, tried hard to interest Ryné, the director of Ferrosan, in taking it further. Rosdahl, who had returned to work at Ferrosan after some years spent in chemical research at the Caroline Institute, where he had devoted much of his time to the chemistry of respiration, was very interested in Lehmann's proposition. In his own free time, he began to experiment with the creation of the PAS molecule. To his surprise, when he attempted to make the molecule using the technique advocated by the standard chemical text, Beilstein, it did not work.

Rosdahl would not be the only chemist who would encounter

this difficulty. We now know that Bernheim, brilliant as he undoubtedly was, had tried to make it himself and failed. On a visit to the United States some years later, Lehmann met a chemist from the American Cyanamid Corporation who told him that they could not manage the synthesis. In September 1946 Lehmann heard from a Norwegian friend that Nyegards had also failed miserably in their attempts to produce it. On trips to France, Portugal and Spain, he would hear the same story repeated over and over. Even the giant pharmaceutical company, Squibb, in the United States, met with failure. It was all the more remarkable therefore to hear, in October 1943, that Karl Rosdahl had succeeded where so many others had failed. The synthesis had proved astonishingly difficult but, in a complex process involving five different chemical steps, this inspired chemist had synthesized para-aminosalicylic acid for the first time.

Yet, by 1 November, and still having had no supply of the drug from Ferrosan, Lehmann read an article by Hans von Euler, which set out to examine the way in which aspirin worked. Lehmann was worried that von Euler, a brilliant Swedish physiologist and Nobel laureate, must have spotted the implication in Bernheim's short report. He wrote an urgent letter to Ferrosan:

"It seems likely that Professor von Euler thinks as I do. We are possibly a little ahead concerning this research, but it can be assumed that von Euler has already started to produce the very same substance. I need hardly emphasize that the utmost urgency is now essential. Engineer Rosdahl has informed me that the first supply is on its way. I have fifty guinea pigs ready and waiting."[6]

The synthesis of PAS was however proving so difficult that Rosdahl could only produce minute quantities. Nevertheless, the management of Ferrosan, accepting that there really was "a fire round the corner", now took a courageous step. They gave Rosdahl the backing he needed for his manufacturing process and the company agreed to provide Lehmann with some PAS for some preliminary studies. It wasn't until December 1943 that he received his first precious supply, thirteen grams of para-aminosalicylic acid (PAS). Four days later he began the most important of the test tube experiments, testing PAS against cultures of BCG bacteria, the live attenuated tuberculosis germ used in vaccination. In a letter, dated 7 December, he reported back to Ferrosan: "The great bacteriological experiment has begun."[7]

Lehmann grew his BCG bacilli in the same jade-green slopes as Albert Schatz in America and Gerhard Domagk in Germany. Now, during the preparation for each slope, he added various dilutions of the para-aminosalicylic acid he had received from Rosdahl, then waited several weeks to see how this would affect the growth of the germs. He diluted the drug to one in a hundred, even one in a thousand – the new drug dramatically blocked any growth of the type of tuberculous germs he was testing. With growing excitement, he diluted it to almost trace levels, one in a hundred thousand. Even at such extreme dilutions, it still inhibited the bacteria from growing and dividing. On 5 January, he wrote an excited letter to Ferrosan, who were by now experimenting with a wide range of alternative chemicals based on the original PAS molecule: "The inhibition by 4-aminosalicylic acid is so effective that all further work should be concentrated on this compound."[8]

Ryné took the news to Rosdahl personally. He burst through the door of the chemist's office, throwing his arms about him and presenting him with a huge bouquet of flowers.[9]

Given Lehmann's drive and energy, it will not surprise anybody to discover that, within just weeks or so of starting, the pace of testing was already frenetic – and this in spite of the fact that difficulties with the synthesis meant that over the next two months Lehmann had to perform all of the early experiments using a pitiful 18.5 grams of drug. At Ferrosan, Ryné gave Rosdahl five assistants to speed up production. On 7 January the drug was first tested for side-effects in rabbits. None of the rabbits showed any signs of toxicity, even when examined very closely for effects on their blood and urine. This was followed by longer term studies, when guinea pigs, rats and mice were given the drug for several weeks: while the mice and rats showed no ill effects, after six weeks or so the guinea pigs became ill, they lost weight and some even died at about eight to ten weeks. This alarmed Lehmann until, to his immense relief, he found that if milk was added to their diet, the guinea pigs fared much better. It wasn't an effect of the drug but some curious problem with their diet.

By 15 January, guinea pigs infected with a virulent strain of human tuberculosis germs began a trial of treatment with PAS. Many tuberculosis researchers had contracted the disease as a result of accidental inhalation of the germ used in such studies. Nevertheless, Lehmann, who was no bacteriologist, carried out these studies himself, with the advice of Anders Wassén, the head of bacteriology at the hospital. Two weeks later it was already clear that those guinea pigs given the drug were dramatically better than the control animals.

For Jorgen Lehmann, wild spirit and scientist, the opportunity that lay before him was a fantastic dream. Nobody could doubt that he had the nerve and the genius to pit himself against the most dangerous disease in existence. But just like so many others, doctors, nurses, scientists, who had made that same courageous decision before him, the struggle would exact a heavy price.

iii

THE SWEDISH WINTER of 1943 was bitter. Deep snow blanketed the streets of Gothenburg, and the Kattegat sea, which separates Gothenburg from Denmark, froze over so that you could walk out for a distance of three miles and fish off the ice. Jorgen Lehmann continued to make his daily journey to the hospital either by tram or his robust black bicycle, setting out early in the morning and rarely returning before the early hours of the following morning. Lehmann's wife, who like Dubos', was called Marie Louise, was a "strong character in her own right",[10] and with Jorgen's total preoccupation with his research, she felt miserable and neglected.

No sooner had he returned from America and the family were just recovered from the upheaval of the move from Lund than he was involved with the vitamin research. Then came another upheaval with the move back to Gothenburg and no sooner had they settled into their new home than he was immersed in the anticoagulant discovery. Now, with the anticoagulant research only just waning, and while Jorgen was still running a busy laboratory at the Sahlgren's Hospital, he was spending all of his spare time on a new inspiration, an idea so immensely important that she hardly knew when she would ever see him in a normal capacity again. Unless she stayed out of bed until two or three in the morning, she did not manage to talk to Jorgen these days, and his arrival home in the early hours of the morning brought arguments and recriminations.

To make matters yet more difficult, Marie Louise, who had been deeply hurt by some earlier family experiences, had involved herself with the refugee problem. Her maiden surname was Walloon and she had escaped her native Belgium, struggling through battle-torn Europe during the first war, taking sanctuary in Sweden as a refugee, accompanied by five sisters and two brothers. These painful experiences had so impressed her that, from the outbreak of the second world war, she had thrown herself body and soul into running two or three voluntary women's groups for peace and freedom. These were desperate times and the villa in an attractive quarter of Gothenburg was always bulging with war refugees, usually Jewish, from occupied Denmark. These organizations would help them escape across the frozen Kattegat under cover of night, arriving in Sweden with nothing more than a toothbrush. Jorgen himself was equally sympathetic and tried to find work for the doctors amongst them in his laboratory. But there was nowhere at home where he could find peace, nowhere he could think, and he was in desperate need now to think often, long and clearly. He would later point out how much he needed such peace: "I must work completely independently and undisturbed. Nobody must interfere with my thoughts, which are as delicate and as easily disturbed as spiders webs."[11]

But with two sons now at high school and such pressures at home, the atmosphere was explosive. Who could blame the neglected Marie Louise if she sought refuge in other arms. This was certainly the impression of her son, Orla, who deeply resented his mother. The situation had become quite unbearable for the whole family and, tragically, the marriage disintegrated at the heart of the tuberculosis research.

After he and Marie Louise agreed to separate, Jorgen Lehmann moved into the basement of his laboratory, taking no more than a table, a chair and a bed with him. He was accompanied for a time by his eldest son, Orla, who would for the rest of his life feel especially close to his father while the younger son, Klas Erik, chose to remain with his mother.

Lehmann was now forced to struggle on with his research while living in a single room in his laboratory, cooking for himself and his son, and washing his own clothes. Witnesses from those difficult years remember him hanging his own socks across a line in the cellar. Even here he could not escape the refugee problem, since he was flooded by Jewish friends escaping from Denmark, their need so desperate that they were willing to help him with the mundane tasks of taking blood from patients or assisting his secretary with typing and filing. It heralded two years of unrelenting hardship in Lehmann's private life. While he himself, no matter his private anguish, could bear the personal distress and the ridicule of his opponents amongst the other staff, it was unacceptably hard on Orla and soon afterwards he left for the home of Lehmann's old teacher and friend, Professor Thunberg at Lund. Throughout this painful period, the research continued unabated.

Now like Dubos and Domagk before him, the intoxication of discovery carried him through these difficult days. With his bespectacled figure, racing down the long hospital corridors on his "Danish" bicycle, ferrying his precious drugs in the basket under the handlebars, he became well known at the Sahlgren's Hospital, where he was the object of affection from those who loved him but the butt of ridicule for the more conservative of his colleagues, who had opposed his appointment in the first place, and who savagely resented both his original genius and his insistence, as a mere laboratory doctor, on fulfilling a bedside role with his patients.

When, during the anticoagulant research, he would arrive on the ward with a tape measure to assess the swelling of the mothers' legs they would scoff: "Here comes the tailor!" Now seeing him pedalling his black bicycle down the main corridor of the hospital, one of the longest hospital corridors in Europe and measuring 1.6 kilometres from end to end, the haughty professor of medicine, whose students were instructed not to salute Lehmann, would exclaim, "Step aside for the eccentric Dane!"[12]

Lehmann gave little thought to these barbs of jealousy and resentment, which he would fend off with a characteristically brilliant and irascible wit. All that interested him was the great experiment.

iv

ALTHOUGH HE HAD been well trained in animal research, he felt less than competent with the bacterial studies. Those first experiments had been conducted in a miniature bacteriology laboratory he had partitioned off within the crowded confines of his chemistry department, using equipment he had cobbled together with his own hands, with clothes pegs acting as clamps and every manner of Heath Robinson invention using glassware and pieces of wood. Lehmann was desperately impatient with the animal experiments, which were taking too long. He set up new experiments in rabbits, which now ran simultaneously with those in the guinea pigs and mice. In fact things were moving at such a pace that the initial animal experiments were completed as soon as February. Overall PAS was wonderfully free of poisonous side-effects. Even while the animal experiments continued, Lehmann decided that the time had come to try out PAS in human sufferers at least as a topical therapy. As with dicoumarol, he decided that the first human guinea pig should be himself.

Only when he himself had survived taking the drug by mouth and injection, did he turn to the surgeon who had helped him with the anticoagulant research, his old friend from Lund, Dr Gustaf Pettersson, head of surgery at the Children's Hospital in Gothenburg, who also looked after Finnish children suffering from tuberculosis of their bones in a special annex on Amund Island.

To the modern clinician, versed in the protracted course of new drug trials, it is astonishing that by March 1944, a bare three months after the research began, a child with a tuberculous infection was treated at the Children's Hospital by Dr Pettersson. The unfortunate child was suffering from a type of blood cancer called lymphoma, which depresses the immune response to infection, and had developed tuberculosis in the bone, which was discharging through an ugly inflamed hole in the skin. Balls of gauze, wetted with 10 per cent solution of PAS, were inserted by Pettersson into this open wound, which had for many months been discharging tuberculous pus. Within eight days there was a dramatic improvement, the unpleasant grey lumps around the wound disappeared and were replaced by clean red healing edges. A second child with a tuberculous infection in a leg bone was treated in the same way – again there was an almost magical improvement.

On 29 March, Lehmann took the clinical testing a vital stage further. He approached Dr Gylfe Vallentin, head of Renström's Sanitorium in Gothenburg, and asked him if he would be prepared to test the new drug in patients suffering from pulmonary tuberculosis. For the tempestuous and single-minded Lehmann, it would never be easy to work other than on his own. In an interview with Jarl Ingelf, the historian for Ferrosan, he would confess that all of his life he had "hunted as a lone wolf". But now he was forced to admit that he was no sanitorium doctor. Tuberculosis was an immensely complex disease and he had no choice but to work with such an experienced physician who could assess PAS in its most difficult and important challenge: the testing against human tuberculosis in all of its dread manifestations. In Vallentin he had made a fascinating choice of partner.

Few doctors knew more about tuberculosis than this calm deep-thinking man. Gylfe Vallentin had himself survived the deadly embrace of the disease not once but twice. He had first suffered tuberculosis as a boy living in his home town of Norrköpine, after contracting it from his uncle, who had returned from the United States dying from consumption. It seems likely that the experience left such a mark upon the boy that he was imbued with a lifelong sense of mission. He would become a doctor and help others who were suffering from this frightening disease. As if to mock this admirable purpose, in 1914, while still under the stress and long hours of work and study as a newly graduated doctor, his tuberculosis burst into a new and dangerous reactivation and he was forced to accept the old-fashioned treatment regime at the Hålahut Sanitorium.

How terrifying it must have been for this slender hazel-eyed young man, with his intimate understanding of the disease processes taking place within him, to suffer the torment of lying on his back, month after month, powerless to help himself, while that life and death battle was fought out in the intimacy of his own breast. Vallentin must have been well aware that his subsequent recovery owed less to the science of medicine than to the whims of a disease that had all of the despotic unpredictability of a Miltonic Satan.

Even during his convalescence at Hålahut, he began to assist the sanitorium doctors in their day to day work with other sufferers. An unassuming and softly spoken man, after his appointment in 1931 as chief physician to the prestigious Renström's Hospital, he established a working routine, six days a week, that began at seven in the morning and did not finish until eight in the evening or later. He would often go in and work a full day on Sundays too, calling on every one of the 200 patients in the entire hospital. It would have been hard to find a doctor more devoted to his patients than this hardworking Swede, with his kindly face, too long and gentle, it seemed, for his medium height and small frame. If Vallentin had a fault, it was his tendency to worry over his patients and what this terrible disease was doing to them, when he would on occasion be overtaken by a deep melancholy, instantly recognizable to those who knew and loved him.[13]

This was the man Lehmann had now engaged as his partner, to test PAS in human sufferers. Two more diverse personalities it would be hard to imagine.

v

IT WAS EXPECTING too much for Vallentin to accept Lehmann's claims for PAS without question. Like so many of the sanitorium directors, and with his own profound awe of the disease, Vallentin could not bring himself to believe that tuberculosis would ever be curable by drug treatment. He had tested all of the so-called wonder cures during the past twenty years, from arsenicals to gold, and he had been disappointed on every occasion. Even with Lehmann's persuasive charm, Vallentin was not prepared to try the new drug except in the most cautious of circumstances.

He agreed to try PAS as a local application, in a similar way to that used in the children. The condition he had in mind was called empyema, where tuberculosis has infected the delicate membranes and fluids surrounding the lung, filling the chest space with a thick cheesy pus. On 29 March, Vallentin began with his first patient, introducing a wide needle through the chest wall, draining out the pus, and then injecting a dilute solution of PAS every second day into the infected cavity. To his astonishment, when he measured the size of the cavity on X-rays, it gradually got smaller. Even more importantly, the patient felt better.

Vallentin now tried PAS as a treatment of empyema in a second patient. By the end of the summer, ten patients with empyema had been treated in this way. With a disease as devious as tuberculosis it was necessary to watch developments for many months, yet there seemed little doubt that the drug was having a beneficial effect. Lehmann now persuaded the sanitorium director to try something more adventurous: "I proposed that Dr Vallentin sluice 300mls or more at the same time over the pleura". The pleura was the delicate membrane within the chest that lined the entire lung and it was within this pleural space that pus accumulated in empyema. Vallentin tried this with two patients. The results were remarkable. Within just a few days their temperatures had returned to normal and they felt better.

Surely, Lehmann insisted, this fall in temperature must mean that the PAS was being absorbed into the blood stream from the membranes lining the chest cavity! In effect, the drug was having a beneficial effect throughout the patient's whole body. Lehmann used this argument to persuade Vallentin to give PAS by mouth to a patient suffering from pulmonary tuberculosis.

vi

ON 4 FEBRUARY 1944, Sigrid, a twenty-four-year-old woman, had her first baby at the Women's Clinic, in Gothenburg.[14] The obstetrician looking after her was concerned to find that both her mother and her brother had suffered from tuberculosis and arranged a chest X-ray, which was thankfully clear. The birth seemed to take a lot out of her and afterwards she felt persistently feeble. However, all seemed well otherwise and, after an uncomplicated confinement, her handyman husband took Sigrid and the baby home. There was a minor difficulty with breast feeding, and she was forced to abandon it. In early May, Sigrid started to feel sick and suffered bouts of vomiting. From May to June, she developed a troublesome cough, with a moderate amount of muco-purulent phlegm. But that strange listlessness that had begun with the childbirth had never in fact left her and now it grew progressively worse. She was losing weight rapidly. She had no thermometer to take her own temperature but she noticed no sweats at all and she did not feel feverish.

On 12 June she was seen at the medical clinic in the Sahlgren's Hospital, where the examining doctor thought she looked thin and sickly. The index of inflammation in her blood was raised, a non-specific pointer to something being seriously wrong. In view of the family history, he ordered another chest X-ray, which now showed an alarming change from the previous one. Widespread cloudy shadowing had erupted in both lungfields. The doctor examining Sigrid found her "delicately built, pale and thin, but otherwise in seemingly good general health". Her throat and ears were inflamed and she coughed rather a lot during the examination. The womb had shrunk to the size of a grapefruit, which was satisfactory for this time after the pregnancy. When they stained a sample of sputum and examined it, under the microscope, it was teeming with tuberculosis germs.

It was clear that Sigrid had developed tuberculosis towards the end of her pregnancy, but the infection in her lungs had been so early and mild it had not shown on her X-ray at that time. Now she was seriously ill with acute tuberculosis in both lungs, a very dangerous form of the disease. She was immediately transferred to the Renström's Sanitorium, where she came under Vallentin's care. To make matters more dangerous still, she was found to be pregnant again. The pregnancy constituted a grave threat to both the mother and the foetus and Sigrid had no choice but to suffer the additional distress of having the pregnancy terminated. This was performed on 26 June at the Women's Clinic and on 3 July she was brought back to the sanitorium for reassessment. Her chest X-ray already showed a rapid worsening. Sigrid was now suffering from a widespread tuberculous pneumonia.

She began the usual sanitorium regime of strict bed rest, following which there was some lessening of her cough and an improvement in her appetite. But she had a swinging temperature, which continued to climb at night, the inflammation index in her blood was persistently raised, and the tuberculosis germ was invariably seen in the stains of her sputum. By October Sigrid had entered the steady decline that was all too familiar to Gylfe Vallentin. In recent weeks this thin young woman had lost a further half stone in weight, her temperature was spiking above thirty-nine degees Centigrade every night, and she had developed a large hole or cavity at the apex of her right lung on the chest X-ray. Ominously, she had developed diffuse pains in her abdomen, felt sick after she had eaten any food, and by early October had developed diarrhoea. Her abdomen was now diffusely sore to touch, and had become swollen and tense. Vallentin was quite certain that her tuberculosis had spread to involve the intestines. He was in no doubt that Sigrid would soon die from her disease.

Vallentin discussed her case with Jorgen Lehmann. There was no longer anything to lose from trying out the new experimental treatment. Sigrid would be the first patient in history to be treated with PAS for pulmonary tuberculosis.

On 30 and 31 October 1944, a month before the young woman from Austin was given the first treatment with streptomycin for pulmonary tuberculosis, in Gothenburg, Sweden, Sigrid received her first cautious dose of PAS by mouth over just two days, a total of six grams, in divided doses the first day, and nine grams the second day. The drug had never been administered by mouth before and Vallentin could only guess at the dosage and duration of the course of treatment. Now, hardly daring to hope, and with an anxious Lehmann looking over his shoulder, he carefully observed her progress. There was a progressive but steady fall in the peaks of temperature over three or four days. But by 10 November the high swinging temperature was back and she was treated once again with PAS, but in larger doses by mouth, and for five consecutive days. The two doctors could not believe what they were observing. Sigrid's temperature progressively fell over five days or so, until it was normal. It remained well below the limits of normality for a full twelve days. More significantly, she felt much better, her cough decreased, eventually almost disappearing entirely, she felt noticeably stronger, and the sickness, abdominal swelling and diarrhoea all went away. She had, however, been nauseated while taking the tablets of PAS and it was quickly realized that this must be a side-effect of the new medication.

For Lehmann, there was an almost unbearable relief mixed with an ecstatic sense of jubilation. But the experienced Vallentin advised him to temper his celebration. Even though the inflammation index was slowly settling, the tuberculosis germs were still present in her sputum. Her tuberculosis was not yet healed.

Over the next two months she was treated with successive courses of PAS, each course of treatment resulting in a dramatic reduction in temperature and improvement in her general health, cough, appetite and increase in body weight. The blood tests also showed a dramatic improvement, and, most significant of all, the tuberculosis germs could no longer be seen in the stains of her sputum, so that, by March 1945, she was deemed fit enough to have an operation to close down the cavity at the apex of the right lung. Sigrid continued to receive longer and longer courses of PAS treatment, following which she made a sustained recovery. By April 1945, even the restrained Gylfe Vallentin felt able to write a single historic sentence in her case notes: "I am hoping for a complete cure!"

In December 1944, two further patients suffering from the extremely dangerous blood-borne tuberculosis were treated with PAS by Vallentin and both made a complete recovery, returning to normal health. In February 1945, Vallentin put a second patient suffering from pulmonary tuberculosis onto PAS treatment by mouth. A man aged thirty-five, he had a potentially fatal pulmonary tuberculosis with large pleural effusions over both lungs (fluid in the normally empty spaces between the lungs and the inner layer of chest wall). Guinea pig inoculation of the fluid from the pleural effusions confirmed the diagnosis of tuberculosis. Vallentin began PAS treatment on 16 February 1945, following which the man improved dramatically, gaining a stone in two months. On 26 June 1945, following the success of PAS in several patients with pulmonary tuberculosis, the drug was given by direct injection into a vein in two patients with tuberculous meningitis.

In a further major step forwards, a patient dying from tuberculous meningitis was also given PAS by direct injection into the cerebrospinal fluid, by means of a lumbar puncture. The recovery of this patient was every bit as miraculous as that of the first baby treated with streptomycin.[15] Jorgen Lehmann was now in a position to astonish the world.

vii

IN MARCH 1944, Professor Runnstrom of the Wenner-Gren Institute in Stockholm had invited Lehmann to take part in a meeting to discuss the current therapy for tuberculosis. Lehmann participated in the meeting but he did not mention PAS. At the time, he explained his thinking in a letter to Ferrosan.

"If I am going to say anything about para-aminosalicylic acid in order to establish priority, I shall be obliged at the same time to publish the experiments I have done. I think it wiser to remain silent until the clinical results are available."[16]

In retrospect this seems incomprehensible. Even at this early stage, he already had as much evidence from studies of the effect of PAS on cultures of tuberculosis germs as Schatz and Waksman had prior to their first paper on streptomycin. But Waksman's life revolved about bacteria and therefore, in his view, the bacterial experiments were his very aim and purpose. Lehmann, who was medical and a biochemist rather than a bacteriologist, inevitably saw benefit in human sufferers as his only interest. Indeed his words, in that letter to Ferrosan, make this abundantly clear.

There were additional pressures upon Lehmann which may have contributed to his curious caution. Ferrosan was having difficulty with patenting the new discovery. In the words of Karl Rosdahl: "As soon as we could confirm the results on the tested materials, we tried to apply for a patent. The first compound tested, PAS, appeared to give the best results. But PAS had already been synthesized in the nineteenth century for an entirely different purpose. Nobody seemed to know its formula, we only knew how to make it – and to get a sole patent (world rights) for the manufacture appeared impossible. It was, however, still possible to register a patent for the manufacture in several countries."[17]

In other words, if Lehmann published the results of his research too early, any other pharmaceutical company in the world could have jumped on the bandwagon. For Ferrosan's investment, this might have proved ruinous.

Yet, by the end of 1944, no less than twenty patients had been treated with PAS by mouth and by February, 1945, afraid that rumours about the success of PAS were already circulating, Vallentin was pressing Lehmann for publication. Lehmann declined the opportunity. "We had an agreement, Vallentin, Ferrosan and myself, to keep the PAS project secret for as long as possible, this being the reason behind my failure to publish the bacteriological and animal experiments, which were by now a year old."[18] By March, 1945, worried that other scientists must surely be working along the same lines, he had changed his mind.

Ferrosan could not prevent Lehmann publishing at this time or indeed at any time earlier, although they were still having difficulty patenting the discovery. There was nothing unusual in the company wishing to patent its discovery but in sad consequence, Rosdahl's name was omitted from the paper that first communicated the discovery of PAS to the world.[19]

On 9 April 1945, Lehmann wrote a two-page article to the journal, *Nature*. But *Nature* refused to publish it on the grounds that they could not accept the illustrations that were part of his article. In this way, an editorial rule not only cost *Nature* a first publication of global importance but, more importantly, it caused a further delay in the global perception of the discovery. On 25 August, Lehmann sent the same article back to *Nature* without the illustrations and this time it was accepted for publication in the spring of 1946. On 24 November 1945, an important forum was open to him, with the yearly meeting of the tuberculosis section of the Swedish Medical Society in Stockholm, but once again he lost the opportunity. He had left it too late to apply to present a full lecture. PAS was not presented in a formal manner, only broached during the discussion.

By this time, forty-five patients with pulmonary tuberculosis had been treated, thirteen with local treatment of empyema and thirty-one treated with PAS by mouth. PAS had been given to its first patient by intravenous injection. Where at first Vallentin had only given the drug by mouth to advanced cases, the lack of harmful side effects had encouraged Vallentin to try the drug in less advanced cases. Even on this small stage, during the discussion at the Swedish Medical Society meeting, Gylfe Vallentin felt he had to present those first successes in the most conservative case imaginable:

"Without reservation, one could state that PAS was not harmful. Obvious benefit has been seen from the point of view of wellbeing, body temperature and sedimentation rate. In some cases we have seen clearing up and diminishing of the X-ray appearances but whether these effects would have occurred anyway or whether they resulted from the drug we cannot say"[20].

Lehmann would later bemoan how Vallentin shook his head even as he spoke with a downbeat tone: "The improvement may be due to spontaneous remission." Lehmann could not resist an ironic aside: "It is curious how these spontaneous remissions so often occur just after giving the patient PAS!"[21]

Vallentin, though of a melancholy disposition, was highly regarded by the tuberculosis specialists throughout Sweden. Sadly, his ultra-cautious conclusions jangled an identical chord of pessimism in the minds of his audience. Dr Beskow, who was present, would later remark how Vallentin's presentation evoked little interest. "On so very many previous occasions, we had experienced nothing but disappointment from so many of these new 'effective' anti-tuberculous drugs. This had been emphasized during the introductory lecture at this very same meeting. Nobody attending this meeting realized that this discovery by Lehmann was the beginning of a new era in the history of the fight against tuberculosis."[22]

To be fair to Vallentin, the first assessments of streptomycin by Hinshaw and his colleagues were every bit as conservative, and for precisely the same reasons.

At last the first definitive paper that would describe the revolutionary potential of PAS in tuberculosis, albeit a preliminary report, appeared in the *Lancet*, on 5 January 1946.[23]

It seems extraordinary that the world at large had to wait two whole years to learn about the remarkable bacteriological and the animal experiments first performed in January 1944. Para-aminosalicylic acid had been first synthesized at precisely the same time streptomycin was discovered by Albert Schatz. It had been administered to the first human sufferer from pulmonary tuberculosis a month earlier than streptomycin. But the world knew nothing of this. As far as history was concerned, and the inevitable consequence of this delay, PAS appeared to have been discovered some two years later than streptomycin. Although such recognition did not matter a jot as far as suffering patients were concerned, it would have profound repercussions for Lehmann some six years later. Anybody reading this paper can see that Lehmann was solely preoccupied with the human studies. He quickly moves through the animal work, pointing to the fact that it appeared to rule out serious side-effects, before moving on to discuss the results of treatment with PAS in twenty patients suffering from tuberculosis.

Sigrid and the thirty-four-year-old man with tuberculous pleural effusions were presented very briefly as part of this paper. Two very dramatic stories of human sufferers who would have died from the disease without the intercession of PAS, the drug was now catapulted into the sensational world of miracle cure.

Newspapers in many countries carried the story. As with streptomycin some eighteen months earlier, passionate appeals for help flooded Lehmann's office at the Sahlgren's Hospital in Gothenburg and the offices of Ferrosan in Malmö. In the words of Karl Rosdahl: "I received many tragic letters, often the last cry for help from patients and their families, some even from doctors who were themselves sick with tuberculosis. Two were pleas to help a very highly placed person in China during the leaderships of Chiang Kai-Shek and Mao Tse-Tung. They arrived from all over the world."[24]

16

Storm Clouds over Gothenburg

I'd like to mention a funny incident. Professor Berglund from Stockholm was visiting Gothenburg and I told him in confidence that I was trying to find a cure for tuberculosis. He replied: "Can you tell me of any garage where they are not trying?"

Jorgen Lehmann

i

FROM THE MOMENT of its first inspired creation, the PAS discovery would be dogged by cynical Cassandras. As early as 1944, when the very first whispers of the discovery were rippling outwards amongst medical circles in Sweden, the Ferrosan director, Ryné, was subjected to doomladen predictions, which often took their origins from highly respectable members of the medical profession. One such typical prediction took the form of a telephone call from an eminent professor of chest diseases: "All work towards finding a cure for tuberculosis is senseless because the bacteria are encapsulated in such a way that they are out of reach of such therapies."[1] Nothing could have been so conspired to cause alarm.

For Ryné it resurrected all the old fears of the Sanocrysin débâcle. He immediately called Rosdahl to his office and told him that "Lehmann's excesses" could not go on. Controlling Lehmann, however, was not going to be an easy matter. He was not only brilliant, he was also wickedly impulsive. Rosdahl was told in no uncertain terms that if Lehmann's imagination stayed in the clouds, then he – Rosdahl – would have to keep his feet on earth. He would be responsible for safeguarding Ferrosan's investment.[2]

Towards the end of August, 1945, Ryné called a meeting with Rosdahl, Vallentin and Lehmann. Lehmann wondered what was going on since, in the clinical stage of testing they were obtaining spectacular results. But in fact it was the very success of the PAS research, at a time when the drug could only be manufactured by the complex and very expensive five stage synthesis devised by Rosdahl, that was putting the small company under increasing financial pressure. The PAS research had already cost Ferrosan 370,000 crowns and still there was nothing definite: the results were insecure, and many doctors were expressing frank disbelief.[3] Rumours were circulating that the drug was not really a cure at all and the anxious management was hardly reassured by Vallentin's cautious interpretation of the early clinical results.

To Ryné, who had committed his company to the enterprise, this looked suspiciously like a lack of faith on the part of the very clinician testing the drug. He gave them an ultimatum: if Vallentin could not provide him with a written statement to the effect that PAS would cure tuberculosis, the product would be abandoned. "Our costs," he insisted to the dumbfounded Lehmann and Vallentin, "have been disastrous."[4]

Vallentin however was not a man to be easily coerced against his own judgement. Unassuming he might appear, but this same stoical man had joined the International Red Cross in 1918, risking his life to protect returning prisoners of war. In Russia, caught up in the aftermath of the October Revolution, he had had to be rescued from a firing squad at the very last minute. Now, in response to Ryné's ultimatum, he reacted violently. "No!" he declared, adamantly. "Not under any circumstances!"[5]

Rosdahl and Lehmann did their best to persuade him to change his mind. They protested that his excessive caution was endangering the entire future of the research. But Vallentin would not write the statement. Rosdahl took Ryné at his word. In some alarm, he approached the company president,

Weissman, at Ferrosan's headquarters in Copenhagen, who supported the continuing research and sent a communication to Ryné affirming his full confidence in Rosdahl and the project.

Though Ryné was somewhat mollified, the threat was not lifted. In desperation, Rosdahl sat on the staircase outside a lecture hall where Lehmann and Vallentin were lecturing, blocking their exit in order to persuade both doctors to put their signatures to a written statement he had prepared. This was to the effect that they unanimously regarded PAS an important medical breakthrough and that it would be tragic if the development of the drug were to be abandoned.[6] This letter, together with the promise of the funds raised by Lehmann and Vallentin's efforts, was enough to reassure Ryné and he recanted. To Lehmann . . . "the decision not to close down production of PAS was a great relief to me. Now we could go on working peacefully and present our results with PAS at the tuberculosis meeting in Stockholm, on 24 November 1945." Then, out of the blue, on 20 December, Lehmann was once again summoned by letter to Malmö to meet up with the company director, on "questions concerning PAS which demand an immediate decision".

Fearing the worst, he arrived at Ferrosan on 20 December to be informed, on the contrary, that Karl Rosdahl had devised a more efficient chemical process of making the drug. In place of five major chemical manipulations, the new method involved four. Not only did Ryné feel more secure with cheaper production costs, but Rosdahl could now promise Lehmann that from February 1946 Ferrosan would be able to provide him with much larger quantities of the drug, as much as 16 to 20 kg of PAS a month. Following such a period of alarm, this was magnificent news. It gave the ever increasing trials a tremendous new impulse. Their scope could now be widened to include many more doctors and sanitoria.

Following the Stockholm meeting, two professors, Kristensson and Westergren, had already requested supplies of PAS for testing in their patients. Now Vallentin could include them, together with Dr Törnell at the Vasterasens Sanitorium, greatly increasing the numbers of patients that could be tested.

Each centre was allowed at least 1 kg of PAS per week. Soon another doctor, Selander in Malmö, was also provided with small amounts for testing. However, with the widening of clinical application, a new danger was at once apparent.

Any news of a cure for tuberculosis was dynamite as far as the press was concerned. Exaggerated claims made too early in the research could jeopardize the reputation of the drug with the conservative medical establishment. This applied in particular to the directors of the many sanitoria throughout Sweden, who felt that the treatment of tuberculosis was their sole prerogative, and who had good reason to fear a new false messiah, having seen many such cures raise great expectations in their patients only to end in heartbreak after proper scientific assessment had been carried out. It was therefore an avowed common policy that the doctors participating in the PAS research would not communicate with the media and particularly not with the press. Everybody remotely concerned with the research was sworn to secrecy, a blanket of silence that extended even to their families.[7] This need for secrecy was particularly important in anticipation of the first national presentation of their findings at the thirteenth meeting of the Nordic Tuberculosis Physicians in Gothenburg, in June 1946.

Lehmann had been joined, in January 1945, by a colleague called Sievers, newly appointed as chief bacteriologist to the Sahlgren's Hospital, and who from then on had taken over all the test tube and animal research studies. Hjalmar Richard Olof Sievers[8] – addressed as Olof – was forty-seven-years-old and the son of Richard Sievers, who had been an eminent professor of internal medicine at Helsinki University. Richard Sievers had been dismissed from his post as Surgeon General of Finland by the Czar Nikolai, because of his anti-Russian and pro-Finnish sympathies at a time when Finland was ruled by the iron fist of Moscow. In 1918, Olof Sievers had himself taken to the streets of Helsinki with a gun in his hands, when the Finns threw off their Russian overlords, and he had served Finland throughout most of the second world war as head of biological services to the armed forces. During the last year of the war, Sievers, who was now being victimized in his own country because he was Swedish speaking and married to a Swedish wife, was delighted to move to Gothenburg, his wife's native city. Lehmann, the Danish immigrant, took to this rebellious Finn from the moment they first met. Soon they were not only working colleagues but the closest of friends.

In the spring of 1946, during their preparatory discussions about the forthcoming Nordic Physicians Meeting, it was decided that each of the three doctors involved in the research, Olof Sievers, Gylfe Vallentin and Jorgen Lehmann, would deliver a formal lecture. They were determined to present as full and up to date a picture of the PAS researches as they could to this very important meeting, which attracted all of the leading tuberculosis doctors throughout Scandinavia and Finland. Lehmann would begin with the discovery of the drug, describe the early experiments on tuberculosis in test tubes and laboratory animals and then go on to their experiences with the first few patients. Sievers would follow with a more general exposition of the drug's potential action against various disease-causing bacteria. Vallentin would close with the most auspicious lecture of all and the fulcrum about which the entire presentation would revolve, the comprehensive results of the treatment of pulmonary tuberculosis in human sufferers with PAS.

All three doctors felt nervous in anticipation of Gothenburg, which would be crucial in telling the world about the drug's great potential.

ii

ALTHOUGH THE *Lancet* paper had appeared a few months earlier that year, this had been no more than a preliminary communication. The media still knew virtually nothing of the true importance of the drug. Lehmann, who was still anxious to avoid public overreaction, was well aware that the presentation at an open meeting to hundreds of colleagues would end the secrecy that had up to now cloaked their efforts. Rather than wait for the inevitable hysteria, it seemed prudent to supply the media with some carefully-worded statement, which would present the drug in a rational and conservative light. "At the conference I proposed that a written press release on the effect of PAS on lung tuberculosis should be prepared by Vallentin and left with the press the day before the meeting. This was issued with a specific promise from the newspapers not to publish until the congress was over."[9]

This is the statement provided by Vallentin, under the terms of the above embargo, to the press.

"When trying to evaluate the results of any sort of therapy for tuberculosis, you are inevitably faced with great difficulties. The disease process is very enduring so that the effect of a specific treatment cannot be assessed until a prolonged period of observation has elapsed, extending for years and even decades. Often there may be unexpected natural remissions. If these spontaneous remissions coincide with treatment, it is very easy to infer a mistaken relationship between treatment and such spontaneous remissions. But with a full understanding of such margins for error, we have during our treatment with PAS at the Renström Sanitorium witnessed improvements that we think might be interpreted as an effect of the drug. This effect is not so dramatic as to allow us to say we have 'cured' tuberculosis with this agent. We have just seen a change in the course of the disease which has made it possible for the body itself with its natural healing capacity to begin the healing process.

"The agent is totally safe and we have found no side-effects at all. The effects we have witnessed are a reduction in fever, improved general condition, the disappearance of tb bacteria from sputum and the clearing of X-rays. The agent has proved beneficial only in certain forms of the disease. It cannot be used generally but must be tested in certain selected cases. For this reason and because it cannot be manufactured other than in very limited amounts, further testing must be reserved to certain hospitals. At the Renström Sanitorium we have so far treated eighty-two cases. Some of these have not as yet completed their courses of treatment. We believe that we can conclude that there has been an effect which in some cases is temporary, yet nevertheless an effect in fifty-three cases."[10]

No pronouncement could have been more guarded or prudent. Yet in spite of Lehmann's carefully worked plan for a judicious press release, it was only natural that those journalists who had received a copy of Vallentin's statement would want to rush into print. A potential cure for tuberculosis was news on a world stage. In today's terms, Vallentin's statement was tantamount to a doctor announcing, no matter how cautiously, that he had found the universal cure for cancer. Indeed the journalists only need make a few discreet local enquiries in Gothenburg to discover patients who regarded themselves as miracle cures. With news of such momentous importance, it was a little optimistic to have leaked a word of it to the press a day before a meeting where they planned to present those same facts to their medical colleagues.

To their credit, the vast majority of the newspapers kept their promise. Sadly, one Stockholm newspaper, *Stockholmstidingen*, broke with the story the following morning. On the 26 June, when they came down to breakfast, the conference delegates could hardly miss the headlines that glowered back at them from their morning papers: A REMARKABLE SWEDISH EFFORT IN THE STRUGGLE AGAINST TUBERCULOSIS. A NEW DRUG, the paper declared, PREPARED BY PROFESSOR LEHMANN ... SCIENTIFIC BREAKTHROUGH AT THE SAHLGREN'S HOSPITAL.[11]

The impact upon the conservative medical establishment can well be imagined.

A day later, with the embargo already broken, every other newpaper in Scandinavia followed the leader. In the *Göteborgs Handels*, the *Göteborgsposten*, *Svenska Dagbladet*, *Ny Dag*, *Dagens Nyheter*, A NEW DRUG AGAINST TUBERCULOSIS ... A NEW SWEDISH DRUG AGAINST TUBERCULOSIS ... A NEW WEAPON AGAINST TUBERCULOSIS ... All through the conference Lehmann, Vallentin and Sievers would be embarrassed by such headline disclosures.

When it came to the formal lectures, Vallentin presented his findings in much the same tenor of understatement that had characterized his press release.[12] After acknowledging the vital role of Lehmann in discovering the drug and the help he had had from his assistants, Ingvar Råman, Stephen Aminoff and Leo Blecher, in the clinical testing, he continued: "We found very soon that the agent (PAS) was entirely harmless. Thus we observed no symptoms of toxic damage to the blood or internal organs. The most troublesome effects of the treatment have been a few digestive upsets, which did not generally cause serious inconvenience... It has not yet been possible to prepare the agent except in limited amounts, so that it has not yet proved possible to set up larger series of experiments. We have found it necessary to limit the number of cases, which were then followed up as closely as possible. Even now the period of observation appears too short to permit a definitive evaluation of the impression which in certain cases amounts to an appreciable beneficial effect, based upon the usual clinical findings, the general condition, temperature course, blood picture, sedimentation rate (blood index of inflammation), X-ray picture, bacterial count, etc."

Although the more fiery Lehmann was critical of such a conservative introduction, in fact, given the press reaction, this was precisely what was needed. Vallentin now went on to give a clear indication of the drug's potential.

"Firstly, the general condition of our patients has shown a definite improvement in all cases. The general wellbeing has increased, the appetite improved, and the tissue turgidity has improved. Even in cases which followed an unfavourable course this improvement in wellbeing has necessarily been transient, nevertheless the impression has been that the agent had a certain general strengthening effect."

He went on to describe how, in combination with the usual sanitorium regimen and in some cases together with surgical measures such as collapse treatment, he had seen the course of the disease inclined towards recovery in some cases which, in his opinion, would have otherwise been destined to die. In Vallentin's words: "It seems highly probable that the reduction of temperature observed in the patients is not merely an effect on the patient's temperature without other importance for the course of the disease. The fall in temperature has rarely been associated with sweating (usual with aspirin's nonspecific effect), while signs of a more far-reaching effect have been demonstrated simultaneously. The sedimentation rate has declined, the X-ray picture has cleared, tuberculosis bacilli have disappeared from the sputum, and the haemoglobin values have risen. When one has seen in case after case how an appreciable and favourable change in the course of the disease has occurred with the initiation of the use of the drug, one is unable to avoid the impression that the agent has had a certain favourable effect on the disease picture."

Vallentin went on to present more detailed case reports in a series of patients: all of twelve patients tried with either tuberculosis affecting the glands at the root of the lung or frank pulmonary tuberculosis had improved; nine of seventeen with long-standing fibrotic tuberculosis of the lungs had improved; twenty-four of thirty patients with exudative pulmonary tuberculosis had improved. There were, admittedly, types that did not improve and he listed six patients with blood-borne (miliary) disease and meningitis, all of whom had died. There were others, with long-standing disease and existing damage, which was well-known to be irreversible, who did not benefit much or not at all.

His concluding words were typically modest. "If we have been lax or mistaken in our assessment of these results, then future research will show. Our experience has in any case been encouraging. We think that with all the necessary reservation it is justified to put forward these experiences."

Then it was time for his audience to comment and put questions to all three speakers.[13]

iii

To ALLOW FOR what followed, one must take into account the fact that previous wonder cures had universally failed, that the trials described by Vallentin were not measured against a control series of patients carefully matched with the PAS patients in terms of severity of condition, and, most vital of all, that the drug was a derivative of aspirin, perhaps the most commonly abused medication in history.

Dr Alf Westergren, a senior physician from St Gorans Hospital, Stockholm, who had achieved world eminence in the field of blood examination, was one of the very few who had kind words to say: "I congratulate Professor Lehmann on what he has done with para-aminosalicylic acid in tuberculosis treatment. Even if this takes us no further than the sulphones – and I think it will – I believe that Professor Lehmann's research represents a bigger scientific contribution than that of Waksman." Westergren, however, went on to express how dismayed he was to see how publicity had been stirred up in the press about this.

Other members of the audience were not so kindly disposed towards the speakers. Dr Erik Hedvall (Uppsala) began cordially enough: "It is a good thing that such a prominent researcher as Professor Lehmann should turn his attentions to the chemotherapy of tuberculosis. We can expect a long series of such preparations in the near future which promise as much yet, after close examination, prove to be ineffective." No doubt, influenced by the memory of sanocrysin, reinforced by Hinshaw and Feldman's recent report of toxicity with Promin, Hedvall added his devastating conclusion: "In my opinion, PAS is just another example of such a preparation." He too regretted the sensational publicity and felt compelled to comment upon it: "Have these people been primed by the drug company which has no doubt been involved in major expenses developing the drug? It is a serious cause of regret that physicians should lend their dignity to this type of thing, particularly since the medicinal value of the preparation is extremely doubtful." It was, he added, a pity that patients would now have their hopes raised only to suffer disappointment. "Ladies and gentlemen," he concluded, "let us continue our work against tuberculosis and go about this energetically but let us not go to the press before a proven agent against tuberculosis has been found."

Professor Heimbeck (Oslo) was of the opinion that these experiments showed precisely nothing. "I should like to ask Vallentin if the only objective influence of PAS on tuberculosis has been the fact that the temperature has gone down – surely this is just an effect of salicylic acid. Have you used PAS against other febrile diseases. Does PAS merely work as an antipyretic?" Lehmann would later remark that this appeared to deliver a knockout punch to Vallentin. Heimbeck, who went on to dismiss utterly the benefits of PAS: "The experiments Professor Lehmann reported concerning the injection of PAS intraperitoneally in guinea pigs in fact showed us nothing . . . It is no more than we would expect from other old medicaments such as Turbans pill, which contains a small dose of salicylic acid and arsenic."

Heimbeck had misunderstood the entire presentation. It was tuberculous bacteria and not PAS Lehmann had injected intra-peritoneally in guinea pigs. And Vallentin had taken care to dismiss the temperature lowering effects of aspirin during his presentation. In reply to Heimbeck's dismissive comments, Vallentin stressed once again that he was in no doubt that the results he had presented for PAS encouraged further research. However, on behalf of Lehmann and Sievers, he very much regretted the press intervention.

Lehmann interrupted to counter the Norwegian doctor's assertions, and to make absolutely sure that every single member of their audience understood very clearly that PAS was not having an aspirin-like effect. This was the most important source of confusion. Lehmann had tried PAS in children suffering from acute rheumatic fever and only in one patient had he seen a slight lowering of temperature. As to the malici-ous suggestion of Hedvall with regard to Ferrosan, he defended the company, which was in truth entirely innocent of any in-volvement in the press release. "We have been performing these experiments for over two years and with some difficulty have managed to keep it secret." Lehmann, who was deeply upset about the newspaper intervention, would, later that day, make a telephone call to the offending newspaper in Stockholm and complain about the ethics of their journalists.[14]

But this was now water under the bridge: the meeting which should have been the flagship for PAS had ended in disaster.

iv

THE DRUG HAD attracted an undeserved opprobrium at a time of maximum vulnerability, when nobody in the country except Vallentin and two colleagues, Difs and Alin, from Kristen-sson's clinic, had had the opportunity to treat any patients with it. The controversy did not end with the ill-fated Gothenburg meeting. Dr Forsgren, a senior chest physician at Svenshögens Sanitorium, forty miles north of Gothenburg, openly attacked PAS in a series of articles published in the Swedish physicians' journal. In Lehmann's opinion, Forsgren's articles, though expressing no more than this one man's opinion, nevertheless ... "give an impression of the psychological environment on the tuberculosis front in those days."

In 1947, Forsgren opened battle with an article: "Para-aminosalicylic acid treatment of tuberculosis proves fatal".[15] A woman with tuberculosis of both lungs had been treated with PAS for two months. One year after completing chemotherapy, she was readmitted under Forsgren with cavities on one lung, one of which was the size of a hen's egg. She was treated once more, at her own request, with PAS, following which she improved, though she was never completely free of fever. She suddenly died of a pulmonary haemorrhage, a known complication of lung cavitation. Forsgren however claimed that PAS had caused the haemorrhage and therefore her death. The basis of his claim probably lay in the fact that aspirin, which has well-known effects on blood clotting, is also known to cause a slight risk of haemorrhage from the stomach.

He went on to report a second case, in which tuberculosis of both lungs and throat had appeared to be cured with PAS. Treatment had been discontinued when supplies of the drug had run out. The patient had to be readmitted some three months later with cavities in her lungs. At this stage, PAS, administered in smaller dosage because of side-effects, did not prevent deterioration and the patient died. Forsgren now had his own theory that PAS might also hasten the formation of cavities.

Forsgren's arguments were nonsense and Vallentin's riposte in the same issue of the journal made clear that the frequency of haemorrhages in the many patients he had treated with PAS was not increased – it was considerably reduced.[16] Forsgren responded, with the bit well and truly between his teeth.

In another article in the same journal, he returned to the attack, with, in Lehmann's words, "a blossoming sarcasm so funny, it was truly inspired".

"On the back of a little PAS you add a little streptomycin here, a little Conteben, or penicillin, or aureomycin, or chloromycetin there. The doses and the duration of treatment changes from year to year and from artist to artist. Some like to exhibit their works of art for public inspection and admiration. Then the public demand more of the same, which makes it difficult for the critical and sceptical painter, who is afraid to damage the greatest work of art of all – the human being"[17]

Forsgren, who was only getting warmed up, issued article after article, discrediting PAS which he now refused to prescribe for his patients, meanwhile the patients themselves, following the tidal wave of publicity, continued to demand the drug of him. To an extent, of course, Forsgren may have been ahead of his time in foreseeing actions of aspirin that would later assume global importance in the prevention of blood clots. He was correct too in baldly stating that PAS was not the total cure for consumption. No more was streptomycin. Unfortunately, this imaginative doctor, in the grip of monomania, could admit no benefit from PAS that was not totally outweighed by side-effects that in reality did not exist. It was a black comedy, in which, in Lehmann's typical reflection, Forsgren . . . "was the cat playing with the mouse. He takes a jump and makes a stab at his booty and then lets it run away in order to jump again and bite it."[18]

Although Forsgren was the only doctor who wrote about the drug in this rabidly disparaging manner, the physicians' journal was a paper read by every physician in Sweden; inevitably it gave a very bad impression. Other doctors would later confess to Lehmann that they had no confidence in PAS until they had tried it for themselves on their own patients. Lehmann sighed: "What could the tuberculosis physicians as a whole think of PAS after this congress? It could be summed up in two words: common disbelief."[19]

Vallentin returned home from the meeting in the deepest pit of melancholy. In spite of the encouragement of friends such as Törnell, this terrible depression would weigh upon him for many months to come.[20] The incredulous reaction of so many sanitoria doctors to PAS, which was reported in detail in several newspapers, had an even more disastrous impact on the Ferrosan director, Ryné. On 14 September, a month or so after the Gothenburg meeting, he called an urgent meeting with the doctors involved in the research, when he told them that Ferrosan could not afford to supply the drug free of charge in any more quantities than currently used in the trials already under way. Meanwhile more and more sanitoria doctors were requesting supplies for testing. Lehmann advised Ryné that any hesitancy now would be seen by enemies and competitors alike as a sign of weakness. The threat was so alarming that he volunteered to go out with "the beggar's staff", and raise charitable donations.

This was the confused situation in the autumn of 1946, when Lehmann, Sievers and Vallentin were compelled to approach every possible charitable source for money to keep the research programme on its course of expansion. By November, they had managed to raise 65,000 crowns. On 8 December, a single grateful patient handed Vallentin, the caring doctor who had saved his life, the magnificent sum of an additional 35,000 crowns. By this time they had raised sufficient money to guarantee a further year's supply of the drug for testing. This was a vital intercession, which would take the struggle for recognition forwards to the spring of 1947, when on 26 April, the Swedish National Board for Tuberculosis assembled all of the PAS researchers for a meeting of fundamental importance for the drug. Present at this meeting were Berg, as chairman, Lundquist, the secretary, Kristensson, Westergren, Vallentin, Törnell, Beskow, Carstensen, Difs and Lehmann himself.

The purpose of this gathering was to initiate a major new trial of PAS, involving six different sanitoria, in which patients with active pulmonary tuberculosis would be treated in the first scientifically controlled study, comparing the effects of PAS with those of a control regime (the normal sanitorium rest and nutrition).

Meanwhile the real sufferers from tuberculosis gave Lehmann heart with letters of thanks. In a card from the Solbackens sanitorium, sent to him in 1948, a cured patient wrote the words: "Professor Lehmann, Gothenburg. Thanks for new hope. Congratulations and hope for further success in your work." And another – "Good news. TB bacillus has dined and died without leaving a will, bereft of new generations to inherit its mantle."[21] On May day 1948, in a heartbreaking demand for treatment with the wonder drug, an unprecedented demonstration took place at Kronoborgs Sanitorium, where a gathering of emaciated patients marched round the grounds with placards, reading: "We want more PAS" and "Hoorah for Lehmann!"[22]

One such patient would subsequently recount his extraordinary experiences.

In the autumn of 1941, a young man called Åke Hanngren, living in Stockholm, first discovered that his life had entered the nightmare of pulmonary tuberculosis.

In 1941, I found myself in the Swedish army, a young man of twenty years of age, standing guard on our borders, when I contracted tuberculosis. I was admitted to hospital, the Savsjo Sanitorium, and treated with an artificial pneumothorax. Before my military service, I had already been studying medicine for one year. Now, discharged from the army with tuberculosis, I tried my best to get back into medical school to follow my career but I developed a tuberculous empyema (pus in the chest cavity). In 1946 tuberculosis spread to my other lung too and soon it also involved my intestines and my throat. I was just a skeleton, lying in a hospital in Stockholm.

In those years, from 1945 to 1946, my mother would come and sit by my bed weeping. I was so upset about her, I asked if I could be transferred somewhere in the country where she could not follow me. I was sent up to Osterasens Sanitorium in the north of Sweden, which was regarded as the best, the "Davos" of Sweden.

I couldn't sit up. I had cavities in both lungs. I knew I was dying. Being something of an amateur painter, and while I still had some strength left, I painted my self-portrait, which, I think, shows much of how I was feeling.[23] At that time I read about PAS in some experimental journal. I had never heard of Jorgen Lehmann until then.

I wrote to Jorgen Lehmann in Gothenburg, telling him I was a medical student and that I was very, very ill. Couldn't he perform his experiments on me? He answered that he had already performed his experiments on patients in Gothenburg. PAS was so contaminated with impure products and people were suffering some side-effects . . . but it also cured these people. I wrote to him again and said I didn't care about these side-effects. Lehmann wrote back that he would speak to Ferrosan and after a week or so I received a parcel containing half a kilo-gram of PAS, together with Lehmann's personal instructions. It was rather a big parcel.

I started to take this and within two days started to vomit. But when I saw all the people around me dying, whenever I vomited the drug, I just took another dose of exactly the same. I had been suffering fevers of 41° Centigrade for three months and now, just one week after starting the drug, I was free of fever. My throat hurt me to eat before; now I could eat. I took PAS three times a day, after each meal. I didn't dare to tell the chief physician at the hospital for he was against all new things. He had tried sanocrysin and seen so many disappointments, he couldn't believe it would work.

When I was free of fever and could sit up in the bed, I had to tell him and he said: 'All right! All right! Continue to take it. I can see you are better. But don't tell anyone else about it. I know we can't get hold of this medicine. At this present moment, we cannot obtain any supply at all.' He was afraid his patients would kill him if he didn't get hold of this medicine for them.

After only one week or so, I could use the toilet in the corridor. I had been placed in a cubicle because I was dying. Now people could see me in the corridor. They realized that some miracle had happened. The physician was surrounded in his room by patients clamouring for the new treatment. He had to telegram Lehmann and after about six months he managed to get some PAS for his other patients.

But I was healed. I recovered with no other therapy.[24]

Åke Hanngren went on to become the professor of chest medicine at the Caroline Institute in Stockholm, and later on Director of the Swedish Heart-Lung Association. Yet in spite of such wonderful successes, the initial delay in publishing the discovery of PAS, the difficulties in production of the drug in larger quantities, the disastrous negativity of so many of the Swedish chest physicians, all conspired to detract from the true and wonderful potential of the Swedish discovery. Meanwhile streptomycin had taken the world by storm.

17

Life and Death

Who was this guy, Schatz? Most people have never heard of him. But I knew him well, because he was a graduate student returning to Rutgers the very time that I got there – a poverty stricken, brilliant, Jr Phi Beta Kappa, who worked with a burning intensity, and brought Waksman's attention to focus on his thesis isolate, Streptomyces griseus.

Doris Jones: fellow researcher at Rutgers
during the streptomycin discovery.

i

ON 29 JANUARY 1945, William Feldman sent Selman Waksman a telegram: "Long term crucial experiment streptomycin terminated today. Incomplete results indicate impressive therapeutic effects."[1] A letter from H. Corwin Hinshaw was to follow, remarking on the progress of two patients on longer term treatment, including the young woman. "The results are sufficiently encouraging to be tantalizing, and we cannot avoid the feeling that if we could give a million or more units a day we might have something more impressive."[2]

From those early trials of streptomycin in the first few human sufferers, the testing of streptomycin now accelerated dizzyingly. The wonder drug was needed in ever larger amounts for an escalating series of clinical trials. Astonished by the rapidly accelerating pace of the tests yet simultaneously alarmed by the difficulties they were having with supplies of the new drug,

Hinshaw made a personal plea to Dr Chester Keefer, of the American National Research Council, on 23 January 1945, to see that everything possible was done to expedite the production of the drug in large enough quantities for more tests.[3] Keefer was so concerned with the insatiable demand, his committee recommended rationing of the drug. There would be no further supplies sent to the huge miscellany of petitioners. For the moment it would only be made available for the most important of scientific requests.

On 25 August, Hinshaw reported even more favourable results in thirty-three patients, including many with very severe and extensive disease. They were planning to extend their treatment to tuberculosis in the army, setting up research stations at Fitzsimons General Hospital and at Burns General Hospital, when they were pre-empted by the War Production Board, which took over the allocation of streptomycin.

On 5 September 1945, scarcely a year after the first trials of streptomycin in guinea pigs, Hinshaw and Feldman published the results of streptomycin treatment in the first human sufferers from tuberculosis. This report, appearing in the bi-weekly journal of the Mayo Clinic,[4] made it clear that they were still awaiting completion of full and detailed studies; nevertheless the results to date were so important they felt obliged to share their limited experiences of streptomycin with their colleagues. Thirty-four patients suffering from tuberculosis had now been treated with streptomycin. Hinshaw was receiving the drug in a much purer form and in larger quantities from George Merck & Co. At first they had proceeded over-cautiously, with inadequately small doses, but, following a more detailed pharmacological evaluation of the drug, they now had a much clearer guide on the doses needed and any problems that might be encountered.

"Streptomycin," they wrote, "is a drug of low toxicity for man and the doses described . . . have rarely caused any serious reactions, even continued for several weeks without interruption. There is usually some pain at the sites of repeated injections but this is no more severe than that caused by penicillin." They went on to list an array of minor side-effects before mentioning that one patient had suffered a temporary deafness while three other patients had suffered a disturbance of balance, which appeared to result from damage to the vestibular organ in the inner ear. This suggested that, in a minority of humans, streptomycin might have a selective poisonous effect on the nerve of hearing and balance.

Sixteen patients with pulmonary tuberculosis had now been treated with the drug and eight of these observed after treatment for periods of up to four months. In the majority, there was a steady improvement of their clinical condition, with slow clearing of the abnormalities on the chest X-ray. "It is important to note that streptomycin did not appear to have any rapidly effective curative action in these cases but that extensive and progressive lesions of known recent origin have tended to improve promptly in a manner which resembles the natural process of healing". Long-standing tuberculosis, with its destructive scarring and cavitation in the lungs, was a different matter and the sputum of these patients "may remain positive indefinitely".[5] In the dramatically fatal blood-borne tuberculosis, which had often resisted PAS treatment, Hinshaw reported apparent cures in two patients with early forms of the disease. Tuberculosis affecting the kidneys and bladder seemed to benefit dramatically and the germs disappeared from the urine. Six patients with tuberculosis of the skin had shown dramatic improvement, while the results in the most horrific form of skin infection, a facial involvement called "lupus", were too early to assess. Nevertheless, like Vallentin in Sweden, Hinshaw was cautious in his summary and comment, acknowledging that they were describing very small numbers and a very short period of observation: "From preliminary impressions obtained from the study of thirty-four patients who had tuberculosis and were treated with streptomycin during the last nine months it appears probable that streptomycin has exerted a limited suppressive effect, especially on some of the more unusual types of pulmonary and extrapulmonary tuberculosis in this small series of patients."[6]

On 12 June Waksman received a telegram from Feldman and Hinshaw: "Our streptomycin studies . . . were fully confirmed experimentally and clinically, establishing this as first effective chemotherapeutic remedy for tuberculosis. Hearty congratulations."[7]

In June, 1946, the longer term results in these early cases were presented to the National Tuberculosis Association meeting in Buffalo. Just as for Lehmann, Vallentin and Sievers, who presented the PAS results in Gothenburg that very same month, this presentation in Buffalo was a nervous moment for Hinshaw and Feldman. It was the first opportunity to gauge the reaction of a national audience. "We feared that disbelief of the results would be expressed because of the many previous false hopes raised by other 'cures' throughout all previous medical history."[8] Hinshaw's nervousness was all the more acute for the fact that, prior to the meeting, he had heard rumours that the Cornell group would report their own experiences of streptomycin. He had no idea whether their report would confirm or contradict his own. The excitement prior to speaking was an occasion Hinshaw would never forget.

His report was brief, but the potential effect of every word had been carefully weighed by Dr Feldman and himself, mindful of that ever-present worry about exciting false hopes in the public. Hinshaw described ten patients with the normally fatal blood-borne tuberculosis, with or without meningitis, four of whom had survived after treatment with streptomycin.[9] In fact, although many sanitoria doctors remained somewhat sceptical, Hinshaw need not have worried. His reputation, together with that of Feldman, based upon their previous work with tuberculosis, was enough to persuade most of their audience to take streptomycin seriously. His audience was so enthralled that, immediately after the Buffalo meeting, a conference was called in Washington, where he was asked to present the streptomycin findings all over again to the military and veterans authorities. Here he received an even more overwhelming endorsement.

Where PAS had suffered a humiliating setback following the Gothenburg meeting, the immediate acceptance of Hinshaw's findings in America led to plans for a massive expansion of the streptomycin research in human sufferers.

The pharmaceutical company, Merck & Co., now played an even more vital part in furthering the streptomycin production and supply for clinical testing. Following the two meetings, and especially that with the military and veterans authorities, George Merck himself was so impressed with the reaction of the medical world to the drug and with the clear importance of the drug to humanity that he made a free gift to the American Medical Research Council of a million dollars worth of streptomycin. This generosity was timely and crucial. Barely a year after its first testing in experimental animals, streptomycin was now the focus of the most extensive medical trial in history. Hundreds of investigators were enrolled in a multicentre study and many thousands of patients. There was an atmosphere of expectancy never seen before in medical research.

By September 1946, the newly created Committee on Chemotherapeutics of the American Research Council were able to report the results of streptomycin treatment in no less than 1,000 cases, suffering from a number of different infectious diseases. By 12 December that same year the first conference, devoted entirely to streptomycin, was held by the Veterans Administration in Chicago. Streptomycin was already established as a pioneering advance in formal medical circles. It was also hailed in popular folklore – and far beyond America.

Within two years of its first discovery, streptomycin was proven to be a breakthrough in the treatment of tuberculosis in virtually all of its manifestations. Not every patient with tuberculosis was cured by it. Predictably the long-standing fibrotic lung disease proved the most resistant. No doctor, no matter how sceptical, could ignore the fact that streptomycin was capable of arresting the dreaded tuberculous meningitis – though it had to be given early in the development of the disease and it often meant that the drug had to be given by repeated lumbar puncture injections. For doctors who had long regarded these conditions with the sort of awe we regard terminal cancer today, the advent of streptomycin was, quite simply, miraculous.

Within months of the first clinical trials, ten, twenty, thirty papers appeared in rapid succession in the prestigious medical journals. Within five years 1,200 articles about streptomycin would be published in the world literature, most of these referring to individual scientific studies, much of which would be summarized in a scholarly book, published in 1949 and edited by Riggins and Hinshaw.[10] By 1952, no less than 10,000 studies on streptomycin would be published in the world literature. This very success brought formidable problems.

In Hinshaw's words: "When we saw even slight evidence of clinical improvement, or a reduction in fever, or change in neurological manifestations, we were utterly delighted but appropriately cautious in interpreting these results. It was our greatest concern that information of this sort would leak out and result in undue publicity and unjustified optimism on the part of the public. Indeed it was the policy of the Mayo Clinic to avoid any media publication that might be regarded as inappropriate or unprofessional. Because of fear of publicity, we kept our activities secret, even among our associates in the Clinic."[11] Such secrecy, which so echoed that of Lehmann and Vallentin, may, in retrospect, seem burlesque but one has to realize that tuberculosis at that time was a death sentence for most sufferers. Five million people would die from the disease worldwide every year throughout the 1940s, not just the poor, but government leaders, distinguished scientists, artists, writers. Under such circumstances – when stories of unprecedented cures were beginning to filter into medical journals, when parents were writing to newspapers about children who had been saved from certain death from tuberculous meningitis – it was impossible to keep streptomycin completely out of the news headlines. In Hinshaw's own words:

"Publicity was unavoidable when evidence appeared that a specific drug had been developed against the most important infectious disease of the human race: tuberculosis. Newspaper and magazine writers appeared sympathetic with our desires to avoid the cultivation of false hopes by patients, yet each assignment to get the latest story on streptomycin had to be fulfilled. We adhered consistently to a rule that no personal interview would be granted. All press conferences were those conducted by medical and scientific societies, with as many participants as possible, hoping thereby to dilute the personal factor. Unfortunately, many societies permit the release of popular articles before scientific publications have made the

information available to physicians who are called upon to inter-
pret the facts to their patients"[12]

A few leaks occurred, which quickly became a torrent. Those
early newspaper articles, at the prompting of the medical
authorities, were couched in that same language of caution.
"We didn't want to create a demand for drugs which were
unobtainable." But even the hint of a cure for tuberculosis was
so sensational that within weeks of the first responsible articles,
the tenor very dramatically changed. The drug was no longer a
promising treatment: it was the miracle cure. Inevitably the
streptomycin researchers were overwhelmed with requests
from people dying from tuberculosis, their relatives and
friends, or the physicians and surgeons trying to save them.
These requests were addressed to whichever name was mentioned in the media, to Waksman in New Jersey, to the Merck
pharmaceutical company, or to Hinshaw at the Mayo Clinic. At
the same time, the pitifully inadequate supplies of drug had to
be placed under the control of a central governmental committee, to which all streptomycin was now entrusted and by
which all allocations were now made. In the eye of this tragic
maelstrom, one man, H. Corwin Hinshaw was empowered by
this committee to make each fateful decision, a decision which
would often make the difference between life and death. "It
was thus established that any use of streptomycin in the treatment of tuberculosis had to be approved by me personally."[13]

This was a heavy burden to place on a single doctor, who was
expected meanwhile to carry on as normal with his everyday
clinical duties, in ward rounds and outpatient clinics.

ii

SUFFERING PATIENTS WROTE to Waksman, begging for the
wonder drug to be offered to them: servicemen who had contracted tuberculosis while fighting for their country, or tragic
parents desperately trying to save their dying children. All such
requests eventually found their way to Corwin Hinshaw,
whether by telephone, telegraph or letter, from South America,

from Australia, from Europe, from Asia, as from every corner of the United States itself. In those very early days, when no streptomycin had officially been shipped abroad, he received a telephone call from an eminent doctor in Moscow. She had somehow obtained a supply of streptomycin and wanted advice on how to use it. While marvelling at how streptomycin had found its way onto the Russian black market, Hinshaw nevertheless instructed her how best to treat a child with tuberculous meningitis, the first to be treated in Russia. Following this, he received a weekly progress report on the child's improvement. In a curious twist of fate, Selman Waksman would subsequently meet a girl, believed to be this very patient, during his visit to the Children's Hospital, in Moscow, in 1946, where he found ... "Ninotchka, a little girl barely nine-years-old, the daughter of a famous mathematician, sitting up in bed having her breakfast on the eighty-third day of her admission to the hospital. She should have died nine weeks earlier from that deadliest of microbial killers, tuberculous meningitis, which never spared any of its victims. The doctors surrounding Ninotchka looked upon her with awe, as upon a child Lazarus."[14] Waksman does not mention the fact that she had, however, become totally deaf, as a result of the streptomycin treatment.[15]

On occasions the pressures upon Hinshaw came from the highest echelons of society. "I was forced to interrupt the treatment of one important case because Eleanor Roosevelt, the wife of the President of America, had intervened in such a way as to interrupt a shipment of streptomycin, so that it could be supplied to some friend or acquaintance who had influenced either Mrs Roosevelt or the President himself."[16] This intervention to save a friend's life would subsequently become all the more poignant for the fact that Eleanor Roosevelt herself would die in 1962 from blood-borne tuberculosis. It seems that the true nature of her disease was masked by the fact that she was taking cortisone for a rheumatic complaint. It would prove the greatest of ironies, that she herself did not receive the streptomycin that might have saved her because her tuberculosis was not diagnosed until the postmortem examination of her body.[17]

A typical letter of heartbreak, dated 10 March 1946 and from Warwickshire, England, was addressed to Selman Waksman by the father of a child with tuberculous meningitis:

> *I would like to express my deepest thanks for your readiness to send, upon the request of the London Daily Express, some of your new drug, streptomycin, in an attempt to save the life of my little child as she lay dangerously ill, with tubercular cerebral meningitis.*
>
> *I have every faith that if streptomycin could have arrived in time it would have saved her, but unfortunately she died on the Sunday evening that we received news from you that you would supply the drug. . . I feel the loss very greatly as she was an extraordinary intelligent child, showing great promise, and I have only just returned to England after five years abroad.* [18]

Corwin Hinshaw saw it as his humane duty to reply to every letter, telegram or call, requesting the drug. But it was all too often a bitter duty, having to tell them that he did not have sufficient supplies, that he hoped more of the drug would soon be available, or being forced to tell them they should apply for it through the department of public health. In reality, nearly all such petitioners died. It was an impossible situation. According to the medical writer Harry Dowling, by 1948, even with eight separate companies now producing streptomycin in the United States, and with an annual output of the drug of over 80,000 pounds weight, yet if this had been used exclusively for patients with chronic pulmonary tuberculosis, it would have treated just 1,000 patients. This was only one in four hundred of the numbers suffering from tuberculosis in the United States alone. The result, as Hinshaw sadly observed, was that "desperate patients, their relatives, and physicians from many countries sought to obtain streptomycin where none was to be had". [19]

The burden was unbearable and, within six months or so, Corwin Hinshaw was relieved to hand it over to the National Institute of Health. But in spite of this, because of his very eminence, many people worldwide continued to petition him. Some two years later, in August or September 1948, Hinshaw would become involved in a fascinating vignette of modern history.

"I received a series of telephone calls of a somewhat mysterious sounding nature from the Pakistan Embassy in Washington, DC. I was asked to make an emergency trip to Karachi, Pakistan, to be consulted in the case of an unnamed person with an unnamed illness. All efforts to determine the nature of the problem and what I might be able to accomplish were in vain. Within a few days, I received a call informing me that my services were no longer needed because the patient had died. Two or three years later, after I had moved to San Francisco, I was visited by the physician who told me that he had been responsible for these calls and the patient was none other than Jinnah. He had been Jinnah's personal physician. The reason for the secrecy was now obvious. This doctor had heard me give a lecture at the Pasteur Institute a few years previously and had read some of my publications."[20]

Mohammed Ali Jinnah was suffering from a chronic cavitating pulmonary tuberculosis, which had been first diagnosed by his physician, Dr J.A.L. Patel, in June 1946. If his enemies had known this, they would have realized that Jinnah was living under a sentence of death. The importance of keeping the true nature of Jinnah's illness a state secret was later revealed in a book, *Freedom at Midnight*, by Larry Collins and Dominique Lapierre.[21] "If Louis Mountbatten, Jawaharlal Nehru or Mahatma Gandhi had been aware in April 1947 of one extraordinary secret, the division threatening India might have been avoided." All they needed to do was to wait a little longer and the one immoveable obstacle to pan-Indian unity would have been removed. "That secret was sealed onto the grey surface of a piece of film, a film that could have upset the Indian political equation and would almost certainly have changed the course of Asian history." According to Collins and Lapierre, the secret was so well kept that even the British Secret Service were entirely unaware of it. Jinnah was so determined to win his fellow Moslems a nation of their own that he forced the last Viceroy to the most important decision the British ever made in India – to accept the division of the subcontinent, the unity of which they had so carefully nurtured for three centuries.

In fact, Jinnah, who was well aware of his fate, refused to rest from the exhausting pressures of politics, and died from

pulmonary tuberculosis on 11 September 1948, barely a year
after the partitioning of India and three months after Gandhi
had died from an assassin's bullet.

From the very first clinical studies at the Mayo Clinic, streptomycin had captured the imagination of the world. Why,
when we compare it to the messianic excitement that surrounded streptomycin's discovery, did Lehmann's simultaneous discovery of PAS fail to take its share of the limelight?

iii

JORGEN LEHMANN, IN an editorial twenty years afterwards,
drew pained attention to the claim of Pfuetze and his associates,
that streptomycin alone was the first chemical agent found to be
practical in the treatment of tuberculosis.[22] One has to sympath-
ize with Lehmann. The article which so offended him was a
personal history of streptomycin in which Pfuetze, who was of
course the sanitorium director who collaborated with Hinshaw
in the first human trials of streptomycin, claimed that Waksman's discovery of streptomycin laid claim for the priority "for
all time".[23] We may assume, since there was nobody else to lay
an alternative claim to the mantle, that this was specifically
directed towards Lehmann and PAS.

In 1953 René Dubos, together with his new wife, the laboratory assistant Jean whom he had married after a protracted and
agonized depression after Marie Louise's death, would write a
masterpiece, *The White Plague*, relating the history of tuberculosis to humanity and society. In this book, written with a
brilliance and literary fluency equal to Waksman's, Dubos
would make a brutal point. A French army doctor, J.A. Villemin, had discovered the infectious nature of tuberculosis
more than twenty years before Koch discovered the precise
germ that caused it. For a time Villemin enjoyed the limelight,
only to be eclipsed when Koch made his world shattering discovery. "Villemin suffered much in his pride from seeing his
work contemptuously ignored by Koch and all but forgotten by
the rest of the world. He would have been wise to accept the
cruel law of scientific life. He becomes the true discoverer who

establishes the truth: and the sign of the truth is the general acceptance ... In science the credit goes to the man who convinces the world, not to the man to whom the idea first occurs." [24]

It is illuminating that Selman Waksman should see fit to quote this passage from Dubos' book in his own publication, *The Conquest of Tuberculosis*.[25] That Waksman had other more personal reasons for quoting Villemin, we shall shortly discover. He also quoted a letter from Villemin to Pasteur, written in 1887. "I do not hope to gain a place beside you but – you will see that I am less modest than I appear – I have been so much discussed, so often attacked, that I suffer a certain amount of distress in thinking that the leading scientific academy still gives, at least, a sort of toleration to my former enemies ... Koch will enter the Academie des Sciences through widely flung doors, in the triumphant way that has made a conquest for him of all the honours of his country."[26]

Scientists, we should not be surprised to discover, are humanly vain.

To be fair to the PAS researchers, the progress with PAS was far from slow. If anything, it was very nearly as fast and furious as that of streptomycin. Compare the progress of PAS with the long barren years that separated Fleming's first discovery of penicillin and its application to infection in human beings. There were two important catalysts in the unprecedented development of streptomycin, the first of which was the fortuitous intervention of Feldman and Hinshaw, whose earlier researches had paved the way to a lightning-quick clinical evaluation. The second catalyst was the pre-existing link between Waksman and the pharmaceutical firm, Merck & Co., whose subsequent generosity facilitated the almost immediate escalation to large scale clinical trials.

PAS was born out of the aspirin molecule and aspirin, by itself, was too well-known as a non-specific treatment of fevers. Partly as a result of this, it took longer for Lehmann's medical colleagues to accept that PAS really was curing their patients and not just bringing down their temperatures. Swedish doctors, like all too many of their colleagues worldwide, simply could not believe that "the Captain of the Men of Death" was curable. These were the circumstances, which, rather than Machiavellian plotting, saw to it that in those two early years, from 1944 to 1946, PAS did not match progress with streptomycin.

In fact, if still somewhat in the shadow of streptomycin, recognition of the importance of the Swedish drug was rapidly growing. At first the only clinical experience of PAS was restricted to Sweden but with the results of the first large scale multi-centre trials, begun under the Swedish National Board in 1947, medical authorities in every developed country were asking for supplies for testing. Ferrosan found themselves competing on the world stage in the company of such giants as Merck & Co. in the States and Bayer in Germany. Notwithstanding their initial nervousness caused by fear of bankruptcy, it is to their great credit that the small Swedish company, employing just seventy-five workers, now committed themselves, success or bust, to the titanic struggle.

The greatest problem faced by Ferrosan from the very beginning was the chemical manufacture of PAS, a complex, slow and expensive process. It was impossible to manufacture the drug in more than limited quantities. The earliest manufacture had taken place during wartime, when the company could obtain no basic materials from their usual suppliers, which were based in the USA. Nevertheless the brilliant Rosdahl, together with a young assistant, Sven Carlsten – later they were joined by a third young man, Hans Larsson – searched tirelessly for a more effective chemical formulation, based upon the PAS molecule.[27]

In Carlsten's own words: "It was a very exciting time, so exciting that you don't know it when you are in the middle of it. We were young people. Rosdahl was thirty-eight and I was just twenty-five. We worked night and day, very long hours. The factory had stopped working on anything else other than PAS."[28] The hard-working Ferrosan chemists created a vast array of alternative drugs, based on the parent PAS molecule, but not one of these proved better than the molecule first prophesized by Lehmann. The answer did not lie in that direction. While banner-holding patients marched through the grounds of sanitoria, demanding the drug, and while their physicians begged Ferrosan for larger supplies of PAS so they could treat them, the tiny band of chemists knew there was only one solution: they had to find a more efficient process of manufacturing the drug.

In 1947 Rosdahl's young assistant, Sven Carlsten, made a breakthrough. Using a chemical technique of carboxylation under water at a very high pressure, and contradicting the chemist's Bible, Beilstein, he found a way of manufacturing PAS by a single step. For the young chemical assistant, this was the greatest moment of his professional life. "I was utterly elated. I had proved the literature wrong."[29] But instead of rushing off to tell Rosdahl, he prudently went back to his laboratory bench and repeated the experiment and made absolutely certain that he was right. Only then did he inform a jubilant Rosdahl, who realized immediately what this must mean. It was the breakthrough they had been seeking for three years. The new process took just six hours and gave a wonderful yield of 50 per cent.

This discovery, perfected a year later to a dry carboxylation method that would give a phenomenal yield of 90 per cent, revolutionized the mass production of PAS. Where, during 1944, the production of PAS had barely increased from 10 to a mere 400 grams a month, now the drug could be produced by the ton. By 1964, using this same process, the production of PAS would rise to an incredible three million kilograms a year.[30] The manufacturing breakthrough could hardly have been more timely. Two years after the generosity of Merck had enabled large scale American trials of streptomycin, Gylfe Vallentin could now initiate the first large scale trial of PAS, incorporating 378 cases of pulmonary tuberculosis from six Swedish sanitoria.[31]

During those first three years, from 1944 to 1947, streptomycin had undoubtedly overshadowed PAS in global recognition. But by 1947, thanks to the mass production made possible by the new manufacturing process, doctors worldwide could now receive large quantities of the Swedish drug for testing. For their patients, suffering and dying from the disease, the issues of personal pride and priority of discovery, were irrelevant. What mattered now, in the rational light of science was, firstly, whether, in much larger trials of human sufferers, PAS really did cure tuberculosis, and, secondly, how its efficacy compared with streptomycin.

In the United States, streptomycin had so swept the board before the arrival of PAS from Sweden that, in this very important arena, it would never see a large scale assessment as a single primary therapy. Elsewhere, particularly in Sweden and the United Kingdom, large scale trials, which could not be read for more than a year, were begun to assess precisely that.

iv

DURING THE HECTIC concatenation of experiments during 1944 and 1945, Albert Schatz had volunteered every mote of his energies to the streptomycin research. Physically and mentally exhausted, and with an income of just $40 monthly, he could hardly afford to run a car or to take girls out on dates. Betty Bugie, who worked with Waksman in the third floor laboratory, saw nothing of Albert Schatz at the parties which were held at the house of Mrs Zimmerman, a generous hearted landlady, who ran a boarding house on the university campus for graduate students. All Betty ever saw of Albert at work was the huge mound of used culture plates and test tubes in the sink, awaiting cleaning from the Trojan efforts of the night before. For Albert, there was a single escape, available because it cost nothing and useful because it helped to clear his head from the night-time labours over the laboratory bench.

In his own words: "The discovery of streptomycin was a major event in my life. But I also found something much more important about the same time. I liked to walk. There was a woman who lived in one of the dormitories on campus and I went out with her once. We didn't go anywhere, just walking. One day I called her up only to find she wasn't there. It was her friend, Vivian, a student at Rutgers studying agriculture, who answered the phone. So I asked Vivian if she would like to come instead and she agreed, because she too liked walking. I later discovered that she was always trying to persuade people to go walking with her. After that, Vivian and I would regularly go out together. These walks, however, presented me with a problem. This girl customarily walked very rapidly. But I was usually quite tired when we went out for an evening walk because I had worked in the laboratory all day long beginning at five or six in the morning. So, it seemed to me, I was always running to keep up with her."[32]

Vivian Rosenfeld had dark hair which fell over her shoulders in thick curls and she had beautiful mauve eyes. Her parents, Jewish refugees from the Ukraine, had been given their German surname by the US immigration authorities when they had arrived in Philadelphia, unable to speak English or write their names.[33] During these walks, Vivian discovered a mysterious novelty to this tired young scientist. "He knew how to find slime moulds and slime bacteria and that really was a wonder."[34] Slime moulds may sound an unprepossessing vehicle for romance, but for Vivian they held an arcane fascination. "Tiny things interested me. And slime moulds are lovely. Their fruiting bodies are incredibly beautiful. But you need keen eyesight to see them and you have to look in the right places to find them." The same vision that had enabled Albert to pick out the colonies of *Streptomyces griseus*, had opened her eyes to a fairytale world invisible to all but the initiated. Here, in the unpromising gloom of the underside of decaying logs and organic dank of the woodland floor, the tiny fruiting bodies of the moulds were miniature gardens of delight, a new voyage of discovery for Vivian, who had had a passion for wild flowers since her childhood in Northern New Jersey.

They fell in love and were married a year later, on 23 March 1945, when Albert insisted on taking his cultures of actinomyces with them on their honeymoon.

This was still a wonderful time to be involved in the streptomycin research. Even before the honeymoon, streptomycin was becoming rapidly established in the clinical trials co-ordinated by Corwin Hinshaw. The discovery had captured the headlines and the American press had become frequent visitors to Rutgers. But with the growing public attention, signs of strain began to show in the relationship between Selman Waksman and Albert Schatz.

Selman Waksman was without doubt the mastermind

behind the entire programme of research at Rutgers. He had
been very fair when he had allowed Albert's name ahead of his
own on all three of the first streptomycin papers. But now, with
the fissile excitement surrounding the streptomycin discovery,
Waksman had reaffirmed his status as the man in charge of the
streptomycin research. There was a striking parallel between
the developing situation at Rutgers and the sense of betrayal
and bitterness felt by René Dubos towards Oswald Avery,
some fourteen years previously.

In the case of Dubos and Avery, a deep and lasting affection
had bound the two men, a mutual trust so powerful that it
overrode René's disappointment and which, given several
more years working together, would allow their true affection
and mutual respect to re-emerge all the stronger for being
tested. It had seemed up to this moment that an equally powerful bond of trust and affection existed between Waksman and
Schatz, which has been confirmed by Betty Bugie. "Even in our
everyday conversation, Dr Waksman would remark to me:
'Look at this. Schatz did this.' I got the impression that Waksman was very proud of Schatz. I think he thought of him as his
brightest student."[35]

At first, when the reporters called to the laboratories, Waksman would bring them down to meet Schatz in the basement.
However, the photographs that would subsequently illustrate
these articles would usually have Waksman posing with a test
tube or plate, while Schatz watched with the eyes of an enrap-
tured apprentice. In Schatz' own words: "I guess it was about
this time, as Betty Bugie came into the picture (checking some of
Schatz' results), Waksman didn't introduce me to people who
visited him. Even when reporters visited him, I generally learnt
about it from other postgraduate students who were working
on the third floor, and from others, after the fact. That was
when I really began feeling uneasy."[36]

As one magazine or newspaper article after another relegated
Schatz to a background role, he felt progressively more
resentful. That there really was a deliberate policy operating,
and not just a quirk of Schatz' fevered imagination, would
subsequently be confirmed by Doris Jones, who was working
in that same basement laboratory at the time.

"About the publicity, let me interject at this point an interesting and revealing comment that Dr Waksman once made to me. It so happened that during 1946, Al had been assigned to the anti-viral project with me, so we found ourselves in the same laboratory (by that time an additional building with a newly outfitted lab.). I was very possessive of my research thoughts and soon got worried that Al would be swamping me and I'd not be able to use my own head. So I went to Dr Waksman to see how I could get the problem settled. I suppose I made some ugly complaints about Al's bossiness, because Dr Waksman soon got to discussing the streptomycin publicity. He told me confidentially that he thought Al was too immature and that all this publicity would go to his head. Therefore he was keeping him out of it. Whereas, he, Dr Waksman, was mature and he could handle it."[37]

In 1946, less than two years after he had started work on the research that would lead to streptomycin, Albert Schatz, still just twenty-six years old, left Rutgers to take up a job at the New York State Department of Health in Albany. "I left Rutgers for various reasons, the most important of which was the fact that my relationship with Waksman was deteriorating."[38]

In this sad fashion, the young graduate left New Jersey, virtually penniless and bitterly resentful of the man he had formerly looked up to as a father.

v

MEANWHILE THE FAME and the glory of streptomycin continued to spread. Within the space of months, following the first success of streptomycin in the infant with tuberculous meningitis, the drug would be used to treat similar cases throughout the world. The subsequent death rates for this appalling disease tell their own story. In New York, in the year 1930, 400 people died from tuberculous meningitis, by 1953 this had been reduced to 47. The steady stream of letters arriving at Rutgers had now become a deluge, thanking Waksman for saving their lives or the lives of loved ones, conveying a sense of gratitude that Waksman, who was not a medical man at all, had never experienced before. From Chicago, Illinois: "It was with great interest that I read that you are the discoverer of streptomycin. To me this is a magical name because the doctors tell me that this is the drug that was responsible for saving my baby's life." From Charleston, South Carolina: "So you see, because you laboured and discovered the drug streptomycin, and because of the prayers of all the good people who heard of our baby's illness, our son is with us today, healthy, happy, and a normal boy in every way. Yours is God given work."[39] Waksman received invitations from all over the world to come and visit. These came uninterruptedly for a period of ten years, from the end of the war until 1955. Although he could accept only a minority of these, he felt compelled to pack his suitcases again and embark upon a world tour. Nobody could express his feelings better than he did himself:

"How can I describe the impressions left upon me by the first sight of a child, no matter in what country and in what position in life, who had been saved from certain death by the use of a drug in the discovery of which I had played but a humble part? For the first time in human history, these children, afflicted with tuberculous meningitis and miliary tuberculosis, which once would have meant certain death, now had a chance to survive. They were being restored to life by a drug produced by a soil-inhabiting microbe and discovered in a small agricultural laboratory."[40]

He recorded his experiences, travelling from hospital to hospital, from Verona to war-ravaged Berlin, from Rome to Florence, Madrid, Stockholm, Paris. It was the ambrosia of dreams for a scientist, the most sublime culmination of a lifetime's devotion to hard duty. Yet even now, at the pinnacle of glory, two hammer blows fell.

In 1946, during his world tour, Waksman was welcomed back to Russia, the land he had fled after the death of his mother, then bilious with anti-semitism. Now he was fêted, the lost son who had become a famous figure in world history. It was during this visit to Moscow that he met the little girl, Ninotchka, the mathematician's daughter who had been cured of tuberculous meningitis. Four hundred children every year were admitted to this hospital with the same diagnosis and every single one of them had previously died in torment. Although deaf as a result of the side-effects of streptomycin, she recited a little poem in English, which she had been especially taught to honour her American saviour.

Waksman had a second very good reason for embarking on this exhaustive tour of Europe that year – to visit his son, Byron, who was in the American army and stationed in Germany. He had not seen Byron for eighteen months, after he had left America for the fighting front. Accompanied by his wife, Bobili, Waksman had a difficult flight, with delays at Shannon, further delays before they finally met Byron, who met them in full military uniform and with many tales to tell, at Frankfurt. There was barely time to inspect the rubble of Berlin before their flight to Moscow, where they learned the fate of the little town of Priluka in the Ukraine, where Waksman had been born and where he had spent his happy childhood. Of no military or strategic significance with its mud-brick terraces and innocent Jewish civilians, it had found itself no more than twenty miles from Hitler's headquarters in the Ukraine. The town had been completely destroyed by the occupying German army and all but three of the population massacred.[41]

The second hammer blow was more subtle and yet more deadly. Wherever he travelled Waksman was invited to address the leading medical establishments. In May 1946 he lectured at the University of Minnesota; in July he gave that same lecture in Moscow; in October in Liège, Belgium. On occasions he would share the platform with Florey and Chain, who had rescued Fleming's penicillin from a laboratory grave and turned it into a global life-saving drug, or with Lehmann from Sweden, or Domagk from Germany. In 1947, Waksman returned to Europe, at the invitation of the International Microbiological Congress in Copenhagen. He delivered two lectures to the International Congress of Chemistry in London *en route*, before continuing to Denmark, then France, and from there on to Switzerland, to meet Professor W. Loeffler, head of the tuberculosis clinic in the State Hospital, Zurich. Loeffler was sixty-years-old and had devoted his entire life to fighting tuberculosis. His wife had died from it. This famous Swiss doctor had tried every last wonder cure for tuberculosis only to suffer

bitter disappointment after disappointment. At last, in streptomycin, he could believe that the terror might soon be conquered.

From Switzerland, Waksman returned to Paris, where he
visited, among other hospitals, the world renowned Salpet-
rière. After a tour of the wards, under the enthusiastic guidance
of Dr Fouquet, chief of the tuberculosis clinic, the director of the
hospital took him by the arm and said: "We have a little surprise
for you."

Waksman was led into the court in the centre of the hospital,
where two shy children came up to greet him. One was a boy of
about five, named Michael, and the other was Janet, a girl of
about seven. The director explained: "These two children were
brought to this hospital six months ago, from distant regions of
France. They were almost in a state of coma on arrival. We
began at once to treat them with streptomycin. As you see, they
have both made a complete recovery. . . Aren't they pretty!"[42]
The children were dressed in French national costumes and
carried two huge bouquets of flowers. The little girl curtsied
and handed her bouquet to the man whose discovery had
brought them back to life from what had been thought a fatal
coma. Both children kissed his hand and Waksman, overwhelmed with emotion, patted their lovely, curly heads. "As I
leaned over, I felt like crying."

A year later, in a pattern that was becoming frighteningly
familiar, a letter arrived at Waksman's office in New Jersey
informing him that little Michael had relapsed and died. The
tuberculosis germs had resurrected and this time they were
resistant to streptomycin.

18

The Order of the Atoms

The captain of all these men of death that came against him to take him away, was the Consumption, for it was that that brought him down to the grave.

John Bunyan: *The Life and Death of Mr Badman*

i

PEACE CAME TO a battered Europe at 2.41 a.m. on 7 May 1945, with the meeting, in a small red schoolhouse in Rheims, of General Eisenhower, the Allied Supreme Commander, and General Alfred Jodl, Chief of Staff for the German Army. For Gerhard Domagk it meant a merciful release from the bombing that had wrought devastation upon Wuppertal and the adjoining small town of Elberfeld, where the Bayer research laboratories were located. His sole concern during the last eighteen months had been for the safety of his family, particularly his son, Wolfgang.

In the summer of 1943, following the heavy bombing of Wuppertal, all the schools in the town had been closed. Wolfgang, then aged thirteen, had been transferred for safety to a boarding school in Thüringen. Two years later, in March 1945, Wolfgang, together with his entire class, had been handed rifles and, marching through the night, they were ordered to advance upon the Russian army. It was hardly surprising that his parents were alarmed for his safety. When peace was declared, nobody had had word of him for some eight months. Gerhard Domagk did not know if his son was alive or dead. What a blessed relief it was when he turned up safely at the tiny Baltic resort of Dammeshöved, to join his mother for Christmas in their holiday room. Here he told Gertrud of his hair-raising adventures, escaping from the Eastern Front.[1]

The previous Easter, Gerhard Domagk had managed to get his home in Wuppertal organized in a makeshift fashion so that Gertrud could bring the children home. At least they were together again and everybody had a bed to sleep in. Only now, with his family once again safely home, could his thoughts return to the struggle against tuberculosis.

A few months earlier, in October 1945, the British Occupation Forces had allowed the research laboratories in Elberfeld to reopen. Many of the buildings had been destroyed during the bombing but this was minor compared with the devastation in the town surrounding it. There was another problem a good deal more serious than broken buildings. Bayer no longer had a workforce. The dedicated little band of technical assistants were all dead or missing, their homes reduced to rubble. Gradually some of those who had survived began to trickle back from their refuges in the cellars and shelters, and were joined by others arriving from prisoner of war camps. Little by little, a man here, a woman there, they began to pick up the pieces of normality. The thiosemicarbazone experiment stuttered back into life. In Domagk's own words: "We had great difficulty in getting the material and animals for the experiments. The British control officer at our company tried very hard to support us, even though he came from one of our competitors, May and Baker (the forerunner of Rhone-Poulenc Rorer). He normally sat in on our Friday meetings which were also attended by Lutter, the company director and the section heads of all the medical and chemical laboratories."[2]

A defeated Germany, fragmented into zones of conquest and racked by hunger and chaos, had to take full responsibility for the war and its consequences. Not only would Bayer have to struggle for its identity – it would struggle for its very survival in a postwar world that was profoundly hostile, a world which regarded its patents and discoveries as the spoils of war, there for the taking.

Throughout 1945 and 1946, commissioners from any far flung

country that deemed itself to have the right, demanded privileged information from the company's records: the details of past discoveries, copies of company regulations, the most intimate secrets of experimental protocols, photographs and photocopies of anything that might be remotely exploitable. In Domagk's words, Bayer's role in the immediate postwar era was nothing more than "a free information centre for passing foreign chemists". The parent company, I.G. Farbenindustrie, was ordered out of business by the war commission. Only the subsidiary group, Bayer, so long distinguished for its contributions to humanity, was allowed to continue to trade under its former name. It was a tragic interlude in the history of the company which had given aspirin, phenacetin, and Prontosil to humanity.

But slowly the old spirit of German initiative began to reassert itself. For Gerhard Domagk, this was the real Germany, a world apart from the fanaticism and brutality of National Socialism, the Germany of limitless hard work, self-sacrifice and determination. The Bayer pharmaceutical company reorganized itself. In spite of the fact that during the winter of 1945 they had to close the firm from time to time because of lack of coal in an area, the Ruhr, which was built on coal, production rose by degree after painful degree, until they were back to fifty per cent of the prewar years.

In the desperate conditions following the war, the need for a renewed effort against the great killer had never been more critical. Every word of Domagk's prophecy, made to Hörlein during their heated exchange in 1941, had come to pass. Millions of ordinary men, women and children in war-ravaged Europe would come to understand Bunyan's terrible epithet. The "Captain of the Men of Death" was riding through the dispossessed, the poverty-stricken, the starving and the homeless.

In 1937, 77 of every 100,000 people living in Berlin had died from tuberculosis. In 1947, this had leaped to 225 people per 100,000.[3] In neighbouring Poland, which had suffered more than any other country, it was even worse. In tragic Warsaw, with its social and medical infrastructure completely destroyed, no less than 500 people in every 100,000 died from tuberculosis

in 1944 alone.[4] In Yugoslavia, Greece, Holland – even beautiful
Vienna – the wave of suffering and death extended far and
wide. Almost 7,000 people would die from tuberculosis in
Berlin alone in a single year. In Domagk's home town of Wuppertal, one in every fifty people walking the bomb-shattered
streets was infected. There was a grave risk of an ever worsening epidemic. The hospital of Wuppertal-Elberfeld, where his
friend and colleague Klee had his beds and outpatient clinic,
could no longer cope with the tide of tuberculosis sufferers.
Although streptomycin and PAS had already been discovered
in the United States and Sweden, neither drug was available for
treatment of tuberculosis sufferers in Germany. In the words of
Karl Jahnke, who had recently joined Klee as his medical assistant, "Treatment was so ineffective, it was a most fearsome
disease. Every single patient who had contracted it was utterly
terrified."[5] The plight of these unfortunate patients in Klee's
wards was as hopeless as it had been in the darkest days of the
nineteenth century.

Gerhard Domagk did his utmost to focus everybody's attention upon the danger facing them: "As long ago as 1935, when
speaking about the need for chemotherapy of tuberculosis as
well as the acute bacterial infections, I had to make people
realize what masses of tuberculous bacteria are to be found in
the lung cavities that characterize this disease. Only when you
think of the millions of highly infectious bacteria being carried
about by a single person, do you comprehend the danger this
person poses to everybody about him. It might be a teacher in
his classroom or a man or woman at home with the family, or
somebody you meet in a hotel, at the theatre, on a train, across
the table in a restaurant – the menace is everywhere. Yet we did
nothing to stop these primary infections from spreading. The
fight against this terrible disease seemed futile. In those earlier
days, the chemotherapy of tuberculosis was never so urgent as
it is today. The disease was not as common then with better
living standards, better housing and nutrition – if anything
there was a tendency for the disease to decline in frequency. But
now tuberculosis has increased in unimaginable numbers in
Germany.

"In our bombed-out cities, the undernourished population

has been crammed into poor houses. Even in the hospitals that are still standing, there is no space to admit people suffering from open tuberculosis. The prisoners of war have returned home with the most advanced tuberculosis in their lungs. It is not unusual to find a family of three or four children, all similarly infected – indeed in the more overcrowded homes, the numbers would be higher still. Nothing could be of greater urgency in Germany today than to find a cure for tuberculosis."[6]

For the chemist, Robert Behnisch, back at his workbench in the understaffed and still poorly equipped research laboratory in Elberfeld, it was time to focus once again on the great experiment at the point where it had been forced to a halt in the horrific conditions of war in 1944 – to the new family of drugs they had created from the order of the atoms, the thiosemicarbazones.

Of the hundreds, perhaps even thousands, of chemical derivatives the chemists had created, three appeared outstanding. When Domagk administered these in small doses to guinea pigs infected with a fatal dose of the most virulent strain of human tuberculosis, the tuberculosis was inhibited though not cured. When he increased the dose, the effect was spectacular. Tuberculosis, as it spread throughout the blood stream in guinea pigs, caused a mass of abscesses throughout every internal organ. At postmortem examination, these showed up as thick cheesy cavities spoiling the cut slices of the liver and spleen. These were so striking, one could hardly miss them. Now, when Domagk examined slices of the internal organs, the fatal abscesses had disappeared, leaving just scar tissue to show where the deadly disease had been eradicated. He could draw only one conclusion. Fulminant tuberculosis caused by the most vicious of human germs had been cured.

All three drugs were very well tolerated by the experimental animals, even in the doses that were necessary to cure them of their potentially fatal disease.[7] Of these three, a single drug, which they called Tibione (TB-one), which would soon become more familiar under the name, Conteben, seemed to have the greatest promise.

Was this the cure they were looking for? After the heroic

efforts of the small group of workers who had risked their lives during the war years, would Conteben make the sacrifices worthwhile? As early as 1946, in Domagk's own words. . . "our work with TB had made such great progress that I felt we were ready for the first clinical treatment in people suffering from tuberculosis."[8]

ii

OF THE MANY tragic and deadly forms of infection caused by tuberculosis, infection of the skin of the face is the most distressing. In this mutilating disease, resembling leprosy, the tuberculosis germs invade the nose or cheeks, to grow and spread in fungating scarlet masses. In its most severe form, this disease produces a horrible disfigurement, in which by degrees the delicate structures of nose, cheeks, eyes and ears are destroyed, so that the face of the unfortunate sufferer resembles a living skull. The latin term for this tragedy is *lupus vulgaris*, so called because, in its earlier stages, the scarlet corrugations and thickening of the nose and cheeks come to resemble the muzzle of a wolf. This would become the first challenge for the newly discovered Conteben.

The Hornhide Lupus Sanitorium, near to Münster in Westphalia, had long taken a special interest in this dreadful malady. Here the doctors had tried every possible remedy to help their patients, but nothing had ever proved more than palliative. When Gerhard Domagk visited them to suggest they try Conteben against lupus they were extremely suspicious. Here, they mused, was yet another useless therapy. Domagk recalled their reaction in his diary. "When I told Professor Moncorps and his colleague, Professor Kalkoff and their colleagues, about the results we had been obtaining in the laboratory experiments, they expressed considerable scepticism. In retrospect I appreciate the fact that in spite of this they accepted my suggestions for clinical testing. They would become the first to treat tuberculosis of the skin with chemically derived therapies that would have been unthinkable just a year earlier."[9]

They agreed to test Conteben because there was in fact little to lose. The advancing skin manifestations of tuberculosis were so miserable that suicide was not an uncommon end. Yet, once having accepted the challenge, there were enormous difficulties to be overcome. The drug was entirely new. Nobody knew what dose to give. Domagk suggested that they should start with small doses. Higher doses had already been tried in Wuppertal by Klee and these had caused unfortunate reactions. Would it work by mouth or would it need to be given by injection? This again he did not know, no more than he knew what side-effects might be encountered. At first even the patients themselves refused to take the drug, worried it would poison them. The failure of every other treatment made them view their doctors with grave mistrust. But even in these sad conditions, the human spirit can rise above the most appalling misery.

A small group of patients had sufferered so terribly from the disease that they had been forced to live permanently within the sanitorium, shunned by the outside world, which could not bear to look upon the hideous effects of their disease. These patients now offered themselves as the first human guinea pigs for the new and untested treatment, which, even if it could no longer help them, might at the very least save others from a fate such as their own.

One of those first patients, who had the courage to try Conteben, was a woman aged fifty-four, whose disease was so severe that she had become a permanent resident of the Hornhide Sanitorium. Frieda had suffered from lupus since the age of twenty-four. Over those long and tortured years, she had tried the sanitorium rest cure, she had suffered electric cautery, the latest diets, ointments that scoured deeply into the skin – she had even tried the most desperate remedy of all, radiotherapy. Nothing had helped her. Although the rest of her body was perfectly healthy, her face had suffered thirty years of destructive ulceration, leading to grotesque deformity. Her nose had been eaten away by degrees until there was nothing there except two gibbous caverns. Her left eye had been destroyed. Frieda now looked out upon the world from a monstrously scarred mask, cratered with festering sores that teemed with tuberculosis germs. Even the comfort of plastic surgery had been denied to her since every graft that had been attempted had itself become infected and ultimately destroyed by invading germs.

After just three weeks of Conteben treatment, under the caring eyes of Professor Kalkoff, the livid ulcers, resistant to every previous therapy, showed signs of healing. Five months later the scarlet eruptions of inflammation had melted away. In Kalkoff's own astonished words: "For over thirty years this fifty-four year old patient with severe lupus of the face had not responded to any treatment until she was given Conteben. After five months treatment, the disease was halted. She suffered no further recurrence of infection."[10] After thirty years of unimaginable torment, this brave woman could at last be offered the hope of facial reconstruction with plastic surgery. Apart from occasionally feeling nauseated, Frieda had experienced no side-effects from Conteben.

There would be many such dramatic cures. Another woman in her fifties, had suffered this mutilating disease since the age of twenty-nine, with spread to her right shoulder and even down the skin of her arm. Her disease had also resisted every previous therapy. After six months of Conteben, she too was cured. Gerhard Domagk recorded these successes with immense satisfaction in his diary. "The small doses were well tolerated. They were effective even when administered for long periods. There were no side-effects. Patients could now be treated at the onset of the disease. We could prevent the terrible disfigurements."[11]

In May 1947 Moncorps and Kalkoff presented the results of treating twenty-six lupus patients with Conteben to a gathering of skin specialists in Wuppertal. At this same meeting a number of other dermatologists also presented their results using the same treatment. Not every patient had completely healed. These doctors with their profound respect for this disease, warned their audience, as Hinshaw and Vallentin had warned their listeners and readers before them, of the danger of underestimating a disease which had such a fearful capacity to fight back. Nevertheless the results, taken as a whole, were sensational. Those cures were confirmed and widened at the autumn conference at the Rheinisch-Westfalen Dermatology Meeting in

Münster, following which doctors throughout Germany welcomed the new drug as the first successful therapy for lupus in history. In any normal chapter of medical advance, this discovery alone would have been the ultimate success story. In the titanic battle against tuberculosis, it was merely one small skirmish along the way. Like streptomycin in America and PAS in Sweden, the time had come for Conteben to be tested in full battle. How would Conteben perform against the myriad of other manifestations of tuberculosis?

iii

LONG BEFORE THE stage of clinical trials, Domagk had talked about the new discovery with his old friend and colleague, Philipp Klee. The thiosemicarbazones had been the excited focus of many discussions at the Scientific Association meetings that took place in Wuppertal between the Bayer research team and the clinicians from the neighbouring Wuppertal-Elberfeld Hospital. But even Klee found it almost impossible to believe that Domagk and Behnisch had found the cure for tuberculosis. Nevertheless this trusted colleague, freed from the shackles that had so recently restricted his work, was willing to undertake the first very tentative assessments of the thiosemicarbazones.

There were many initial difficulties. Three different types of thiosemicarbazone were given in high dose short-term therapy, which immediately gave rise to side-effects. Patients reacted with disabling nausea and vomiting. They were reluctant to take any more of it and their doctors were not inclined to force them. In June 1946, a young woman aged twenty-five suffering from tuberculous meningitis, as a result of blood-borne spread from a fulminant infection in her lungs, was treated with large doses of Conteben. Two days before her death, the white blood cell count in her blood fell almost to zero, a disastrous complication caused by depression of the blood-forming elements of the bone marrow. Was this a complication of the new drug therapy or was it a direct result of the fulminating disease by itself? Nobody could be sure. They knew virtually nothing about the way the drug was handled by the internal chemical balances of the body. They did not even know how it worked, or what dose it was best to give.

While Klee doubted that the new drug had depressed the woman's bone marrow, he could not be certain. He was forced to slow his programme of research right down until they had a great deal more information on the drug, its side effects, the correct dosage, and the duration of its administration. It was also clear that his 55 hospital beds would be hopelessly inadequate to assess this development. Even with the planned expansion to 280, there would hardly be enough beds to assess this drug.

Tuberculosis was not a single disease caused by a common germ. This strange disease was the leviathan that dominated every medical discipline and department throughout the world. In every field of medicine, whole subcultures had evolved to fight against it, each in its way a distinct theatre of war. For the ear, nose and throat surgeons it was the disease that infested the throat and the voice box, slowly infiltrating, ulcerating and destroying the delicate membranes of speech, making it an agony even to whisper. For the abdominal surgeon it was the disease that so often followed the throat infection, whether as a primary invader that ulcerated, scarred and destroyed the bowel, ruining its digestive ability and leading to progressive emaciation, or, secondary to the well-known lung disease, as the late complication of unrelievable diarrhoea and vomiting, so often the harbinger of a fatal outcome. For the gynaecologist it was the insidious infiltration that destroyed the fallopian tubes and ovaries, engulfing the fine tissues of motherhood in a deformed and distorted mass of inflammation and thick cheesy pus, robbing the young woman, should she survive, of her opportunity for a family. For the orthopaedic surgeon it was the common cause of suppurating arthritis of childhood, the slow incurable torment that destroyed the hip joints, the shoulders, the elbows, knees, invading the long bones of the legs and arms, to cripple children, or to collapse the tender spines of millions of young people into the characteristic hunchbacks.

From meningitis to infections within the eye or the ear, from lupus of the skin to the manifold horrors of consumption in the lungs, tuberculosis was the protean and omnipresent menace. Not a country, a race, or a people in the world escaped its thrall. Hundreds of thousands, perhaps even millions, of scientific papers had been written about the disease in every civilized language of the world, in fear and desperation, all expressing one way or another the determination and the struggle of doctors, nurses, public health officials. Entire medical journals were devoted to it. In every medical library, you could find a thousand or more books that described one aspect or another. No single man, no single department of medicine, could take on the massive spectrum of responsibility that would be necessary in order to test the new drug against all of these diverse manifestations.

Gerhard Domagk began his long and difficult series of journeys, to expand the scope of human testing of Conteben. Early in 1946, with petrol unavailable, this one man with his singular purpose, rode by horse-drawn carriage to Flensburg, in the far north of Germany, to explain the nature of the research to a conference of doctors. From centre to centre, city to city, he carried the urgency of his mission, using any form of conveyance that would carry him, persuading, inspiring, bringing together the best experts in all Germany. Professor Loebell and his assistant, Eickhoff, working colleagues of Kalkoff, would be the first to test thiosemicarbazone against tuberculosis infecting the throat. While Philipp Klee – assisted by a team which included the young Karl Jahnke, Doctors Melzer, Ruhs and Kothe – was working night and day to discover the optimum dosage for the treatment of pulmonary tuberculosis, Professor Kuhlmann and his assistant, Knorr, in Mölln, were already planning the trials of Conteben not only in pulmonary tuberculosis, but also tuberculosis affecting the bowel, and even that famous and most ancient of manifestations of the disease, scrofula, "The King's Evil". Professor Boshamer would test it against the infections in the bladder, ureters and kidneys, as well as the genital infections in women. Dr Kurt Ullmann would test it against the most intractable infections of all, those crippling abscesses of joints, the long bones and spine. Soon many other eminent doctors would join the great cooperative effort: the pragmatist, Paul Martini in Bonn, Ludwig Heilmeyer in Freiburg, W. Catell in Mammolshöhe.

Nobody could accuse Domagk of underestimating his enemy. In his diary, he reminded himself of the need for caution: "We are still a long way from achieving our aim. Let us hope that in spite of all the problems and the obstacles in our path, that we shall achieve them. . ."

iv

FOR A LITTLE while, he could think of getting away from the pressures of work. It was time for his annual holiday when, despite the frugal postwar limitations, he could look forward to some light amusement. In August Gertrud and he took the long slow train to Dammeshöved where the children were already enjoying their school holidays with their grandfather. After a few weeks' relaxation, Domagk and his wife carried on to Partenkirchen to join a university week organized by Professor von Shücking.

In Hamburg, the train was so crowded that they nearly cancelled the trip. . . "Eventually we were allowed into a private compartment but soon this too became quite unbearable. As soon as the train had left Hamburg, people pushed their way from the overcrowded corridors into this compartment and in the end our small compartment, meant for eight, was bulging with fifteen to twenty people. In Lüneburg, at the last minute, an old mother came in huffing and puffing – and since she couldn't find any other room, she sat on my wife's lap. My wife was getting so distraught with the pressure and lack of air that she started to cry. The old woman couldn't care less, she unpacked her handbag and started to stuff herself. Tomatoes, apples, tomatoes, apples – it went on like that for a while, then she wanted to get out to the toilet, which was impossible because the corridors were chock-a-block with a human wall. She returned unable to carry out her purpose.

"After a while she started to stamp her feet on the floor. 'I've got to go, I've got to go.' She pushed out towards the toilet – again in vain – and every foiled attempt was followed by energetic stamping of her feet. Finally, the woman jumped to her feet in the dark compartment, exclaiming, 'Well it's too late now. I've done it." So saying, she pulled her skirt over her head and took off her pants – at least so one gathered in the dark – and packed them into her handbag. Soon after this, the atmosphere became more and more unbearable until a few hearty chaps declared, 'The old girl has got to go'. At the next station, Würzburg, they forced the unfortunate and loudly protesting woman out through the window. Hardly had the window been lowered to eject her than two others climbed in. They were fumbling their way round in the dark compartment, when, feeling their clothes, they suddenly squealed in horror: 'Ooh, there's something sticky'. It seemed that when climbing in through the window, they had wiped up the trail made by the woman as she was being passed out of the window! That's how the people travelled in 1947, in the supposedly most cultured of the 'Western Zones', some two years after the ending of hostilities."[12]

At the conference there was the opportunity, between lectures, for the participants to sit in a genuine Bavarian restaurant, drinking large glasses of beer, which were quite drinkable though hardly as good as those before the war. Following the meeting, Gertrud returned home while Domagk travelled on to Mölln where he discussed the treatment of pulmonary tuberculosis with Professor Kuhlmann. Kuhlmann had for some short time been conducting a small pilot study of Conteben in just a few patients.

That November, in 1947, a new tuberculosis hospital was opened in Flensburg, under the directorship of Dr Delfs, an old friend and colleague of Kuhlmann's. To mark the occasion, Domagk returned to Mölln, to make an historic journey, in the company of Professor Kuhlmann, bringing the first five patients treated with Conteben for pulmonary tuberculosis to the meeting in the old town. The weather was bitterly cold and the patients had to travel under a flimsy canvas cover in the back of a lorry. Yet the meeting was a vital step in convincing the sanitorium doctors that here at last was a therapy worth taking seriously. In Domagk's own words, "A lot could be said about this trip. We travelled in a wood-gas lorry as no petrol

was available for Germans and Professor Kuhlmann and I took
turns at stoking the boiler with wood. The patients sat in the
back of the lorry, insulated with straw. Mulled wine was available during the entire trip, to keep up the temperature as much
as the spirits."[13]

The response of the sanitorium doctors was disheartening if
altogether predictable. Kuhlmann and Domagk were subjected
to exactly the same disbelief as Lehmann, Sievers and Vallentin, a year earlier in Gothenburg. In spite of the histories, in
spite of the long series of chest X-rays, in spite of presenting the
very patients themselves, who were able to describe their harrowing experiences and then the dramatic improvement in
their health as a result of taking Conteben – in spite of the fact
that Delfs himself, and a handful of his assistants had seen
those same patients prior to their treatment back in Mölln –
nobody else would believe that they had been cured by the
drug. "We had to listen to many more accusations by the 'TB-
popes.' When we said that only a few months ago these
patients had been dying from severe pulmonary and bowel
tuberculosis, they looked at us as if we were either out of our
minds or imposters."[14]

Upon his return from Flensburg, Domagk found a more
pleasant reception awaiting him. He had received a letter from
the Swedish Consulate. Would he be willing to attend the
Nobel Prize ceremony on 10 December in Stockholm where, at
last, he would be presented with his Nobel Prize?

                                   V

"I AGREED BY telegram. To get an exit visa I had to fill in
three questionnaires in German and English. When I thought I
had completed them and took them to the passport office, I
was told they were far from complete. First I needed a priest or a
doctor to certify that my answers to the questionnaire were
truthful. Then they needed a character reference from the
police, which should be obtained from room 224 at the Town
Hall. When I went there, the official was very polite – he carefully made a note of all the details. 'Contact us,' he suggested,

'in three months.' When I said I needed it immediately he just laughed and added, 'First we have to make enquiries at your place of birth.' I pointed out to him that Lagow, my dear old home town, was now in Poland. 'Then,' declared he, 'it will take a good deal longer.'

"Eventually we came to an agreement. Since I had lived in Elberfeld since 1927, I would get a certificate of good conduct for the time I had lived there, in other words from 1927 to 1947. Back I went to the passport office but still they were not satisfied. Now they demanded a health certificate. The official was quite indignant when I suggested that since I was a doctor maybe I could write one myself. No, that certainly was not possible. I must get one from a doctor in the community health service. This doctor was not to be found. He was out of town. Eventually one of his younger colleagues examined me and in the evening I held in my hand a certificate personally signed by the community health manager that I was free of infectious diseases and parasites.

"A few days later, after I had sent off all these papers, a courier arrived from the Swedish Consulate in Hamburg and brought me my passport, together with an invitation for my wife. Ridiculous as it might seem, we had to start with the same story all over again. Finally, by Friday we had permission for a joint passport. I thanked the General Consul for all his help. Then they asked me, very sympathetically, if I had a Danish visa. Unfortunately I had to say no. In order to get one we would have to stop in Hamburg on Monday on our way to Stockholm, but if we had to stop on Monday in Hamburg it would be too late to get to Stockholm by 9 December. So we sent a personal messenger to Hamburg on Friday night. On the Saturday morning, I had to give a lecture in Münster. When I returned in the afternoon, there was a discussion on the treatment of tuberculosis of the skin at the Wuppertal-Elberfeld Hospital, attended by the dermatologists of Münster as well as Professor Klee, Professor Sturm and the paediatrician, Dr Gehrt. Professor Hehring from Cologne joined us later. Afterwards, pea soup was served by Professor Koch in his flat. It was midnight when I got home and the passports had arrived. I knew that we could travel the following day.

"I had arranged that the driver should come and pick us up and take us to the ten o'clock train to Düsseldorf, but he had misunderstood and did not arrive. We tried to ring him but the line was engaged, so one of our sons ran up to his house. He arrived with a coat over his nightshirt and raced at 100 km per hour across the fields on the highways and byways to Düsseldorf.

"We arrived ten minutes before the train was to leave but when we tried to get on the platform we were told this platform is out of bounds to Germans – it was an international train. Showing them my passport to Sweden made no difference. We needed to get special permission from the English authority, which was located back in the foyer. But when I went to their office and asked for permission, they declared, 'It is impossible for you to travel on this train. Perhaps you would like to make an application? Maybe in a fortnight? Good morning!'

I could try my luck with the long queue in front of the counter, where they were doling out special dispensations. Five minutes to go before the train leaves. I joined the queue, not at the back but in front. I showed them my pass and was allowed to travel as far as Osnabrück. At last we could sit down peacefully on the train, in the second-class compartment. Ironically, it was nearly empty. We were grateful for every stop we were able to pass without being checked beyond Osnabrück. All we needed now was another bureaucrat who would make us get out before Flensburg and demand renewed admission. So, fortunately at midnight, we arrived at Flensburg. Our foreign ticket should have been left at the first station in Denmark because with German money we were only able to buy a ticket as far as the German border. Because I was feeling a bit uncomfortable about travelling into a foreign country without a ticket, and without foreign money, I asked the stationmaster at one of the stops if he would he be so kind as to make a 'phone call to the town beyond the border and ask if our tickets and money had been left there. Just as the train was about to leave he came back and informed us, 'No, there are no tickets'.

"So there we were, at midnight, my wife and I, together with one suitcase, standing on the station platform in Flensburg. It was raining. The counters were all closed, so we couldn't even deposit our luggage. Eventually we managed to rid ourselves of it, with the help of a sympathetic station official, who deposited it in a refugee hut, smelling strongly of disinfectant. The friendly official also offered us his modest bed, but since we have relatives in Flensburg, we decided to try and get in touch with them. We arrived there after a short walk but the factory door was locked. Their home was in the garden behind. So we called, 'Edda!' At last there was a reply: 'Who is it? Oh it's you! How many of you are there then?'

"'All of us,' we said, 'parents and four children,' just to give them a bit of a fright. The pleasure of meeting again was wonderful. There was so much to talk about. The Amberlangs had been forced to leave Liegnitz when the Russians entered the city. Mr Amberlang had left behind his life's work, his sawmill, and his beautiful home in his beloved Silesia. Many memories dwelt on the homeland he had left behind.

"This forced break in the journey brought an unexpected bonus. Before my departure, I had tried everywhere to find a white tie and waistcoat to go with my evening suit. It had proved impossible. The Americans had found my new evening suit when they took over our house. Neighbours told me that they had played football in front of the house, wearing my dinner jacket, and had finally draped the remains of the suit over the trees. So now I had to make do with my old wedding suit, together with a borrowed waistcoat and white tie. During the latter years, my old wedding suit had barely reached halfway round my chest, which is why I had sent it, together with the old dinner jacket, to Dammeshöved, where Gertrud had gone to stay with the children during the later bombing. All I had in mind for it was the gardening. When Gertrud returned home at the end of the war she had brought it back with her thinking that perhaps she could make something for the children out of it. After so many lean years, the suit fitted me again like a glove. Now my brother-in-law, Hermann, helped me out with a waistcoat. He had rescued his evening suit by hiding it in his car. At least, now, with my borrowed white waistcoat, no matter that my old suit did not look altogether smart, it showed that the spirit was willing.

"After a good breakfast, which was possible because Flensburg was so close to the Danish border, we went back to the station and the friendly station employee telephoned Padborg again. Wonderful news – our tickets were there. At twelve o'clock we stepped calmly and confidently into our train. But when I tried to get out at Padburg to get the new tickets, the whole train had been locked up. I ran along the length of the train until I found the stationmaster. I tried to tell him that I had to get out to collect our tickets. When they finally opened the doors, the train was ready to leave again. Now we felt the drawback of having a joint passport. Either I stepped out of the train having left it with my wife and she could carry on in the train with a pass but no ticket, or I would have two tickets and both our passports and she would be left, if the train pulled out, with nothing at all.

"But we managed to meet up in time and finally we journeyed onwards together through the snow-sprinkled Danish landscape until we arrived in Copenhagen that same night. There we had to change to a sleeper that was going to Stockholm. When I got out of the train to look for it, I noticed men with cameras and flashlights coming along the platform. I guessed this meant an assault. As soon as we stepped on to the platform they were already rushing forwards. 'Professor Domagk, may we take a photograph – we are from Stockholm – may we speak to you on the train?' Over the last part of our journey, Gertrud and I found ourselves being asked more questions than we knew how to answer. At last we found our sleeping cabin and arrived at about eight o'clock in the morning in Stockholm.

"Professor Henschen, who seemed to tower over everybody else on the platform, came smiling towards us accompanied by a young diplomat who was going to be our guide during the festivities there. So many questions to and fro. So much had happened since we last met Professor Henschen in May, 1939, in Rome. In the car on the way to the hotel, the young diplomat asked me whether I had my tails. I confessed that all I had was my old suit. Whereupon he answered very genially, 'Our king also knows old tales and he loves old tails.' He offered to have a suit cut in time for the presentation. But I did not feel a particular need to be seen, as a present day German, in a new evening suit. Why conceal reality behind a pretence!

"The big occasion, for which I had waited so very long, was in the afternoon on the following day. Our young diplomat picked us up in the car. We went to the Concert Hall where there were big columns with flaming torches overhead and where, in the falling snow, a large crowd was gathered to see our arrival."[15]

vi

ON 10 DECEMBER 1947, a thin-faced man, weary from a lifetime of struggle, stood on the platform of the Festival Hall in Stockholm, to receive the Nobel Prize medal and certificate from King Gustav V of Sweden. At last, more than ten years after Prontosil had cured its first patient, Gerhard Domagk waited his turn to receive the highest accolade in the scientific world. Two years earlier, on 7 December 1945, Alexander Fleming, together with Howard Florey and Ernst Chain, had been presented with this same high honour for the discovery of penicillin.

Having waited eight years already, he could bear to wait a little longer as the other laureates for 1947 were presented first. In his gaunt face, his haggard appearance, Domagk personified the postwar hunger and suffering of much of Europe. In a final irony, because the award was being presented retrospectively, he was denied the cheque which was customarily presented with the medal. "My wife was escorted by the young diplomat to a box from where one got a particularly good view of the whole festivities. The people who were awarded prizes had to go backstage first. Every prize winner was escorted by a Swedish scientist in the same field. With me was dear Professor Liljestrand. So we lined up in pairs. First there was the English physicist Sir Edward Appleton, then the chemist Sir Robert Robinson, then the married couple Gerti and Carl Cori followed by Professor Bernardo Houssay. Finally it was my turn – the leftover from 1939."[16]

In a way he was too unassuming to acknowledge, the award signified more than the recognition of academic or scientific achievement. One man was now outstanding in the world, the representative of a wholly different Germany and Germanic tradition, the Germany of Beethoven, Schiller, Handel, Einstein, and Schubert. Two great German doctors, Robert Koch and Paul Ehrlich, had received Nobel Prizes for what could now be seen as stages in that same odyssey. What did Gerhard Domagk think about during that long wait, as all the others rose in their turn, made their brief speeches, and were presented with their Prizes? Nobody present in the Hall realized better than he did that the odyssey was far from over, that at this very moment it was surging forwards in those myriad trials of Conteben now taking place throughout the length and breadth of Germany.

At the ball after the ceremony, Domagk danced with an attractive young brunette, the daughter of Sir Edward Appleton. They were captured in a photograph as they were dancing, when Domagk appeared pale and fragile, emaciated, yet preserving the dignity of a humane and compassionate man.

vii

GERHARD DOMAGK CAME home to a mushrooming excitement with the Conteben results, which were astonishing doctors, scientists and patients alike in every corner of Germany. In 1948, at a conference of Rheinisch-Westfalen doctors held in Düsseldorf, Klee had acquired enough experience of the drug to recommend much smaller doses than they had used in the beginning. With such doses few if any patients suffered the nausea and vomiting that very often accompanied high doses. Still they knew virtually nothing of how the drug worked, how it was absorbed into the body and dealt with by the liver and kidneys. Women called the drug the nine months' wonder because they sometimes experienced the most curious sensation when taking it, as if they were nine months' pregnant. High doses of the drug resulted in side-effects in a minority of patients, the most serious of which was liver damage. Such large doses, Klee suggested, should be reserved for the fulminating infections such as blood-borne tuberculosis and tuberculous meningitis, where the higher doses need only be given for relatively short periods.

The solemn Klee, with his Goethe-like piercing blue eyes and the white nimbus of hair encircling his domed forehead, went on to give them all wonderful news. He reported striking cures of blood-borne tuberculosis using Conteben. Those wonderful initial results against tuberculosis of the skin had been dramatically reproduced by Loebell and Eickhoff in tuberculosis affecting the larynx. The agony of speaking, the hoarseness of the voice, had disappeared within a few days of starting therapy. Hitherto hopeless cases were able to swallow again without discomfort. The same dramatic benefit had been obtained in dozens of intestinal sufferers, where Kuhlmann was frankly amazed at how it alleviated the otherwise uncontrollable and exhausting diarrhoea, allowing the patients to return to eating normally and to put weight back onto their skeletally wasted bodies. Time and time again, the emaciated patients, often thought to be in their terminal decline, went on to make a good recovery. Kuhlmann, like Klee, and indeed every other investigator, presented his results formally and warned that Conteben did not cure everybody. It had, however, worked the same miracle for Professor Malluche in that agonizingly painful condition, tuberculosis of the bladder. Even in that most intractable form of infection, tuberculosis of bones and joints, Ullmann now added his stories of extraordinary recoveries. Spinal vertebrae that were being slowly eaten away, had solidified into strong new bone. Incurable infections of the small joints in the hands, the pelvis, the sterno-clavicular joints at the junction of chest and collarbones, all had shown dramatic improvement, with high temperatures falling to normal, the intense inflammation disappearing. The delighted surgeons could now reconstruct those bones that had already been damaged beyond repair. In report after report at the meeting, Gerhard Domagk listened with pride to stories of Conteben bringing new hope in place of sickness, deformity, maiming and death. But what of the greatest challenge of all, the commonest manifestation of tuberculosis, and the form in which it spread in epidemic form, afflicting millions?

In pulmonary tuberculosis, the painstaking trials of Philipp Klee in Wuppertal, Ludwig Heilmeyer in Freiburg, Paul Martini in Bonn and the pioneering F. Kuhlmann in Mölln, showed marvellous promise.[17] In this, the most devious and unpredictable form of the disease, as with Hinshaw in relation to streptomycin and Vallentin in relation to PAS, Klee tempered his good news with caution. Interpretation of the pulmonary results would never be easy. With pulmonary tuberculosis, it was always difficult to be sure that the drug was curing patients. The disease fluctuated naturally, the body's own defences played an important part. Given the many different presentations and manifestations, from the tiny primary spots that typically presented in childhood, to the galloping consumption that swept through both lungs like an acute bacterial pneumonia, it was difficult to get enough sufferers within each subgroup to draw accurate comparisons. As had been the case in the United States and Sweden, Klee informed Domagk that it would be necessary to test literally hundreds, perhaps thousands, of patients, before they would really know the drug's full potential.

In spite of this understandable caution, Domagk's friend, Hoff, would subsequently capture the prevailing sense of wonder. "In 1948 I was put in charge of the Medical Clinic at Aachen. This hospital had, as was usual in those days, a big ward for patients suffering from tuberculosis. These patients were full of bitterness. They made cynical jokes about themselves saying that the moths were eating up their lungs. Many of them suffered from high fever, they had diarrhoea from involvement of the intestine, they suffered much pain and those who had tuberculosis of the larynx could not speak in more than a whisper. Often a massive haemorrhage from the lungs ended their lives. I wrote to Domagk and very soon he sent me a package of Conteben. This brought about a miracle on our tuberculosis wards. The fever was gone, the bacteria could no longer be found in their sputum, their weights increased and in many cases the symptoms of intestinal tuberculosis and tuberculosis affecting the throat disappeared. At last there was hope for the future. Prior to this, most patients had looked upon us, their doctors, with eyes filled with suspicion: now they were filled with a new confidence in the ability of their doctors to help them. I must say that this was one of the most uplifting experiences I had in my medical career."[18]

In two years, from 1947 to 1949, no less than 20,000 people were treated with Conteben. At a time when Germany was suffering a massive resurgence of tuberculosis, there can be no doubt that many thousands of lives were saved. For Karl Jahnke, Klee's young assistant, it was a glorious time to be a young doctor.

"Before 1948, tuberculosis wards and tuberculosis clinics were depressing places. To enthusiastic young doctors, who like to cure people, tuberculosis was the Cinderella of diseases. The sick lay there exhausted, feverish, breathless, racked by an intractable coughing. Only the lucky few, well-wrapped against the cold, were allowed to lie out on the open balconies. Apart from collapse therapy, we doctors could offer them very little apart from opiate drugs to relieve the coughing. When they suffered the much-dreaded lung haemorrhages, we would try to help them with some rather dubious therapies, such as Sangostop or Clouden. We were well aware that all we were doing for these people was offering psychological support. In spite of the hopelessness, these tuberculosis wards were popular with young doctors such as myself, because here we could get plenty of experience, percussing and auscultating chests.

"Everywhere there was more pathology than you could cope with. We could look at an endless variety of abnormal chest X-rays. In their desperation, the sufferers would pay anything to obtain secret remedies. One I remember was concocted from a witch's brew of dog fat and sand from the Sahara Desert, and sold to them by unscrupulous businessmen with the promise that here was the latest wonder cure. I had seen the despair of these unfortunate people, often they were such beautiful young women, before the advent of Conteben. Now I saw those same beautiful young women lying in their beds suffering from exudative tuberculosis. Only now we could give them the new treatment, now we could see how they blossomed. The most dramatic effect was on the infections in the throat and the bowels. Here we saw the most exciting and dramatic improvements within just a matter of days. Day by day, we could see how they lost their fever and gained weight. The improvement in them was all the more wonderful to a young doctor such as myself for the fact they were so young. It was exhilarating to observe how the horrific death rate from the disease was at last falling. Klee, in his extensive reports, could draw attention to a halving of mortality in Wuppertal in just three years, between 1945 and 1948."[19]

Such youthful enthusiasm would have a price to pay. Karl Jahnke, like so many of his young and equally enthusiastic colleagues, attracted to the tuberculosis research by its wonderful new promise, contracted tuberculosis himself from his attendance on his patients. One of the techniques for healing the big cavities that formed in the lungs was to place a long thin tube, called a Monaldi catheter, through the chest wall and then through the diseased lung until the end of the tube lay in the cavity. The cavity would then be sucked dry before the young doctor connected his own mouth to the upper end of the catheter and blew Conteben powder deep into the cavity, teeming with bacteria. The dangers were obvious. Many of Jahnke's friends contracted pulmonary tuberculosis. Jahnke contracted the disease in the lymph glands of his neck, the age-old scrofula. The greatly swollen glands were lanced so as to allow the cheesy pus to discharge and streptomycin was instilled into the abscess. But the abscess refused to heal. At the suggestion of his physician, Karl, together with his young wife, travelled to the Alps to be treated in one of the famous sanitoria.

Here his doctor permitted him to walk out of doors but with the caution that he must at all costs avoid direct sunshine. "From then on, I walked only in the shadows. One day, in overcast weather, I walked to the top of the Nebelhorn, in the Allgaeu. Suddenly, to my consternation, the sun came out from behind the clouds and, looking round, there wasn't a tree at this altitude to offer me the slightest shade. I got well and truly sunburnt. But from that moment on, my tuberculosis began to improve. The enlarged glands grew smaller and smaller until they finally healed up altogether."[20]

At the very heart of the great discovery, the disease might have been sounding yet another warning. When you thought you most understood it, it had a tendency to take you by surprise.

19

Premature Celebrations

I have been horribly ill the last few weeks. I had a bit of a relapse, then they had another go with the streptomycin, which previously did me a lot of good, at least temporarily. This time only one dose of it had ghastly results, as I had built up an allergy or something . . .

George Orwell

i

THE WINTER OF 1947-8 was the coldest on record in England, and rationing, which was still in force since the war, was actually being tightened. The previous spring, Eric Arthur Blair, better known as the iconoclastic novelist, George Orwell, had moved to the remote Scottish Island of Jura in order to write his masterpiece, *Nineteen Eighty-Four*. For Orwell, it was a courageous act, for he was already in poor health with bronchiectasis, a chronic lung problem. He had contracted this mysterious chest complaint during an eccentric and eventful life in which he had dressed in rags to share misery with the poor in the East End of London and had served in the Republican Militia in the Spanish Civil War. Now this world famous writer embraced another spartan lifestyle, living in a rough cottage, with few comforts and sleeping in a bedroom that was heated by a smoky grate. He also forced himself to a marathon effort of writing, day and night, completing a gruelling 5,000 words a day. In the words of his friend and biographer, Tosco Fyvel, "From a letter in October 1947, I

323

gathered that his new book was going well... He also wrote that his chest troubles were afflicting him again – and then came disaster."[1]

Bronchiectasis is a relatively inactive disease of the lung, with thick fibrous-walled cavities which are often infected by the common respiratory germs. This had been diagnosed during Orwell's stay in Preston Hall Sanitorium in 1938, when X-rays had shown a cavity at the apex of the left lung.[2] Tuberculosis is also a common cause of bronchiectasis. At the time he had been repeatedly tested for tuberculosis but the tests had proved negative. Orwell, however, had long suspected the true nature of his complaint but refused for several months to see a doctor because it would interfere with his writing. Now he was so sick that he was forced to call a chest specialist, Dr Bruce Dick, all the way from Glasgow to see him. Dr Dick confirmed that he was suffering from pulmonary tuberculosis.

He was admitted to the Hairmyres Hospital in West Kilbride on 20 December 1947, where he began the usual sanitorium regime of enforced bed rest. In an attempt to close the cavity at the top of his left lung, the nerve to his left diaphragm was crushed, followed by twice weekly sessions when air was pumped into the abdomen, the so called pneumoperitoneum. To his personal worries were added the concern that his adopted son, Richard, was in danger of contracting this ghastly disease from him. The little boy was allowed a single visit, after which Orwell had to be content with photographs. A great fighter, who refused to bow to his illness, while in the hospital Orwell wrote a letter, dated 1 February 1948, to his friend, David Astor.

"Dear David ... before anything else I must tell you something Dr Dick has said to me. He says I am getting on quite well, but slowly, and it would speed recovery if one had some streptomycin."[3] Orwell, who was normally given to understatement, spelled out the name of the drug once more, in capitals.

At this time, when the British Medical Research Council had just begun a crucial trial of the drug, streptomycin was more precious than gold dust. Astor, who had been arranging food parcels for Orwell from America, now cabled New York for a supply of streptomycin. He also spoke personally to Nye Bevan, the Minister for Health in the postwar Labour Government, to make sure there would be no problems with importing it. By the end of February, Orwell had received his first injections of the drug, with dramatic effectiveness. Orwell wrote to Julian Symons, "I have been having the streptomycin for about a month and it is evidently doing its stuff. I haven't gained much weight, but I'm much better in every way."[4]

Out of the blue, Orwell suffered strange complications, which he noted in his diary. His skin turned red, itched continuously and peeled, and he developed a severe sore throat with blood-filled blisters in his throat, cheeks and lips. At night, while he slept, these would burst so that his lips were caked in blood and stuck together in the morning. His nails disintegrated and his hair began to fall out. Ominously, after fifty days, the injections had to be discontinued. But his tuberculosis was so much improved that by July 1948 he was back on Jura, working even harder during the six glorious summer weeks on the final revision of his book. In November, he suffered a relapse, during which, racked by an unremitting cough and fever, he sat up in the old iron bed, dressed in his seedy dressing gown which was held together with a frayed belt, and forced himself to re-type the entire lengthy typescript.

He completed the task in one heroic month. But it proved disastrous. He suffered an overwhelming relapse of his tuberculosis which caused him to be taken to Cranham Sanitorium, 900 feet high in the Cotswold hills, between Stroud and Gloucester, where he was treated once more with streptomycin. The following April, in a letter to Fyvel, Orwell recorded the grim message that presages this chapter.[5] What had gone so dangerously wrong?

The streptomycin, which had previously saved him was no longer helpful. A single dose almost killed him and the drug had to be stopped at once. It is certain from Orwell's description that he had developed a true allergy to the drug. From this point onwards he deteriorated rapidly. He was transferred to Dr Andrew Morland, a Harley Street chest physician who had also attended D. H. Lawrence. Morland admitted him to the private wing of the University College Hospital in London, where, despite the fact he survived through 1949, he died on 22 January 1950.

The overwhelming evidence would now suggest that even if he had not been allergic to streptomycin, a second course of treatment would have made little difference. In his death, some six years after the first appearance of streptomycin, Orwell was all too typical of hundreds of thousands of sufferers worldwide. Why was this happening?

ii

A BACTERIOLOGIST CALLED William Steenken Jr attempted to explain it. He looked very closely at patients who were treated with streptomycin at the Trudeau Sanitorium and the Veterans Administration Hospital at Sunmount, New York. Although the vast majority of these people had germs that were sensitive to streptomycin at the beginning of their courses of treatment, drug resistant germs began to show in their sputum by the fourth week of therapy. If streptomycin was continued for four months, a staggering ninety per cent of patients were coughing up germs that were now resistant to streptomycin.[6] The implications of this were very frightening.

Clearly streptomycin would have its maximal effect during the first month or two of therapy, after which it would have almost no effect at all. And two months was not long enough to cure pulmonary tuberculosis.

Even in the horrifically fatal tuberculous meningitis and blood-borne tuberculosis, where the drug had proved most miraculous ... "One streptomycin investigator had admitted in 1948 that 'early enthusiasm concerning the value of streptomycin in tuberculous meningitis was considerably dampened as one after another of the patients who were considered to be on their way to recovery ... gradually lapsed into a comatose state or developed other complications and died.'"[7] In their frustration, doctors were in danger of overreacting. Streptomycin was still a discovery of phenomenal importance. But it had limitations which needed to be clearly understood.

The wonderful results of the early American trials had not been obtained in strictly controlled scientific experiment. Following those first reports of Hinshaw and Feldman, doctors in

America were understandably reluctant to include a control group of patients who would, by design, be given no drug treatment at all. British doctors however could only obtain very small quantities of the drug so that very few of their patients could be treated with it anyway. The Medical Research Council had nothing to lose in asking a mathematician, Bradford Hill, to invent a trial in which chance alone would decide who would be treated and who would not.

Fifty-five patients with acute pulmonary tuberculosis were treated with streptomycin and the outcome compared with that in fifty-two patients with a similar degree and extent of acute pulmonary tuberculosis, treated with just the sanitorium regime. The results, published in 1948, were not only illuminative, they were also heartbreaking.[8]

Most of the patients treated with streptomycin showed clearing of the tuberculosis on their chest X-rays, while only eight per cent of those treated with the conventional regime showed any improvement. Fourteen of those treated with the sanitorium regime were dead within six months compared with just four of those treated with streptomycin. One could scarcely imagine a more poignant demonstration of the potency of streptomycin – or of the inadequacy of the sanitorium regime in treating acute pulmonary tuberculosis. But when another group of doctors analysed those same patients some five years later, there was an even more harrowing tale to tell. Thirty-five of the original fifty-two patients denied the drug were dead, which was perhaps not too surprising. More disturbing was the fact that thirty-two of the original fifty-five patients treated with streptomycin were also dead.[9]

The conclusion was inescapable: few of the patients treated with streptomycin had been cured by the drug. What it had achieved was a temporary reduction in the severity of the disease. The deaths following streptomycin were almost invariably due to the germs becoming resistant. For resistant germs to emerge took only a period of eight weeks. Once resistant, the germs remained so, indeed the resistant germs proliferated rapidly. In a further chilling demonstration of the power of this disease to fight back, it was possible in the laboratory to find germs which were no longer just resistant to streptomycin: they had developed a partiality to it, preferring it to their customary food.[10]

Streptomycin would be no panacea for pulmonary tuberculosis though it remained the single most effective therapy for tuberculous meningitis and blood-borne tuberculosis, where the short course of the disease did not give the germ as much time to develop resistance. In the excited media reaction to the drug's first arrival, and in spite of the warnings of Hinshaw, people had expected too much of streptomycin. They had taken the words "miracle drug" too literally.

Yet another source of unease was growing. In a small but significant number of patients, streptomycin was poisonous to the delicate nerve mechanism of the ear. It made people deaf, permanently dizzy or gave them disabling noises in their ears. This toxicity, which affected about ten per cent of those treated, was lessened by giving smaller doses; and the relatively high frequency of bacterial resistance was avoided to a certain extent by giving the drug for shorter periods of therapy. But such small doses and short duration therapies were not as effective in curing the disease.

Why did the bacteria develop this resistance in some patients and not in others? Nobody knew. Why did the drug exert such serious side effects in a minority of patients while not in the majority? Again it was a mystery. Nobody had the slightest idea how the drug worked. In William Feldman's honest acknowledgement: "It would be highly gratifying intellectually to have said that our attack on the problem of chemotherapy for tuberculosis was based on a complicated and astute understanding of the chemistry of the tubercle bacillus. Unfortunately, such was not the case. Instead our approach was similar to that of countless others: a formula consisting largely of enthusiasm, hope, faith, persistence, and luck. Perhaps the latter was the most important ingredient."[11]

Tuberculosis chose this uncertain moment to fight back in a deeply personal way. In December 1948, William Feldman attended Corwin Hinshaw, who had long been his personal physician, for his compulsory annual medical examination. On all previous occasions he had been found fit and healthy. This time, however, things were not so reassuring. In Hinshaw's words: "I saw Bill's chest film and I was alarmed because the right upper lobe was largely consolidated and heavily infiltrated. My first thought was that Bill had developed cancer of the lung from the years of his smoking cigarettes. However the first examination of his sputum revealed tuberculous germs and culture of these germs indicated that they were probably of the H37–Rv strain, which he had been using in the guinea pig experiments."[12]

At the same time that George Orwell discovered the true nature of the disease that would kill him, William Feldman was also seriously ill with pulmonary tuberculosis. He had developed a fever, a racking cough and his weight was falling. The fears of Albert Schatz' colleagues, who had refused to work with such a dangerous bacterium, were now amply justified.

Given what was now known about streptomycin in the long term treatment of pulmonary tuberculosis, Feldman must have been well aware that streptomycin alone would not save him. Nothing could more dramatically have focused Dr Hinshaw's attention onto the drug that had been largely ignored in America during those heady first years of the streptomycin miracle, Lehmann's para-aminosalicylic acid.

iii

THE EARLY TRIALS of PAS in pulmonary tuberculosis had all too often been performed in people suffering from extensive and advanced forms of the disease. How could anybody really expect a fair assessment of any drug in such patients, with extensive fibrosis, cavity formation, pleural thickening and the after-effects of surgery! In Sweden, a sanitorium doctor, Bo Carstensen decided he would test the drug in more representative circumstances. He gave PAS to twenty-two people suffering from severe pulmonary tuberculosis of recent onset. These were not cases with cavities and fibrosis but desperately sick people suffering from an acute fulminant disease, rather like an acute pneumonia. All of them had additional bowel tuberculosis and it was likely that without effective treatment they would die fairly soon from their disease. The results, which he presented to a tuberculosis meeting on 26 November 1947, were as miraculous as in any of the early streptomycin trials.

In nineteen out of the twenty-two cases, the clinical symptoms of the intestinal tuberculosis had completely disappeared and even the remaining three cases had shown definite improvement.[13] These dramatic cures were much better received than Vallentin's early results a year previously in Gothenburg. Dr Alf Westergren, who had been one of the very few to respond favourably in Gothenburg, and who was once again in the audience, made a very important observation. Surely the dramatic response of the intestinal disease was due to the high concentrations of the drug in the bowel, a major advantage of PAS, which, unlike streptomycin, was taken by mouth.

In 1948, Carstensen published further details of these patients together with some additional cases in a medical paper.[14] People with fresh exudative tuberculosis who had not been previously operated on, people with intestinal tuberculosis or with tuberculosis affecting their kidneys and bladder, a patient with blood-borne tuberculosis, another with meningitis that was deemed hopeless – every one of them had lost his or her high temperature, and had gone on to make a wonderful recovery.

Carstensen's study in a single stroke won over most of his sceptical colleagues in Sweden. It also coincided with the newly improved techniques of drug manufacture as a result of the inspiration of the Ferrosan chemists. Soon, further Swedish and American studies would amply confirm his findings.[15,16] But there was an additional very worrying outcome of these trials. The tuberculosis germs had also shown themselves capable of becoming resistant to PAS. Though this was not so dramatically seen as with streptomycin, by the end of their treatment one in three patients was growing resistant germs. If it was not obvious already, simple comparisons between streptomycin and PAS were no longer relevant.

In 1948, the British Medical Council performed a new and very different type of study involving PAS and streptomycin.

This compared the results of treatment in three groups of patients: one given PAS alone, one given streptomycin alone, and a third given the two drugs simultaneously. The plan was to assess the results of the trial some time in 1950. On 31 December 1949, in an unprecedented manner, the trial was interrupted when only half complete by a dramatic announcement in the *British Medical Journal*.

> The trial is not yet completed, but certain results already obtained are of such importance that the joint committee responsible for guiding the trial has decided to issue the following preliminary statement... The trial has demonstrated unequivocally that the combination of PAS with streptomycin reduces considerably the risk of development of streptomycin resistant strains of tubercle bacilli during the six months following the start of treatment.[17]

The same urgent conclusion would be drawn from huge trials simultaneously conducted in the United States, in the veterans hospitals.[18] Combination therapy, with PAS and streptomycin, was as important a breakthrough as the pioneering discovery of each of the two drugs themselves. How fitting too that it arrived just in time to help save the life of the wonderfully unassuming William Feldman.

After a month's treatment in the Methodist Hospital in Rochester, he was transferred to the Presbyterian Hospital, in Albuquerque, New Mexico, before moving on for a longer stay in Nopeming Sanitorium, near Duluth, Minnesota. Here he stayed for a year or so, receiving streptomycin and PAS in combination, together with Promin for additional security. Where Orwell, given single therapy, had died, Feldman, given the combination treatment he had helped to pioneer, made a good if slow recovery.

Even now the brave Feldman had no intention of giving up the battle against tuberculosis. So determined was he to return to work that his physician had the greatest difficulty in persuading him to agree to a further year's convalescence before he insisted on returning to the fray, helping to coordinate the massive tuberculosis research programme, throughout forty-six separate hospitals and institutions, now undertaken by the Veterans Administration.

In that same year of 1949, the life of Selman Waksman would be turned upside down by a bombshell. In his own words:

"The future that appeared so bright and so full of promise in 1949 was headed for a severe blow. This came from quite an unexpected quarter. It came from one of my former students, one in whom I had great confidence as a promising future scientist, one whose name I had placed side by side with mine on numerous scientific papers, one who I hoped would carry on in the same tradition and spirit of research as I had done myself, as Dr Lipman did before me, and as some of my former students were already doing."[19]

iv

ALBERT SCHATZ HAD of course left Rutgers Agricultural College in 1946, convinced that his part in the discovery of streptomycin had been deliberately undermined by Waksman. Whether this was true or not, it had resulted in a tragic deterioration in the relationship between the two men, which had previously been one of mutual respect and friendship.

On 31 January 1945, Waksman and Schatz had signed the American patent agreement as joint inventors of streptomycin. Betty Bugie, the second author on the first streptomycin paper, and a vivacious young woman, had no intention of making science her prime objective in life. "There was a strong belief that a girl could get a masters degree and live normally but if you got a PhD, you didn't get married. I was a young girl when I got my degree. Dr Waksman invited me into his office and asked me if I wanted to go on to a higher degree. I said, 'I don't know.' He told me I might do well if I went to California, where I might get a different view of the possibilities. I told him I had decided to quit anyway. I wanted to have the time to read women's journals. When the patent came up, I met Dr Waksman one day at a meeting and he told me about it. He took me to one side and suggested that I need not sign the patent agreement. My thesis had not been concerned with streptomycin (her antibiotic was Chetomin, which was unfortunately inactivated by blood and so never proved clinically useful) and my part in the streptomycin discovery had been a relatively minor one. I played no part at all in writing the papers, merely being asked to read them and approve them by Waksman."[20]

Like many of his postgraduate students, Betty adored Waksman and accepted his advice without demur. Very soon after her conversation with Waksman, she married another graduate called Gregory. "When the lawyers called me to discuss the patent, I said I wasn't interested. I had moved into the next phase of my life."[21]

Albert Schatz was a very different proposition. Not only was he highly intelligent and ambitious, he had a native New Jersey stubbornness, toughened by his childhood years in the great depression and reinforced by his short spell in the armed forces. It was out of the question that Schatz would accept anything other than what he considered his due share in the recognition for the streptomycin discovery.

Even when working at Rutgers, when Feldman and Hinshaw were performing the first guinea pig trials, and during the subsequent human testing, Schatz heard nothing of these exciting developments, only catching glimpses from what he read for himself in newspapers or in the medical journals. Schatz left Rutgers in 1946 for the New York State Department of Health, to work in their laboratories at Albany on polio and smallpox research. While there, he started the project that would lead to the first drug ever to cure thrush infections, Nystatin. But he felt dissatisfied with the virus field and, in 1947, moving to the Sloane Kettering Institute for a year, working on the notion that if antibiotics cured infection, perhaps he could discover an antibiotic that would work in a similar way against cancer. It was an illusion and he soon came to realize this. Unhappy with the medical direction his research was now taking him, he wanted to get back to his primary interest, soil microbiology. Suddenly there was the opportunity to spend a year in the laboratory of C.B. van Niel, at the Hopkins Marine Station in Pacific Row, California, a branch of Stanford University.

As a veteran, Schatz would receive $90 a month and with Vivian being pregnant, this would increase to $120 when the child was born. Schatz made a successful application for the job. When Waksman heard that Schatz was going to van Niel's laboratory, he invited him to visit him. Schatz did go to see him when Waksman, in recognition of their former close relationship and Schatz' circumstances, made him the generous gift of a $500 personal cheque. Schatz was desperate enough for money to accept it, though with reluctance. Waksman also offered to get Schatz' a grant, based on the streptomycin royalties. For a time the relationship between the two men had recovered some of its former trust and cordiality. Schatz used the money to help move house to California and they maintained a correspondence. On 16 November 1948, Selman Waksman wrote the following letter:

> My dear Schatz,
>
> Enclosed you will find a cheque for $500. I hope that this will help you cover your current expenses during your stay in Dr van Niel's laboratory. As I wrote to you in a previous letter, I hope to be able to do likewise during the first half of next year, at least.
>
> Please consider these cheques as outright payments to you to help you in obtaining advanced training in Microbiology. Should these funds be insufficient to cover your necessary expenses, let me know.[22]

On 26 November, a second letter arrived from Waksman, showing interest in Schatz' new research projects. It continued: "I am enclosing a paper which I would like to have you sign in the place indicated and have it notarized as shown by the attached slip and return it to me as soon as you can."[23]

The paper was an assignation of the rights for the Japanese royalties on streptomycin. Schatz replied that he would only sign it if Waksman would give him a signed statement that he had not personally profited from the royalties. Waksman must surely have been offended by this. Schatz received a reply not from Waksman but from the attorney for the Rutgers Research and Endowment Foundation assuring him that none of Dr Waksman's associates had ever profited personally from any royalties. Schatz wrote back thanking him for the information but pointing out it was not an answer to his question. "I knew then that Waksman had received royalties although I had no idea how much."[24] On 12 January 1949, Schatz received a further letter, asking him to sign away the New Zealand and Canadian patent rights. Schatz was now convinced that Waksman was benefiting from the royalties on streptomycin. This infuriated him. It had been Schatz' understanding at the time he had signed away his rights to the streptomycin patents for $1, that nobody would profit from this assignation. "That satisfied me at that time because I felt that streptomycin, what it did for people, was so important, it should be made as readily available, and therefore as inexpensively available, as possible."[25]

Schatz' reply, dated 22 January 1949, was a lengthy one, covering seven closely typed pages, in which, for the first time he detailed his suspicions and doubts. After a few paragraphs, in which he acknowledged their previous friendship and Waksman's interest in his career . . .

> You will recall that at the time we signed the original patent application for streptomycin, I mentioned to you that I knew absolutely nothing about such matters and was relying entirely upon your judgement. At that time and since then, I have had complete confidence in you, and for this reason I have unhesitatingly and unquestioningly signed any and all documents on which you requested my signature. . . At the time we signed the original patent application, I told you that I trusted you implicitly in this matter. My willingness subsequently to sign whatever documents you have sent me is concrete evidence that this confidence in your sincerity has remained unshaken. I earnestly hope that you will not feel, because I am raising certain issues, that I have stopped trusting in you. Rather, it is because I so very much want our friendship to continue that I am giving voice to what might otherwise become matters of an upsetting nature. You will notice that at this present time I am lodging no complaints at all, nor have I yet drawn any conclusions whatsoever, but will await the benefit of your reply in order to do this most fairly. There are so many things about this whole patent business that I simply do not know and, at this present time, I am doing nothing more than asking about them.
>
> I have slowly been signing myself out of streptomycin completely by affixing my signature to one document after another. . .

I feel a deep and sincere sense of satisfaction from my work which resulted in the discovery of streptomycin. To me, the fact that it has alleviated human suffering means so very much more than whether my name is mentioned or omitted in an article in the popular press. I have always been concerned with my own personal evaluation of myself and my efforts much more than with the evaluation which others have made of me. This is by no means to imply that I have not been interested in opinions from others; I certainly have, am, and will always continue to be. But, you see, I have to live with myself, my convictions, my conscience. Whenever any conflict has arisen, I have been able to disregard all outside criticism and the like as long as "within me" I felt just or correct with respect to what-ever thoughts, attitudes, or actions of mine were concerned. I suppose it's the old story, "This above all: to thine own self be true."[26]

The letter went on to raise many questions about the patent rights and stressed that Schatz had received not so much as "a red cent" from the royalties on streptomycin. Schatz went on to ask some questions about the Rutgers Research and Endow-ment Foundation, to which he had assigned the money from the patents. He reported that he had written to the Foundation and not had the simple courtesy of a reply. He was now de-manding copies of every paper he had signed.

Indeed there were no less than thirteen detailed and enu-merated questions in his letter, all pertaining either to the patents, to the royalties on the patents or to the Rutgers Re-search and Endowment Foundation, to which he demanded answers. The letter continued, "I earnestly hope that you will be good enough to help settle these matters to our mutual satisfaction in the shortest possible time, as unilateral action on my part would be not only difficult but embarrassing. Since I am to a considerable extent personally responsible for the discovery of streptomycin, it follows "as night follows day" that all funds derived from streptomycin are in large part the fruits of my labours. I therefore feel that it is my privilege to have such questions as the above answered. In addition, it is my moral responsibility that I have them answered, for I must know how these monies to which I am legally entitled will be expended should I choose to give them away rather than claim them for myself."[27]

This bitter letter, ending in the language of litigation, had a devastating effect on Selman Waksman. Waksman considered himself chiefly responsible for the discovery of streptomycin, which, in his view, was no more than a step along a path he had personally paved, with the prior discoveries of actinomycin and streptothricin. Schatz could hardly deny that Waksman was the architect of the entire programme of antibiotic research at Rutgers. Schatz had not even wanted to do antibiotic research for his thesis but had been persuaded by Waksman to do so. Waksman had also allowed Schatz to put his name first on the three breakthrough publications, an indulgence that was not only unprecedented in Waksman's association with his post-graduate students, but one which would now have important consequences when it came to the legal interpretation of those patent agreements.

It was an angry and hurt Waksman, hardly behaving with his usual generosity, who declared through the voice of Mr Watson, the lawyer for the Rutgers Foundation, that Schatz' contribution had been no more than that of "a carefully super-vised laboratory assistant."[28]

Schatz received no public acknowledgement of his rights from Rutgers. On 7 November 1949, Selman Waksman's portrait adorned the cover of *Time* Magazine. The relevant article eulogized streptomycin as a wonder drug and Waksman as its discoverer. "Today, the department of microbiology is the brightest spot on the Rutgers campus at New Brunswick, NJ, and its chairman, Dr Selman Waksman, is one of the world's top microbiologists. He has won for his university not only fame but fortune. Streptomycin for a sixty-day course of treatment costs $60 to $80. For every gram sold, Rutgers gets two cents. By last week the university's harvest of pennies had reached more than $2 million." The implications had Schatz' head reeling. Still working in California, he consulted a New York lawyer, who retained Jerome C. Eisenberg of Newark to start a lawsuit.

In March 1950 the scientific community was shocked when the suit emerged into the open. Nobody could believe that the young assistant, Albert Schatz, really was suing his professor, Selman Waksman, and the Rutgers Research and Endowment Foundation. This unique situation was aptly summed up by Hubert Lechevalier: "In brief, Schatz was asking Waksman to refrain from representing himself as the sole discoverer of streptomycin and was asking for an account of the royalties received from licences granted by the defendants. In addition, he was asking that half of the funds so collected be turned over to him."[29]

Although the sums of money involved were potentially very large, money was not the real issue. For Albert Schatz, his exclusion from the media after the success of streptomycin, the apparent denigration of the part he had played, had left him with a smouldering sense of injustice. Now, in the royalties suit, he had the chance to reaffirm his status. For anybody who cared for both men, the situation had the pathos of a Greek tragedy. Selman Waksman was heartbroken. "I endured nearly a year of this nightmare existence. To proceed with the case, or to settle it as amicably as possible? One's pride, one's feeling for justice and for one's friends, all demanded that the first course be pursued. On the other hand, some of the factors listed previously, especially the possible delay in the building of the institute which would culminate my lifetime's work and devotion to science, and finally, the prospect of having to face daily attacks in the press during the days in court – all made me decide that, after all, the second course might be the wiser. The decision to settle was largely mine. . . with a pain in my heart, I agreed to it."[30]

In December of 1950, the case was settled with the approval of the court. Dr Clothier, the President of Rutgers University, stated publicly that it had never been disputed that Dr Schatz was co-discoverer of streptomycin and that Dr Schatz was to receive three per cent of the royalties paid to the Foundation.

Following the court settlement, which also awarded Waksman seventeen per cent of the royalties, he insisted that seven per cent should be shared by everybody who had worked in his laboratory, from graduate students such as Woodruff to the portly Mr Adams whose job it was to wash the dishes. For many impoverished students, it was an unexpected but very welcome windfall. Betty Bugie for example made excellent use of her share in supporting her new husband through his years of postgraduate studies. Of the ten per cent remaining to Selman Waksman, he subsequently donated half for the setting up of a Foundation for Microbiology, which would be devoted to furthering scientific education.[31]

Albert Schatz felt that his case was now vindicated. He had won both public recognition of his role in the discovery of streptomycin and a share in the royalties. The settlement, in which he was awarded an immediate lump sum of $125,000, made newspaper headlines, where Albert Schatz was described as modest in victory.[32] But it would prove a Pyrrhic victory. Albert had intended to use the money to allow him to devote more of his time to microbiology research. But in the wake of the notoriety caused by the settlement, he found it impossible to get work in his chosen field. Although he suspected that Waksman was behind this, it seems more likely that the establishment simply closed ranks, siding with a respected and eminent colleague. Albert Schatz would never work in a top grade microbiology laboratory again, being forced to accept a series of rather menial jobs in small institutions, on substandard salaries.

For the drug company, Merck & Co., the streptomycin success had also proved a fragile edifice. In 1945, when Waksman realized that streptomycin was becoming a very important antibiotic, together with Dr William H. Martin, the Dean of the College of Agriculture, he had approached George Merck & Co. and proposed the cancellation of their earlier agreement. The intention was humanitarian: to allow competition between different pharmaceutical companies which would both reduce the price of the drug and allow its uninhibited development and production worldwide. H. Corwin Hinshaw was also present at this meeting, where George Merck in person, previously so generous in supplying doctors with free quantities of streptomycin for research, now made a gesture of historic benevolence. Without demur he returned the patents to Rutgers, relinquishing the potential for millions of dollars in profits.[33]

V

WITH EVEN GREATER irony, even as the lawyers were de-
bating the terms of the royalty settlement, there had been a very
worrying development in the tuberculosis struggle.

The results of the British MRC trial had now been confirmed
by many others in different countries, all of which proved beyond doubt that combination therapy with streptomycin and
PAS was far more effective than either drug on its own. Combination therapy also allowed doctors to reduce the dose or the
frequency of steptomycin injections, making it easier to avoid
those dreadful side-effects. But the dose of PAS used in the
British trial was fairly high and gave rise to an unpleasant
degree of nausea and bowel upset. Unfortunately, when, as
Daniels and Hill in 1952, they tried reducing the dose, there was
a huge increase in streptomycin-resistant germs.[34] Even more
worrying was the observation, in the very large scale studies,
conducted over two years by the Veterans Administration in
the United States – as in the Medical Research Council trial in
Great Britain – that even with the combination of both drugs,
tuberculosis had not yet been defeated.[35] Overall, about eighty
per cent of sufferers from pulmonary tuberculosis showed
clearing of their germs on the combination treatment. But this
also meant that twenty per cent were not cured, in the main
those with extensive disease, complicated by cavities and
scarring.

Another note of warning had been sounded. At first it was
just a trickle, but with time an increasing number of patients
were coughing up germs that were resistant to streptomycin.
The combination treatment could only be expected to work in
patients whose germs showed no resistance to either drug to
start with. Following the widespread use of streptomycin in
earlier years, many new patients turned up at the clinics and
hospital wards already infected with resistant germs they had
acquired from others with long standing disease. Other
patients had to have one or other of the two therapies discontinued because of side-effects, leaving them vulnerable to the
development of bacterial resistance to the single drug that was
left.

Streptomycin and PAS had been wonderful breakthroughs. But now, in the words of Dr M.E. Florey, "Progress in the chemotherapy of tuberculosis seemed to have come to a standstill."[36] For anyone who understood the awesome capacity of the disease, it could only be a matter of time before tuberculosis became widely resistant to both drugs in combination.

20

The Battle is Won

What matters in science is not the pursuit of power but the knowledge gained. We must realize this afresh every day, just as every true doctor wishes for nothing more than to be able to help his patients even more with every new day.

Gerhard Domagk

i

IN THE AUTUMN of 1949, Dr H. Corwin Hinshaw, now working at Stanford University, California, and Dr Walsh McDermott, a consultant physician at the prestigious Cornell Medical School in New York, and editor of the *American Review of Tuberculosis*, travelled to Germany on board the liner, the *Queen Mary*. In McDermott's words: "We were sent over to Germany to investigate reports that, virtually unnoticed by the occupying powers, the Germans had treated some 7,000 tuberculous patients with a new synthetic chemical of the thiosemicarbazone series under study by Gerhard Domagk, the discoverer of the first sulphonamide."[1]

After docking on the German coast, they travelled far southwards to meet Domagk, together with the Bayer management and chemists, at Elberfeld, where Hinshaw found himself gazing upon the Bayer factory and the surrounding town in undisguised amazement.

The factory and research institute was huge, "an area, covering several blocks. All around it the town was severely damaged by air raids, but our military leaders had known that the big IG Farben factory would be terribly important after the war, and gave the order – 'Don't let bombs hit that place'."[2] Just how far-sighted the Allies had been in preserving the factory, events would soon reveal.

The Allied Control provided Hinshaw and McDermott with a chauffeur-driven limousine, in which they toured Germany from North to South. Neither man harboured any illusion about the true nature of war and they were well aware that the inhumanity of the *blitzkrieg* had been invented by the Luftwaffe as early as Guernica and had been ruthlessly put into effect from the first invasions of Poland and the air raids over London; nevertheless, wherever they travelled, they could only feel shocked at the extent of the destruction. "Going across Germany, it was absolutely ghastly. I remember trying to visit a house where we had stayed before the war, a *pension*, but when we finally found it, it was totally destroyed except for somebody living in the basement."[3]

The main purpose of the trip was to visit sanitoria and this they did, calling on many of the larger institutions still very much involved in the clinical assessment of Conteben. During this tour, Hinshaw and McDermott were impressed to find that in spite of such difficult circumstances, Conteben had already been subjected to a very extensive study. They examined dozens of patients who had been treated with it, studying their temperature charts, the results of sputum stains and cultures, the X-rays before and after treatment. The evidence in favour of the drug was overwhelming. Tuberculosis in all of its dangerous manifestations had healed after treatment with this curious new drug, a drug that was unknown outside Germany.

When Hinshaw and McDermott returned to the States, they took a supply of Conteben back with them for further testing. On 21 November 1949, *Time* magazine, in a tone reminiscent of the *Pathé News*, reported the outcome of the trip, in an article with the unfortunate title, "War Booty".

"When two US doctors went to Germany last summer to check on reports that a new chemical was showing promise in treating tuberculosis, they got an eye-opener. The drug had passed the promising stage, had shown impressive results over

a two-year period in the treatment of 7,000 patients. And behind
its discovery and development was the potent name of Professor
Domagk, aged fifty-four, who won fame and a 1939 Nobel Prize,
which the Nazis would not let him take, as top man in perfecting
the sulpha drugs. The drug was Tibione (Conteben). . ."

The article went on to report on a new trial of Conteben which
Hinshaw and McDermott had carried out on American tuberculosis sufferers, which had been presented a week earlier to a
Veterans Administration Conference in Atlanta. After
explaining that the thiosemicarbazones were a new group of
chemicals entirely unknown to American medicine, the two doctors had compared Tibione to streptomycin and concluded that
while streptomycin was better in treating miliary tuberculosis
and tuberculous meningitis, Tibione was most impressive in the
treatment of tuberculous infection of the throat and bowels. It
was quite clear that Hinshaw and McDermott saw the main
usefulness of Tibione rather as they saw PAS – as an adjunct to
treatment with streptomycin, where it should help reduce the
emergence of resistant germs. In a medical paper, based on those
same findings, Hinshaw and McDermott drew a somewhat disparaging conclusion. "A crude approximation of the current
situation can be made by the statement that thiosemicarbazone
appears to have anti-tuberculous activity of the same general
order as para-aminosalicylic acid and a potential toxicity somewhat like the arsenicals used in the treatment of syphilis."[4]

Domagk would disagree very strongly with such a damning
conclusion, which was, he thought, based upon a very small
series of patients treated with too large a dose of the drug. In his
opinion, while Conteben was toxic to a larger number of patients
than either streptomycin or PAS, its toxicity was less serious
than that of streptomycin, causing mainly loss of appetite, feelings of malaise and skin rashes resembling measles. These side
effects soon cleared when the drug was stopped. In contrast with
streptomycin, the drug could be given for many months and
even years. The *Time* magazine article finished with the pro-
vocative statement: "Because the drug was developed during
the war, the German patents are no good and any US manufacturer can make it. A few patients in US hospitals have been dosed
with Tibione; it will soon be tried on thousands."

The refusal of the Allies to allow Bayer to patent their discovery would have other more important consequences in the very near future.

Streptomycin was not only a pioneering discovery, it was also a singular discovery. In all of the further research at Rutgers and George Merck's pharmaceutical company, there was no stream of streptomycin derivatives, each opening a new chapter of advance against tuberculosis. Even in the case of PAS, where Ferrosan had experimented with a large number of modifications to the molecule, none of these had proved equal to the parent molecule and so not one of these ever came to clinical testing. Conteben, and the class of thiosemicarbazones, born from such heroic efforts in the scorched rubble of Elberfeld, was unique in this respect. The drug was quickly manufactured in America without recompense to Bayer, where it was renamed amithiozone. Meanwhile, the atomic structure of the thiosemicarbazones became the template about which chemists in many different pharmaceutical companies throughout America could allow their imaginations free rein, creating ever newer orders of the atoms.

Over the four years, from 1948 to 1952, thousands of new permutations of the parent Conteben molecule would be dreamed up, brought to creative reality, and tested against the tuberculous bacterium. Many of these would be found to have some effectiveness, but they would all turn out to be either less effective, or more toxic, than Conteben. Leading American researchers involved in this thiosemicarbazone chapter included Herbert Fox of the pharmaceutical house, Hoffman-La Roche, based in Nutley, New Jersey, and Jack Bernstein, of the Squibb pharmaceutical company, based in Brunswick, New Jersey. Sooner or later – and the expectancy charging the atmosphere of the giant pharmaceutical laboratories suggested sooner – the new wonder drug would emerge.

ii

SOME YEARS PREVIOUSLY, in July 1944, a French doctor, Vital Chorine, had infected rats with leprosy, injecting some of them subcutaneously with nicotinamide, a chemical derived from a vitamin of the B group. Those rats given the vitamin derivative showed no signs at all of developing leprosy whereas some control animals given the same dose of leprosy developed obvious disease at the site of injection. Because leprosy and tuberculosis were caused by the same genus of bacteria, the *Mycobacteria*, Chorine now performed a similar experiment on guinea pigs infected with tuberculosis. The effects, while not quite so dramatic, were very interesting. Those guinea pigs given the nicotinamide by subcutaneous injection showed a dramatic lessening of the spread of their tuberculosis. On the other hand, if he gave them nicotinic acid – a common vitamin, and not the nicotinamide which was so closely derived from it – the effect against tuberculosis in the guinea pigs completely disappeared. This was all the more curious for the fact that the nicotinic acid still had some damaging effect on tuberculosis germs growing in cultures. Chorine admitted that he was completely baffled by this.

In January 1945, he told his colleagues at the French *Académie des Sciences* about these curious findings, but they could no more explain them than he could himself.[5] Chorine might not be able to explain them but he had no doubt that they were important: "this action is more efficacious than any experimental treatment available to us at this present time." He had also arrived at another, and quite critical, conclusion: in spite of the fact he was using a chemical that was derived from a vitamin, the activity against tuberculosis was not due to any vitamin-like effect. Instead the effect of nicotinamide seemed to rely on some curious need of the tuberculosis germs themselves.

Chorine's discovery, published in just two small pages in his native French, was not widely appreciated. In that same year, 1945, a second French worker, Huant, drew attention to the very same findings and was again ignored.[6] In the words of the American chemist, Herbert Fox: "In one of those rare and inexplicable circumstances, this notable discovery passed unnoticed in this country."[7]

In June 1948, Kushner and McKenzie, reporting from Geneva, Switzerland, on behalf of the Lederle laboratories of the giant American Cyanamid Company, rediscovered this bizarre effect of nicotinamide on the tuberculosis germ. Without ever having heard of Chorine's work, they repeated his experiment and confirmed exactly the same results.[8,9] If they administered nicotinamide to cultures of tuberculosis germs or if they gave it to mice infected with tuberculosis, the tuberculosis germ was damaged in some way. However, Kushner and McKenzie made a fatal error in their conclusion. "The failure to increase the activity or even to retain the activity of nicotinic acid amide (nicotinamide) by any slight alteration in the molecule led us to suspect we might with dealing with the specific activity of a vitamin". Unaware of Chorine's brilliant observation, they had missed the point.

There is a tantalizing similarity between the atomic structures of nicotinamide and Conteben. There is an equally tantalizing resemblance to para-aminosalicylic acid. But where both Conteben and PAS contain a chemical ring of six carbon atoms, the benzene ring, as part of their structures, nicotinamide has a different ring, with an atom of nitrogen displacing one of the carbons. This mysterious atomic structure is called the pyridine ring.

Sadly, Kushner and his colleagues were now diverted by their false conclusion – but years later this same line of enquiry would lead them to discover an important new anti-tuberculous drug, pyrazinamide. Meanwhile the enterprising Herbert Fox was suddenly very interested in Kushner and McKenzie's experiment with nicotinamide. He created a number of new molecules, all variations on the nicotinamide theme, and all containing this pyridine ring. Sure enough, some of these chemicals had powerful anti-tuberculous effects. How strange that chemicals so closely related to a common vitamin should have these properties! Fox, like Chorine, drew the right conclusion. This had nothing whatsoever to do with the vitamin effects of nicotinic acid. And that really was a puzzle.

iii

ON 8 SEPTEMBER 1951, Gerhard Domagk completed an exhaustive world tour with his first visit to the United States, a venue towards which he confessed to having very mixed feelings. Domagk was suspicious of Americans, whom he largely blamed for the devastating bombing of his home country. More importantly, he was carrying the solution to the nicotinamide puzzle with him.

The flight took an arduous twenty hours, during which he recorded in his diary ... "I am having heart trouble and sweating a little."[10] He was experiencing a recurrence of the chest pain he had suffered after his imprisonment and interrogation by the Gestapo during the war, now more accurately diagnosed as angina. It was a forewarning of the culture shock he would experience from the moment of disembarkation in New York.

"At 19.10 hours we land. Eight dollars immigration tax. The latter appears to be the most important thing, and for which you receive no receipt. Everyone has to pay it, although I say I don't really feel inclined to immigrate at all! I am asked to explain to a distraught woman who does not have the eight dollars, that she must pay. Without pity, the young woman with red painted fingernails, demands payment, although the distraught woman assures her that her relatives have already paid for everything. Not a friendly reception, but a sobre and characteristic one: make dollars!"[11]

The man who carried his luggage out to the airport bus took his dollar note and, with a grin, disappeared without offering a dime in change. Domagk recorded his first impressions as he travelled from the airport to his hotel, which was in the heart of downtown New York, over the bustling Grand Central Station. "First we pass small family houses as you see in London, sober *petite bourgeousie* on both sides of the road, then buildings up to four or five storeys, with shops within them. Now we are surrounded by ten-storey buildings. There is a roar beneath us and the streets shake slightly with the passing of an underground train. These streets are wider than our motorways, with two carriageways one way and two the other, a central reservation with tufts of scorched grass, wide pavements at the sides. The first skyscrapers loom in the distance. New York receives us with an architecture that reaches for the sky. It is pleasantly warm, even in the evening. The women are wearing summery clothes and are all painted, but many have no radiance left in their eyes."[12]

The following morning, up early to deal with his post, he was astonished by "the traffic which now boils many storeys below me. Shrill car horns, cars in glaring colours, yellow, orange, red and sky blue, and in them all manner of mixtures of human races and types, as varied as the colourful ties which men wear here."

On the second day of his stay in New York, he took a cab to the famous Hotel Statler, the venue for the Twelfth International Congress of Pure and Applied Chemistry. This was an important meeting, attended by the most creative chemists in the world.

One of the Italian speakers had dropped out and Domagk was invited by Dr Moseltig, a well-known chemist from the National Institute of Health at Bethesda, to accept the honour of chairing the afternoon session. Listening to the opening lectures on tuberculosis in the afternoon, Domagk, who remembered Hinshaw's and McDermott's caustic conclusions from the year previously, had cause for reflection. "Only a short time ago, these same Americans had shown little interest in the anti-tuberculous effects of the thiosemicarbazones and after a very superficial clinical assessment they were rejected because of the side-effects caused by incorrect and initially overlarge doses. Now, all of a sudden, we see what interest is being shown in this war booty!"[13]

In paper after paper, leading American chemists talked about work that was derived from thiosemicarbazones. Domagk delivered his first ever improvised talk in English, at the end of which he produced a chart showing the Bayer results ... "in order to ascertain from the discussion prompted by the chart whether the Americans had discovered anything better." His chart listed PAS, streptomycin, thiosemicarbazone and a previously unheard of drug, labelled "hydrazone". It must have come as a considerable surprise to the most prominent American speaker, who was none other than Dr Herbert Fox. Earlier that same afternoon, the senior chemist from La Roche had delivered three interesting lectures on new chemical formulations derived from the thiosemicarbazones, all with promising anti-tuberculous effects.

Now, in Domagk's projected table, the four drug groups showed a dramatic stepwise rise in effectiveness against tuberculosis. This in fact was more than a little misleading, since one just cannot compare drugs in such simplistic terms as gram for gram effectiveness. For example, streptomycin could only be tolerated in much smaller doses than PAS, and a more meaningful table would have compared the prescribed doses of each drug for their comparative effectiveness. Nevertheless this chart with its striking tenfold dose-effect leaps, did contain a clue of great moment. Streptomycin was portrayed as ten times as potent as PAS in killing tuberculous bacteria, thiosemicarbazone ten times as potent as streptomycin, but here, in his final column was this new entity, hydrazone, dose for dose a staggering ten times as potent again. If Domagk's information was to be taken at face value, this mystery drug was by far the most powerful anti-tuberculous medication ever found.

The new discovery, which was called isoniazid, had an atomic structure based on the very interesting pyridine ring. It would soon become a sensation throughout the world.

All three of Fox's lectures concentrated on derivatives of thiosemicarbazone, in which that same pyridine ring was prominent. Domagk would record in his diary that none of the other lecturers had produced any formulae he had not come across previously. What he could not realize, however, was that by extraordinary coincidence, Fox had also discovered isoniazid. Fox never said a word about this discovery, although he was well aware of its exceptional potential, and also that it had begun its clinical testing with human sufferers in the Sea View Hospital, New York, some four months earlier.

Herbert Fox would subsequently write a detailed account of his simultaneous discovery of isoniazid, when he made no secret of his debt to the earlier work of Domagk and the thiosemicarbazones. First he had made a detailed analysis of Conteben and its derivatives. Then, when Kushner and his colleagues drew Fox's attention to nicotinamide, he had replaced the benzene ring in thiosemicarbazone by the pyridine ring. It had been just a matter of time and patience, through a complex series of atomic transformations, before this master chemist had unlocked the mystery of isoniazid. Fox concluded his paper with the comment: "Though it is too early to assess completely the role which isonicotinyl hydrazine (isoniazid) and its derivatives will play in the control of tuberculosis, it is already apparent . . . that it is one of the most potent – if not the most potent – single (anti-tuberculous drug) available."[14]

iv

A SECOND AND equally bizarre meeting would take place before Gerhard Domagk said goodbye to America.

He toured the United States for several weeks, enjoying a warm welcome in one university centre after another, delivering lectures, meeting eminent doctors and scientists, paying visits to the pharmaceutical companies and talking to their medical staff and chemists. In Indianapolis, he took part in a televised interview with Professor Thompson, where his discussion, and his fundamental humanitarianism, was hailed by the newspapers. He would depart for Germany in early October, feeling rather more warmly for America than he had on his arrival. "Apart from the scientific meetings, which have the same aim in America as they have in Germany – to make people's lives more tolerable and pleasant – I have wonderful memories of personal discussions and relationships with doctors, with university professors, and industrial scientists during my stay in the USA."[15]

One such personal discussion took the form of a fond farewell to Dr Walsh McDermott of the Department of Public Health, Cornell University, New York. McDermott was of course the tuberculosis expert who, accompanied by Hinshaw, had visited him in Elberfeld and first taken thiosemicarbazone back to the States for testing. We now know that at this time McDermott had only recently started to test another brand of isoniazid in human sufferers. Nydrazid, the brand of isoniazid he was testing, had been created by the innovative chemist Jack Bernstein, and supplied to him by the Squibb Pharmaceutical Company. McDermott would recall bidding Gerhard Domagk that fond farewell with wry amusement. "Neither of us mentioned the exciting promise of isoniazid, which each of us thought he alone knew. I feel certain that each of us walked away from our warm friendly parting with the thought, 'Isn't *he* in for a surprise!' "[16]

This state of blissful ignorance, at least as far as McDermott was concerned, ended abruptly on New Year's Eve, 1951, when Dr Elmer Sevringhaus, the medical director of Hoffman-La Roche, arrived in McDermott's New York office on a confidential visit. To McDermott's astonishment, Sevringhaus asked him if he could cooperate in the clinical testing of a new drug of astonishing potency against tuberculosis. The wonder drug was none other than isoniazid, the same drug McDermott was already testing in patients for Squibb. "We promptly discovered that there were two groups in the field; we did not then know about the third group."[17]

By an extraordinary coincidence, three pharmaceutical companies, Bayer in Germany, and Squibb and Hoffman La Roche in America, had simultaneously discovered the same wonder drug. Doctors Robitzek and Selikoff at the Sea View Hospital, New York, had been testing the La Roche brand of isoniazid, Rimifon, in human sufferers from tuberculosis since June of that year. McDermott had begun testing the Squibb brand of the same drug in human sufferers at Cornell and the New York Hospital three months later, in September. In Germany, Professor Klee had also begun the clinical testing of the Bayer brand of isoniazid at the Wuppertal-Elberfeld Hospital that same September. No group knew of the concomitant trials being conducted by the others. In every case, the discovery had come from the template of the thiosemicarbazone molecule.

Early in January, 1952, the two American companies came together for a somewhat tense meeting. It was agreed that publication of both the drug's discovery and the early animal experiments should go ahead at the earliest possible moment. The date for publication was now decided: the first week in April. It was also agreed that the human testing of isoniazid should be kept secret to avoid arousing hopes that might later prove illusory. On Wednesday 20 February 1952, there was a similar meeting in the research institute of the Bayer laboratories, chaired by Gerhard Domagk. All the famous clinicians who had taken part in the thiosemicarbazone research were present, as was Klee's enthusiastic young assistant, Karl Jahnke.[18] By this time, they knew the results of the test tube and animal experiments on the Bayer brand of isoniazid, Neoteben, and Klee could report the preliminary results of testing the new drug in human sufferers. The gathering of experts heard a story of wonderful promise. Isoniazid was clearly a much superior drug to its parent, thiosemicarbazone. Up to that date, not a word of the discovery had been leaked to the medical establishment or the press. Domagk assured them that their patient silence was over. "It is my opinion that we know enough of this drug and its promise to go ahead and release our results for publication in the scientific journals."[19]

However, unknown to Domagk and his colleagues in Germany, incredible rumours had reached the ears of the press in New York. The rumours emanated from people suffering from tuberculosis, apparently hopelessly incurable cases, who could not keep quiet about the fact their lives had been saved by some mystery drug at the Sea View Hospital, on Staten Island. On the same day that Domagk was addressing his medical colleagues in Elberfeld, the media fever had reached such a pitch that reporters from several newspapers invaded the Sea View Hospital, to check the veracity of the stories for themselves. What they saw and heard amazed them. All those plans for a controlled media release, made by Squibb and La Roche in New York and Bayer in Germany, were thrown into the dustbin. The attention of the world was riveted upon newsflashes. The excitement and misinformation was such that Dr Marcus Kogel, Commissioner of Hospitals in New York City, decided he had better clarify matters with a special press conference on 21 February.

That same morning, the *New York Post* carried the first banner headline: "Wonder Drug Fights TB". The *Evening Star*, Washington, opened with the statement: "Two new wonder pills have saved people hopelessly sick with tuberculosis, their lungs riddled with holes, too weak to get out of bed..." The evening paper had the benefit of the Kogel interview to add credibility to their report. "Whether the two new drugs have actually cured TB, the nation's biggest infectious killer, is too early to say. But they look 'better than anything so far' in treating TB, Dr Marcus D. Kogel, commissioner of New York City Hospitals, announced."[20] Dr Kogel was in fact doing his utmost to control the hyperbole. He warned that there were as yet many unanswered questions. How long would such good effects last? Would bacterial resistance emerge, as it had with every other drug that had been found? But people did not want to listen to such downbeat professional caution. In report after report, the public read of wonder cures, of the successful treatment of people who had literally been at the brink of the grave. One paper carried colour pictures of patients actually dancing with joy in the wards of Sea View Hospital.

v

DOCTORS EDWARD H. ROBITZEK and Irving Selikoff at the Sea View Hospital were besieged by newspaper and radio reporters from all over the world. They too did their best to calm such expectations. There could hardly be a doctor in the world who was not aware of the need for caution when interpreting the latest wonder cure for a disease as deceptive as tuberculosis. Indeed, in the Paris Edition of the New York *Herald Tribune*, on 3 March Dr John Zarit, chairman of the Colorado State Medical Society's tuberculosis control committee, and Dr William Klein, medical director of the Jewish Consumptives Relief Society, deplored the more extravagant claims. Dr Zarit complained that the announcement of the discovery of these new wonder drugs had brought a flood of telephone calls to his office from tuberculosis sufferers, who "think they can stay at home, take a pill like an aspirin and be cured".

In this tidal wave of near-hysteria, where did the real truth lie?

In a twenty-seven-page article, received for publication in the *American Review of Tuberculosis* on 19 January, but not published until April, Robitzek and Selikoff described how they had treated tuberculosis sufferers with the new wonder drug, isoniazid, for the first time.[21] Although worded in the usual scientific language, and cautious in its conclusion, this lengthy paper in fact went a long way towards confirming the sensational newspaper reports.

They had tested two variants of isoniazid, trade names Rimifon and Marsilid, which had been synthesized by Herbert Fox in the La Roche laboratories, at Nutley, New Jersey. The report, which covered only a six-month period, should be seen as no more than a preliminary trial. During this short space of time, they had tested ninety-seven consecutive patients with pulmonary tuberculosis that had presented to their unit. Within this group was a very interesting subgroup, of forty-four consecutive cases, and it was these who formed the basis for this preliminary report. The criteria for including these were without doubt unparalleled in the history of any tuberculosis trial in the world.

These patients were without exception suffering from tuberculous pneumonia affecting both lungs, which would almost inevitably prove fatal without effective treatment. But there was an even more extraordinary entry requirement. "The fundamental criterion which was applied in the selection of each patient was that his disease had progressed so far that he was no longer a candidate for any other standard accepted form of therapy." In other words, they only accepted patients who had failed to respond to every treatment then available, including streptomycin and PAS – "the so-called hopeless case, in many instances close to terminal status." They had even taken the precaution of trying conventional treatment for a "sufficient pre-therapy observation period" to preclude the selection of any patient who was improving either spontaneously or with streptomycin or PAS therapy. In thirty-nine of the forty-four patients, the disease was classified as far advanced on the X-rays. Without a miracle, all of these patients were condemned to die.

Every patient had a high temperature at the start of treatment with isoniazid: within days, sometimes no more than two days, their temperatures had returned to normal. On average, each of the emaciated patients gained 19.7 pounds in weight with therapy. The gain in weight on isoniazid was so striking that it would subsequently prompt doctors to carry out trials quite unrelated to tuberculosis, to see if the drug had some mysterious effect on the body's calorie metabolism. The effect on these very sick people's appetites was described as "ravenous". Three bowls of cereal and five eggs were considered ordinary breakfasts. Appetites were so huge that food offered between meals was greedily accepted.[22] Even such a difficult parameter to measure as improvement in energy and wellbeing ... "has been strikingly obvious to the nursing and medical staff." The return to life was so wonderful, so invigorating, that disciplinary problems were common, a factor "which is obviously attributable to resurgent animal vigour". It was asking rather a lot of the press to expect them to resist the implications of such statements, which suggested that some patients brought back from the brink of the grave had celebrated this unexpected "spring" with an old-fashioned Roman Bacchanalia.

These effects on the various symptoms and signs of the disease went hand in hand with the clearing of bacteria from the sputum, and with a slow but steady improvement in the horrific chest X-ray appearances. Even the cavities on the X-rays, the most difficult feature of all to cure, had become smaller in seventeen cases. Many of these patients had tuberculosis elsewhere – in the throat, the tongue, the bowel. All of these manifestations had completely cleared. Most vital of all, every single patient, hitherto condemned to death, was still alive at the end of the six months period of observation. Indeed they were more than merely alive – every one of them felt dramatically reinvigorated. These patients had already suffered much damage in their lungs prior to therapy. Some, though not all of them, were completely cured while many were sufficiently improved to allow the thoracic surgeons to remove lobes or whole lungs that had been damaged beyond repair prior to starting the new treatment.

The side effects were wonderfully minor. A few patients experienced twitching of the hands and feet, changes in their tendon reflexes, constipation or vertigo.

On 3 May 1952, Mrs Veronica Hall was taken by car from the Sea View Hospital to 114 West 19th Street, New York, where she had a tearful reunion with her family. She was the first patient to be officially discharged from Sea View Hospital. Like the other forty-three patients who had received that first batch of isoniazid treatment, she had been dying from a fulminating tuberculous pneumonia. Like all the others, she had tried every other known method of treatment, including streptomycin and PAS, but all such treatments had failed to cure her. Mrs Hall was well aware that she had looked death in the face. She returned to the bosom of her family firmly convinced that she owed her life to a miracle drug called isoniazid.[23]

vi

FOR PHILIPP KLEE, who had been testing Neoteben, the Bayer brand of isoniazid, since the previous September, and who was poised to report an identical picture of dramatic effectiveness in his patients at the Wuppertal-Elberfeld Hospital, the American trials came as a bombshell. For this cataclysm to arrive in the form of sensational newspaper reports rather than formal medical articles rubbed salt in the wound.

To make matters even worse, many German newspapers now followed the American lead. Although, after the first few days of uncontrollable excitement, they tried hard to comply with the need for caution that was impressed upon them from all sides of the medical profession, not every paper was able to restrain its enthusiasm. Banner headlines, with all of the jangling rhetoric of their American counterparts, would find their way through the net: *Deutschland besiegte Weltangst Nr 1: DAS ENDE DER TBC.* On 1 March the more restrained and respected newspaper, *Stadt Anzeiger,* in an article that would set the tone of the more sophisticated German press some weeks later, distanced itself from this tawdry hysteria while nevertheless communicating a little of its effervescence to its readers. "Even the *New York Times,* not given to exaggeration, speaks of this wonder drug and reports amazing successes. They predict that in a few years' time, one of the world's most widespread and devious of diseases will be completely conquered." The article described in some detail the hopeless cases that had been rescued in the Sea View Hospital trial. It then continued with a note of caution.

Were the numbers of patients involved in the trial sufficient for such optimism? Moreover, this wonder drug was not quite as novel as it seemed. The drug was in fact identical to Neoteben, which had already been created by a young chemist, Hans Offe, working in the Bayer laboratories in Leverkusen. Offe, then forty years old, had taken over the thiosemicarbazone research from Behnisch, and, working in partnership with a second chemist, Werner Siefkin, had come to exactly the same realization as Fox and Bernstein.

The *Stadt Anzeiger* article went on to declaim the sensationalism of the American press: "Here we have a case where a valuable drug through too much propaganda could all too easily become discredited."[24]

Klee had first of all tested Neoteben on himself. At the time of the American press sensation, he already had a series of 126 patients taking the drug, many of whom had been receiving it for five months. He too had seen hopeless cases improve as with no previous medication. He had witnessed that same dramatic increase in appetite – one patient had gained a stone in weight in a single week. One impressive example was a woman, aged thirty-six, who had suffered from open tuberculosis for many years, and had developed cavities in both lungs. She had attended every clinic and hospital her doctor could think of. She had been treated with large doses of PAS and streptomycin without success. Her tuberculosis was rapidly worsening and the cavities were rapidly increasing in size. When she was admitted to the Elberfeld Hospital, the previous October, she was emaciated and clearly dying. Within days of starting Neoteben, she was already showing signs of improving. Her temperature fell to normal and her appetite returned. Within weeks, the enormous holes in her lungs had begun to shrink. Her appetite became so ravenous that she gained a stone in weight in one week. "There is every hope that this success will last and she will be able to go home soon."[25]

This same wonderful story was being simultaneously reported by Elmendorf, Cawthon and McDermott in their trials of the Squibb brand of isoniazid (Nydrazid) at the New York City Hospital.[26] Domagk and Klee would publish their experience with Neoteben a few months later, when it would corroborate the dramatic American findings.[27] But Domagk was far from happy with the coincidental discoveries of the same drug in three laboratories at precisely the same time. He wrote indignant letters to some of the scientists he had met in America, drawing attention to the fact he had disclosed the discovery of isoniazid on his tour of America.[28] It seemed certain that the controversy would boil over into an international lawsuit. But there was a tremendous shock in store even at this late stage in the treatment.

As with the earlier shocks with Prontosil and PAS, now, at this very late stage, all three companies discovered, to their amazement, that isoniazid had been synthesized back in 1912 by two Prague chemists, Hans Meyer and Josef Mally. Meyer and Mally did not have the slightest notion of its potential in tuberculosis. They were not looking for a medical therapy of any sort, merely satisfying a requirement for their doctorates in chemistry.[29] For La Roche, Squibb and Bayer there was no longer any controversy. Not one of them could take out a patent on isoniazid.

For the dying millions, this in no way diminished the extraordinary importance of the isoniazid rediscovery. There was an additional wonderful advantage of the new drug. At the time of their first discovery, PAS and streptomycin had been difficult to manufacture. This had made them more precious than gold. Millions of sufferers worldwide had suffered the appalling torment of knowing there was a treatment available that might cure them, only to be told by their doctors that they could not get hold of it. Even eight years after PAS and streptomycin had been discovered, the cost of treating the average American with tuberculosis was a staggering $3,500. Isoniazid, a simple chemical that could be synthesized from coaltar, brought the cost of treatment down to less than $100. In the hubris of celebration, people really believed that with isoniazid ... "the first of possibly scores of its kind, had been added to the medical arsenal for the fight against mankind's greatest infectious scourge."[30]

Little wonder then that the press and radio continued to follow the isoniazid story with adulation. A typical flavour of the reaction of newspaper and radio news bulletins around the world was the following report, taken from a fifteen-minute radio script broadcast throughout twelve Central American networks under the heading, "Science on the March":

> Tuberculosis – the disease which destroyed more than five million lives last year, whose indiscriminate path through man's recorded history has filled more graves than war, famine, or pestilence – has been stopped. Scientists and clinical physicians have reported "amazing results" in the treatment in New York hospitals of some 200 tuberculosis patients. The results are amazing not only because they worked effectively against tuberculosis, but because they stopped tuberculosis in patients for whom all hope had been abandoned. Every drug and treatment known to the medical profession was tried without effect until Marsilid and Rimifon were administered.[31]

Even this popularly directed broadcast was prudent enough to add a note of caution. "But even now, one great question remains: what will happen after a year or two years? Will some patients develop resistance to Marsilid and Rimifon? Will relapse occur? There is no evidence so far that either of these will happen. Of those first hopeless patients placed on Marsilid and Rimifon, not one has died, not one has had a relapse, and eight months have passed. Not even the most optimistic of doctors can guarantee the future, but to all it appears that the greatest killer of all time may itself now be on the road to complete extinction."[32]

vii

YET, IN THAT first human trial by Robitzek and Selikoff, the sputum had completely cleared of germs in only eight of the forty-four patients treated with isoniazid. Two questions now needed answering. Firstly, was isoniazid as effective as that first clinical trial promised? Secondly, would the tuberculosis germ develop a resistance to the drug that would destroy this great promise? These questions were uppermost in the mind of Walsh McDermott in a discussion he now had with his senior colleague, Dr Carl Muschenheim, who also worked at Cornell.[33]

Between them they decided that the quickest way to answer this and other questions was to study the effects of isoniazid in acute blood-borne tuberculosis. McDermott had performed exactly such a study following Feldman and Hinshaw's first investigations of streptomycin. Quite by chance, a novel opportunity presented itself. Over the new year weekend of 1951–52, Dr Charles LeMaistre, another of the Cornell group, was dispatched to the sunbaked wastes of Arizona's Navajo reservation to investigate an epidemic of hepatitis. These gentle native Americans, living under wretched conditions, were known to be very susceptible to tuberculosis. To his surprise, LeMaistre discovered that tuberculosis was not only very common amongst the Navajos but when they developed blood-borne disease it "had to go untreated". So desperate were the Navajos themselves to get help, their tribal council offered to put up $10,000 towards the costs of a research project that might help their people. The opportunity was too vital to miss and the Cornell group packed their cases and rushed to Arizona.[34]

The first Navajo to be treated with Nydrazid, the formulation of isoniazid supplied by Squibb, was a seven-month-old baby girl, called Patty. When her parents brought her to see Dr Charles Clark, one of the Cornell doctors, at the Western Navajo Hospital in Tuba City, Patty was a wizened starveling weighing just nine pounds. Her temperature was 103 degrees Fahrenheit and she was too weak to swallow. The chest X-ray confirmed the death sentence of blood-borne tuberculosis. After seventeen days of isoniazid, her temperature returned to normal and she took the bottle hungrily. Seven months later, and fully recovered, she was a normal toddler, weighing sixteen pounds.

Soon there was another case, a seventeen-year-old girl, Jean Smith, who also had blood-borne tuberculosis. Jean was also emaciated and dying, with a rattling cough and extreme breathlessness. Her chest X-ray showed a late appearance of blood borne tuberculosis, where the miliary deposits had expanded until they "looked like a snowstorm". She too was treated with isoniazid. On 21 July 1952, *Time* magazine would capture her joy at being rescued from certain death, when she would smile for their photographer, in the company of a delighted Dr Clark. Six months after she began treatment with isoniazid, she was living a normal life and weighed a healthy 114 pounds.

Within five months, McDermott and his colleagues treated ten Navajo patients suffering from blood-borne tuberculosis with no drug other than isoniazid alone.[35] Without isoniazid, they would all have died. For McDermott, it was an anxious time. In 1946, he had conducted an identical trial with streptomycin in ten patients with blood-borne tuberculosis, when all ten had initially responded, only for five of them to relapse and die weeks or months later, from a recurrence of tuberculosis with germs that were completely resistant to the continuing streptomycin therapy. The experience with isoniazid was now following that same initial improvement. Yet, even as the trial was still under way, and as early as April 1952, no less than six separate research studies had shown that tuberculosis readily became resistant to isoniazid.[36] In McDermott's own words, "Once burned, twice shy." All through spring and summer, they waited with mounting anxiety for the deadly bacterial resistance to emerge in their Navajo patients. Alarm bells sounded when, after a hundred days of isoniazid therapy, one patient developed an enlarged lymph gland under the chin. The gland broke down and discharged pus containing live tuberculosis germs. Yet, curiously, this patient, who continued to take isoniazid, made a good recovery and the gland healed. In this admittedly very small trial, all ten patients with blood-borne tuberculosis made a wonderful recovery on isoniazid alone.

When, in July, they sat down to analyse their results in detail under the gleaming tower of Manhattan's New York Hospital-Cornell Medical Centre, McDermott and his colleagues were both delighted and puzzled about this. That same month, when Dr Ralph Tompsett, another member of the group, stood up in "London's cavernous dingy Central Hall" and described their experiences to the 400 experts gathered for a British Empire conference on tuberculosis, nobody knew how to explain it.

That London audience must surely have included tomorrow's pioneers, with such members as John Crofton, Wallace

Fox, Sir Geoffrey Marshall, and Marc Daniels, all now involved in another great MRC trial along the lines of those already conducted into streptomycin and PAS, but this time focusing on isoniazid. On 4 October, the results were published.[37] The isoniazid used was Nydrazid, as supplied by the Squibb pharmaceutical company. In a series of 331 patients with pulmonary tuberculosis, isoniazid on its own was found to have a similar healing capacity to PAS and streptomycin combined. But there was an ominous additional conclusion. "It demonstrated, however, a frequent and rapid development of bacterial resistance to the drug (isoniazid) and showed that this was a serious problem, since it affected the response to treatment."[38]

Once again, the tuberculosis germ had caused those alarm bells clangorously to ring out.

viii

THE VERY ADVANTAGES of isoniazid were now giving cause for concern. It was potent, had a very low incidence of side-effects – above all, it was relatively inexpensive. These made it a very tempting drug to prescribe, especially for treatment outside hospital. Nothing was more certain than that it would be very widely prescribed, and even more widely abused. Yet no such single drug was the miracle cure for tuberculosis.

Even larger scale trials were set into motion. Two months later the American Public Health Service announced their preliminary findings in a huge group of patients who were already infected with tuberculosis germs sensitive to streptomycin at the beginning of treatment.[39] They too found that isoniazid on its own was little better than the combination of streptomycin and PAS, but streptomycin given together with isoniazid was much better. Even in the big American trial, which would eventually include some 1,500 patients with pulmonary tuberculosis, bacterial resistance had proved a problem in a minority of patients. Was this merely a nuisance problem or would it grow in time? Was the combination of isoniazid and streptomycin the global answer to pulmonary tuberculosis?

At the heart of the continuing global intoxication that surrounded isoniazid, a new wave of excitement rippled outwards from its origins in the Caroline Institute in Stockholm. Soon it would ignite an incandescent excitement in the great centres of learning worldwide. Rumour had it that this year the Nobel Prize would be awarded for the discovery of the cure for tuberculosis.

21

Glory and Controversy

When Rutgers University needed to save money during the war winter of 1941–42, a budget official had a bright idea: Why not fire Selman Waksman, an obscure Ukranian-born microbiologist who was getting $4,620 a year for "playing around with microbes in the soil?"

Time magazine, 7 Nov 1949

i

IT WAS INEVITABLE, that from the very moment of its inception, the Nobel Prize would excite great controversy.[1] Under the terms of his will, Alfred Bernhard Nobel, who died unmarried and alone in his villa overlooking the sea in San Remo, Italy, in 1896, left the bulk of his fortune, derived from the discovery and patenting of nitroglycerine, to four separate institutions which would award five annual prizes. The prize in Medicine or Physiology would be awarded by the Royal Caroline Medico-Surgical Institute in Stockholm, according to Nobel's specification: "to those who, during the preceding year, shall have conferred the greatest benefit on mankind in the field of medicine." How can anybody say which doctor or scientist in the world has conferred the greatest benefit on mankind? There can be no truly objective measure of great science or human achievement, no yardstick – the choice, by its very nature, must be subjective.

In the autumn of 1951, the Caroline Institute followed its usual custom of sending out feelers to previous prize winners and a select list of the most prestigious medical and academic institutions worldwide, inviting them to nominate potential candidates. All such proposals had to be returned to the Institute in writing before 1 February of the following year.[2] Nobody was allowed to nominate himself or herself – it is a rule of the prize that self-nomination will lead to automatic disqualification. It is important also to realise that the one person never consulted is the potential candidate himself or herself.

On 1 February 1952, the committee drew up a shortlist of candidates for the prize, and each candidate was then passed to a single member of the committee, who had until the early autumn to evaluate his candidate further. The committee could then call upon the advice of any expert worldwide, when, once again, all such deliberations would be shrouded in secrecy. By September or early October, the committee would have debated the respective merits of each candidate and would have decided upon the name of the winner. This would then be passed to the governing body for ratification. Soon afterwards, in early November, the Nobel Prize winner for Medicine or Physiology for 1952 would be announced to the world. The rules of the prize allowed a maximum of just three personalities to share it in any one year. The decision, once ratified, was final and no further appeal would even be considered.

Because of the secrecy governing these deliberations, we cannot be certain that we know all of the nominees that year. But the potential list is revealingly small. Had Domagk not received the Nobel Prize already, we can be certain he would have been an outstanding candidate. The remaining names in a fast dwindling list include Selman Waksman, H. Corwin Hinshaw, William Feldman and Albert Schatz for the streptomycin discovery and Jorgen Lehmann, Karl Rosdahl and Frederick Bernheim for the PAS discovery. Indeed there would be subsequent confirmation of the committee's interest in four of the names on this list: Selman Waksman, H. Corwin Hinshaw, William Feldman and Jorgen Lehmann.[3] From this point forwards, we enter the maelstrom of controversy.

At the Mayo Clinic, in the words of Corwin Hinshaw, "some of the authorities had been opposed to my continuing the tuberculosis work. As a result I was not given full opportunity to perform experimental work during regular hours. Most of my research was, in consequence, performed out of hours, at night, at weekends and during my vacation periods. The Nobel Prize (for the streptomycin discovery) was originally proposed for Dr Waksman, Dr Feldman and myself. When the Nobel Committee sent their delegates to look into the background of this – and I was given this account directly by a man responsible – a director told them that he did not think that Feldman and I should receive the Prize because he was not thoroughly convinced of the validity of our work and he was disturbed that we had continued to perform the tuberculosis research against advice. I believe that but for this intervention, we would have been included in the Nobel Prize. Indeed I was told by Waksman that he expected that it would have been given to the three of us."[4]

William Feldman and H. Corwin Hinshaw would not share the Prize. If the negative intercession of a director of the Mayo Clinic was truly responsible for their exclusion, this can only be seen as a tragedy. It would not be the only potential injustice in relation to the Prize that year.

Within Sweden itself, where the senior doctors at the Caroline Institute inevitably knew Lehmann personally, the committee's investigation could only be intimate, perhaps almost incestuous. Nevertheless, shrouded in the customary secrecy, delegates from the committee conducted their researches on Lehmann, where, amongst others, they interviewed Karl Rosdahl.[5]

Tuberculosis had not been cured by one drug. It had taken two drugs in combination, discovered at almost precisely the same moment in time, to give sufferers even a modest hope of a cure. Those two drugs were streptomycin and para-aminosalicylic acid, or PAS. Streptomycin had been discovered by Albert Schatz, working under the direct instruction and supervision of Selman Waksman and as a result of a sustained research programme that was Waksman's brainchild. PAS had been discovered as a result of Jorgen Lehmann's creative genius and synthesized by the chemical brilliance of Karl Rosdahl. While, in the United States nobody doubted that Selman Waksman would either receive the Prize or share it, in Gothenburg everybody regarded it as a foregone conclusion

that Jorgen Lehmann would also share it. Close to the time of
the announcement from the Nobel Institute, Lehmann received
a courteous telegram from Waksman, congratulating him in
anticipation of their sharing the Prize. Olof Sievers, Lehmann's
close friend and colleague at the Sahlgren's Hospital, went out
and bought champagne in readiness.

But when, on 23 October, the Committee of the Caroline
Institute made their formal announcement, it was to declare
that Selman Waksman alone had been awarded the Nobel Prize
in Medicine or Physiology for 1952.

Lehmann first heard the news as a result of a telephone call
from a Swedish radio journalist. The purpose of this call, which
was cruel in the extreme, was ostensibly to ask him if he would
like to make a statement on the merits of Waksman's discovery.

Few would dispute awarding the Nobel Prize to the remarkable Selman Waksman, but why had the Nobel Committee
decided that the prize should go to Waksman alone?

ii

ONE FACTOR WHICH may have tipped the scales was the
timing of the first publication. The first paper, by Schatz, Bugie
and Waksman, was published in February 1944, while the
world had to wait until January 1946 for Lehmann's paper in
the *Lancet*. It is a stated rule of the Nobel Committee that only
published work will be taken into consideration. Yet by 1952 it
was abundantly clear – and particularly so in Sweden – that the
two drugs were indeed Siamese twins in the standard treatment of the disease. A decision against Lehmann based only on
the timing of the first paper would appear pedantic beyond the
spirit in which the Prize was intended.

There is a commonly held belief in Sweden that a miscarriage
of justice did indeed take place. It is claimed that Lehmann was
excluded from sharing the Prize with Waksman by a very senior
member of the Nobel Committee, "who persistently opposed
his receiving it". According to common belief, this adamantine
opposition arose from a combination of academic rivalry and
simple jealousy.[6] This is a serious allegation which, given the

secrecy with which the committee operates, is impossible to confirm or refute. In defence of the Nobel Committee of the Caroline Institute, it comprises some of the most experienced and eminent doctors in Sweden. It would be unusual for a man in such a position of trust to betray the very principle of the award. Yet a committee, no matter how exalted, is human and therefore prey to the weaknesses of its members. If prejudice rather than justice excluded Jorgen Lehmann from the Nobel Prize, then no more ironic or tragic parallel could have followed the experiences of Lehmann's beloved teacher, Thunberg.

When he arrived home on the evening of the announcement, Jorgen Lehmann was understandably upset. His elegant new wife, Maja, remembers him anxiously pacing the floor of their apartment. "I thought," she asked him, "that you should have shared it with Waksman?" Even at the moment of his greatest crisis, Jorgen Lehmann retained his sense of humour. "Yes," he declared. "Perhaps you should let them know that, in Stockholm!"[7]

Lehmann in fact behaved very honourably about the Nobel disappointment, refusing to air his disappointment publicly – although he would often ruminate about the cliffs and hazards that would often endanger his work. But was jealousy the reason why Lehmann was excluded from the Nobel Prize? To be fair to the Nobel Committee, no prize is ever without controversy. But circumstance lends some credibility to this popular belief.

Following the discovery of PAS, Jorgen Lehmann was honoured with awards and gold medals from every corner of the globe, including, in 1947 the Société Philomathique de Paris, in 1952 the American College of Chest Physicians Medal for Meritorious Service, the Trudeau Gold Medal in America, the Jahre gold medal from Norway: yet throughout all those years, his achievement was never formally celebrated by his colleagues in Stockholm. Given the importance of his contribution to medicine, this is extremely unusual. Not until he was seventy-seven years old was he presented with a minor medal in this capital city of Sweden, and then it was only granted to him when Åke Hanngren, who as a young man owed his life to Lehmann and PAS, was made Professor of Respiratory Medicine at the Caroline Institute.

To his credit, Jorgen Lehmann insisted on opening the bottle of champagne and toasting Waksman's success with his friend, Olof Sievers, before the two men sat down and together drafted a complimentary notice for the newspapers about Waksman's work and achievement.

Yet even now, after the announcement of the Prize, when he was on the very threshold of receiving it, controversy would dog the steps of Selman Waksman even to the very platform of the most prestigious prize on earth.

iii

IN JUNE 1951, the trustees of Rutgers University, with the happy patronage of the New Jersey state governor, decided to build an institute of microbiology on the site of the humble agricultural college which Waksman had made famous. It was the pinnacle of Waksman's career, and he immediately decided to build a house for himself and his wife, Bobili, close to the institute so that he would not have to waste time travelling to and from work. The cornerstone of the institute was laid on 6 May 1952, when, in a formal reply to the president of the university, Waksman reiterated the faith and inspiration of his lifetime: "This occasion is for me one of the greatest personal significance and satisfaction. You may see before your eyes a mass of brick, mortar, and steel, which is beginning to take the shape of a building. I see in it the realization of a lifelong dream, the fulfilment of my highest aspirations."[8]

On 23 October Selman Waksman had the additional marvellous surprise of hearing he had been awarded the Nobel Prize. His comment was typical: "Thus, the most coveted scientific award was given to a humble worker in the field of microbiological science, primarily in its application to the soil."[9] This "humble worker" had already changed the face of bacteriology. The very name given to the genus of bacteria, now called the *streptomyces*, was a memento to his capability. He had given specific names to more than a dozen newly discovered bacterial species. His election, in pre-antibiotic days, to the National Academy of Sciences of the United States, had given dignity to the profession of soil microbiology. The research programme in his department, which would continue in the new institute, would discover more than thirty antibiotics and anti-cancer drugs, the most important of which after streptomycin would be neomycin, discovered in association with Hubert Lechevalier. Waksman would in his lifetime put his name to twenty-eight books and no less than 500 scientific papers. He would supervise seventy-seven postgraduate students, working towards their higher degrees.

"For several days, my office and laboratory were bedlam. They were swamped with reporters, photographers, radio and television groups. My time was no longer my own. I had to answer all sorts of questions. In concluding my comments, I said: "Out of the earth shall come thy salvation". The newspapers spread the story. Congratulations began to arrive from all over the world. Telegrams, cables, letters, telephone calls, in many languages from many countries. They came from my former students, from colleagues, from well wishers, from tuberculosis sufferers, from foreign groups proud of the accomplishments of an 'immigrant boy'. Altogether too many."[10]

It was at this moment of glory and happiness, and completely out of the blue, that the laurels of success were tossed into a new hurricane of controversy.

Within days of the announcement of the awarding of the Prize to Selman Waksman, Professor Cöran Liljestrand, Secretary of the Nobel Prize Committee, received a formal communication from Elmer S. Reinthaler, Vice-President of the National Agricultural College Farmschool, Bucks County, Pennsylvania, dated 29 October.[11]

It is with a sense of profound satisfaction that the Administration and Faculty of this College has heard of the award of the 1952 Nobel Prize for the discovery of streptomycin. We are particularly gratified by this honour as the original discovery of streptomycin was jointly made by Selman A. Waksman and Dr Albert Schatz who is Professor of Microbiology at this College. We note, however, with amazement that the award was made solely to Dr Waksman, one of the co-discoverers.

We are certain that so distinguished a body as the Council of the Caroline Institute could not have been aware of, and yet ignore, certain most pertinent facts regarding the discovery of streptomycin and the original co-discoverers thereof. . .[12]

The letter drew attention to the fact that the Nobel Prize for the discovery of penicillin had been jointly awarded to Fleming, Chain and Florey and offered documentation to prove the case of Albert Schatz for a joint share in the Nobel Prize for streptomycin.

The Nobel Committee made no direct reply to this letter, but on 31 October, Professor Nils K. Stahle, Director of the Nobel Foundation, issued a statement to the Stockholm news agency, Svenska Dagbladet, to the effect that Nobel Prizes are not subject to review. Professor Hilding Bergstrand, President of the Nobel Committee, also made a statement through this same channel, confirming that Selman Waksman alone had quite properly been awarded the Prize. For Reinthaler, this was unacceptable. In a second letter to Professor Liljestrand, he continued to press Schatz' case. "We think that you will agree with us that mere procedural technicalities should not permit what would constitute a serious injustice to a scientist, and conceal from the scientific and lay world the facts surrounding the discovery of streptomycin."[13]

Dissatisfied with the response of the Nobel Committee, Albert Schatz wrote personally to King Gustav VI, of Sweden, pleading his case. Meanwhile, copies of Reinthaler's letter were forwarded to a huge list of eminent scientists worldwide. These included many previous Nobel Prize winners, such as Gerhard Domagk, Howard Florey and Alexander Fleming. The flames of controversy were now fanned to even greater heat by the fact that the world press somehow became involved. How ironic the copy of Reinthaler's letter must have seemed to William Feldman, who knew that his own employer may have helped destroy his and Corwin Hinshaw's opportunity to share this same prize with Waksman. This is Feldman's modest reply:

"From my knowledge of Doctor Schatz' part in the discovery and development of streptomycin it would seem just and proper that any award recognizing solely this contribution should be conferred jointly on Dr Waksman and Dr Schatz.

However, is it definitely known that the Nobel Prize award was given especially in recognition of the discovery of streptomycin or was it in recognition of Dr Waksman's distinguished achievements of a long professional career devoted largely to investigations pertaining to the microbiology of the soil from which streptomycin finally emerged?" Feldman went on to caution that the widespread circulation of the protest addressed to Professor Liljestrand was most unwise. "I wonder if you don't agree with me that experience has shown that it is quite impossible to correct all the iniquities that are so often involved in awarding prizes, Nobel or otherwise. Rightly or wrongly past evidence indicates that the decision of the constituted committee must be accepted.'[14]

Feldman's assessment would soon be confirmed by none less than King Gustav VI, who replied to Albert Schatz through his private secretary, C.F. Palmstierna:

Having made Himself acquainted with the contents of your letter as well as its appendixes, His Majesty has commanded me to bring the following facts to your attention. The Nobel Foundation is a free and independent institution which by no means is submitted to directions from state authorities. The decisions taken by different organs of the Foundation regarding the award of the Nobel Prizes – in this case by the Council of the Caroline Medico-Surgical Institute – are, according to express instructions, final and thus not liable to alterations by any superior instances.[15]

The issue divided the scientific world. But, although many eminent scientists took up the cause of Albert Schatz, on the whole, the Nobel laureates and senior scientists took the view that Waksman, who had masterminded the entire programme of research at Rutgers, was chiefly responsible for the discovery of streptomycin. In his reply to a letter of support from Professor Stuart Mudd, Waksman made it clear where his opinion lay. He openly suggested that William Feldman and H. Corwin Hinshaw were more deserving of a share of the prize than Albert Schatz.[16] For Selman Waksman, it was a relief to receive the reassurances of the Nobel authorities, and he could now make arrangements to travel to Sweden to receive the prize. He had already made a commitment to travel to Japan in December to deliver an address in commemoration of the centenary of the birth of the great Japanese bacteriologist, Shibasaburo Kitasato, and he refused to cancel this. The Nobel ceremony would have to be fitted in immediately before he travelled further eastwards.

Late at night, and accompanied by Bobili, he arrived by plane in Stockholm, where they were met by a delegation from the Nobel Foundation and the American Embassy, accompanied by an old friend, who was a local professor. There were more newsmen to take photographs and ask questions.

At the suggestion of the American Press Attaché, most of the journalists had gathered in the Grand Hotel for a conference and to take more pictures. This was followed by more discussions going into the night, an early breakfast the next morning, formal invitation to the grand reception, which had to be accepted equally formally in writing, and that evening a dinner given by the National Anti-tuberculosis League of Sweden in a famous old restaurant, where the Queen of Sweden was represented by the Countess Bernadotte, widow of the Count who was murdered in Palestine.

Was Jorgen Lehmann invited to sit with the famous local dignitaries? We certainly know that he had met King Gustav – indeed the King had been one of the first people in Sweden to show interest in the PAS discovery.[17] Whether he was invited or not, the celebration of Waksman's triumph in Lehmann's own country exactly mirrored Villemin's situation of sixty years earlier and could hardly have proved more ironic.

On the morning of 8 December, Selman Waksman travelled by train to Strängnäs, some fifty miles outside Stockholm, where, as a direct result of the release of the world patent rights by George Merck, the Swedish company, Kabi, was opening its first streptomycin-producing plant. In an interesting coincidence, this same company, as Kabi Pharmacia, would one day incorporate Ferrosan with all of its astonishing history into the newly amalgamated company. The trip was a welcome distraction for Selman Waksman, who had felt weighed down with this new controversy upon his shoulders. During the afternoon of 9 December, when he attended the reception at the Nobel

Foundation House, he voiced these worries with Gustav Nobel, Alfred Nobel's nephew, who was himself Russian born, and who had also fled Russia at the time of the Bolshevik Revolution. Waksman was much relieved when Gustav reassured him, "You have nothing to fear."[18]

During the ceremony, he had a conversation with King Gustav, who had for years taken a close interest in the tuberculosis struggle, and who talked to him about "other treatments" for tuberculosis.

At the formal banquet Bobili was escorted to her seat by Prince Wilhelm and she sat between him and the King. Selman escorted Princess Sibylla, the mother of the Crown Prince, who sat to his right. On his left was Mrs Erlander, the wife of the Prime Minister. Preceded by a fanfare of trumpets, the Rector of the university delivered his address, in English and French. As he waited his turn to be presented with the medal and certificate, Selman Waksman must have reflected upon the arcane and circumambulatory journey that had brought him to this unexpected place, a journey that had begun all those years ago with the youth whose life had been saved by chance, shivering over a clay oven in the kitchen of a kindly Russian innkeeper. Soon, in the words of his pupil, Doris Ralston:

"On 12 December 1952, a short man with a bristly moustache and busy, intelligent eyes, stood before the King of Sweden and heard Professor Wallgren of the Royal Caroline Institute extol him: 'Professor Selman A. Waksman, the Caroline Medical Institute has awarded you this year's Nobel Prize for Medicine or Physiology for your ingenious, systematic, and successful studies of the soil microbes that have led to the discovery of streptomycin, the first antibiotic remedy against tuberculosis. Neither are you a physiologist nor a physician but still your contribution to the advancement of medicine has been of paramount importance. Streptomycin has already saved thousands of human lives. As physicians, we regard you as one of the greatest benefactors to mankind.' "[19]

In his answering address, Selman Waksman would not mention the very real role Albert Schatz had played in the discovery of streptomycin. Instead, he made a vivid reference to the humble microbes of the earth that had been his life and inspiration:

"From the moment he is born to the moment he dies, man is subject to the activities of microbes. Some are injurious and some are beneficial. The latter have recently made a great contribution to mankind by producing the antibiotics. Thus has been placed in the hands of the medical profession one of the greatest tools for combating infectious diseases ..."[20]

There would only be one Nobel Prize awarded for the search for the cure for tuberculosis. That search was, however, far from over.

iv

IN SPITE OF the controversies and the bitterly felt disappointments, the Nobel Prize was exactly that, a prize, no matter how prestigious: the tuberculosis story did not revolve about one star, no matter how brilliant, but a constellation of stars, large and small, in what was soon to become a rapidly expanding firmament. In the growing confidence surrounding the cure, many people, including Waksman himself, were already coming to believe that tuberculosis was now defeated. Indeed Waksman would subsequently write a book, *The Conquest of Tuberculosis*. Although this makes fascinating reading, focusing almost exclusively on the streptomycin story, the title was premature: tuberculosis was not yet conquered.

At the time Waksman was presented with the Nobel Prize, isoniazid, though looking very promising, had barely entered the stage of detailed clinical testing. And although streptomycin and PAS had been available for eight years, still nobody had the slightest idea how the drugs worked. The terrifying ability of the bacterium to develop resistance to every new drug was hardly comprehensible at a time when science knew nothing of DNA, nothing of the structure of bacterial cell walls, nothing of the sinister ability of certain bacteria to pass coded information from one to another, without needing any cell division, using mysterious structures called plasmids. Like Dubos with his Cranberry Bog Bacillus some seventeen years earlier, the pioneers had overtaken the scientific understanding of their day. Yet, time after time, those warning bells had sounded out for those who had ears to hear them. In spite of every advance, in spite of all three drug discoveries, tuberculosis had lost surprisingly little of its aura of deadly mystery.

Already the more naive of the optimists, convinced that isoniazid would work against tuberculosis in the same simple way that Prontosil or penicillin worked against acute bacterial infections, had been disappointed. Isoniazid was the most potent of the three discoveries. But the germ became resistant to it with effortless ease so that its future could only lie in combination therapy. Every coupling and permutation of the three drugs would soon be assessed for comparative effectiveness in every clinical manifestation of the disease. As insurmountable obstacle after obstacle was by degrees surmounted, still there remained a nagging anxiety within the hearts of the more knowledgeable doctors around the world. No less a scientist than the distinguished Georges Canetti, director of the laboratory of the Pasteur Institute, could express his doubts as late as 1955: "Short of spectacular progress in one way or another, it is unlikely that chemotherapy will become the exclusive treatment of pulmonary tuberculosis. There are too many factors against it."[21]

v

THE WORLD TEEMED with people at all stages of development of the disease: pulmonary sufferers with huge festering cavities, where all vestige of normal pulmonary function and delicate defence against acute bacterial infection was irrevocably destroyed: intestinal sufferers with section after section of bowel damaged with strictures: people with deep-seated infections in their bones, including the destructive cavitation of spinal vertebrae, chronic festering sores that involved the long bones of the legs or arms, from joint to joint. No drugs could put right the effects of such pervasive destruction. This was the real explanation for the late deaths of millions of tuberculosis sufferers, for example that of Vivien Leigh, the actress, who succumbed to the disease on 8 July 1967. The role for drug therapy, in the thinking of many doctors, was to bring the infective process under sufficient control to allow the surgeons to cut out the damaged lungs, or lobes, or attempt to stiffen the carious spines, or permanently to fuse hip joints that had been macerated by the infection. Nevertheless, in Britain, the United States, Germany, France, Scandinavia, Canada, Australia – throughout every country in the developed world – the wind of change was blowing through the sanitoria, through the long-term sick wards of children's hospitals, as in trial after trial the hopelessness of a death sentence was seen no longer to hold true. Many years after they had first been discovered in America, Sweden and Germany, new trials of the three drugs were being instituted in other countries for the first time.

For Lehmann, Domagk and Hinshaw, it heralded several years of travel, carrying the new gospel from country to country throughout the world. Wherever they travelled, even years after the discoveries, doctors in every country would astonish them by confessing that they simply could not bring themselves to believe those early trials. Perhaps the majority of doctors and patients remained sceptical of the cure until they had seen it happen with their own eyes. The awe of tuberculosis, the ageless leviathan of terror, was so great and the prevailing despair so ingrained, it would take a decade of convincing before the three drugs were generally accepted into medical practice – and even this was solely in the more affluent countries.

On 5 July 1948, Aneurin Bevan, the minister for health in Britain's postwar Labour government, introduced the greatest shake-up of health care in British history, with the Nationalized Health Service. The myriad sanitoria, scattered throughout town, city and countryside, were drawn into this rosy-hued new philosophy of universal right to health. There was no question where the new health service's first priority lay: tuberculosis was public enemy number one, and every enthusiastic ounce would be dedicated to defeating it. In the 1950s Britain introduced global vaccination with BCG, the "tame" living bacterium developed by the French doctors, Albert Calmette and Camille Guérin. Calmette's discovery had known many vicissitudes since its discovery in Lille, in 1931, including a major disaster at the Children's Hospital in Lübeck, Germany, where seventy-three children died following vaccination with a vaccine accidentally contaminated with real tuberculosis germ. Britain had only reluctantly accepted the philosophy of vaccination after it had long been policy in France and Scandinavia and following a Medical Research Council survey of 50,000 children, which showed an 80 per cent reduction in infection rate following vaccination. In America however, the results of their own researches showed the very opposite, so that, in consequence, BCG was never used.

Nevertheless, on both sides of the Atlantic, a new mood of optimism had been growing. People dared to ask themselves a question that would have seemed no more than a pipe dream a generation earlier: could the greatest killer of all time be eradicated from the face of the earth?

In 1960, John Crofton, a Dublin-born tuberculosis expert working at the University of Edinburgh, delivered a lecture in memory of his friend and fellow tuberculosis worker, Marc Daniels, to the Royal College of Physicians in London. Crofton had, as an MRC fellow at the Brompton Hospital in London, been active in the first MRC trials of streptomycin and subsequently isoniazid. The title of the lecture, "Tuberculosis Undefeated", belied its evangelical intent.[22]

At the time of his lecture, it was acknowledged that 12 to 25 million people worldwide were still seriously infected with tuberculosis, with anything from four to eight million in India alone, and 375,000 cases in England and Wales, of which about 45,000 were infectious to others. "Confronted with such an astronomical computation of distress, it is clear that tuberculosis is very far from being defeated, even in economically developed countries. Indeed, in underdeveloped countries it is often said that little can be done until the standard of living is raised. One can hardly accept that."[23]

A resolute and humane man who would subsequently go on to become President of the Edinburgh College of Physicians, Crofton went on to say how, in his opinion, the disease could be conquered, once and for all. He had indeed arrived at an important realization. Given the limited understanding of antibiotics in the early 1950s, much of the early chemotherapy had simply

been inadequate. Working closely with his bacteriological colleagues, Sheila Stewart and Archie Wallace, he looked at what
was really happening and arrived at some surprising conclusions. Germs that had developed only a very mild resistance to one drug had to be seen as highly significant. After a
further year of study, the Edinburgh group were able to show
that with meticulous adherence to effective drug combina-
tions – provided they were dealing with new patients, whose
germs were not as yet resistant to any of the drugs – they were
able to cure every patient. They achieved this revolutionary
success rate by using not two drugs together, but all three, in
the theory that even if the germs managed to develop a resistance to one, the other two drugs would still eradicate the infection. There should be no uncertainty, no ambiguity, to the message that Crofton and his colleagues were now putting to the
world. At last, by treating people with all three drugs at the
same time, streptomycin, PAS and isoniazid, tuberculosis was
completely curable. If the message was taken to its logical conclusion, nobody need fear the terror of the progressive destruction of their lungs, nobody need fear the great fever, nobody
needed to be maimed in spine and limb, nobody need suffer the
lingering death that entered homes and progressively annihil-
ated whole families – nobody need die from tuberculosis any
more.

From this exigent milestone, Crofton and his colleagues took
their studies yet further.

It was still universally believed that, in severe cases, even
following drug therapy, the badly diseased lungs had to be cut
out by the surgeon. "We now realized, and it was later generally accepted, that effective chemotherapy made surgical
treatment redundant." Next, breaking a tradition that had
lasted almost eighty years, they showed that bed rest in the
milder cases was no longer necessary. The unfortunate sufferer
no longer needed to stay in bed for six months, being spoon-fed
like a baby, not allowed up even to go to the toilet. Finally, they
attacked the large numbers of tuberculosis patients in the population of Edinburgh, many of whom had been waiting for treatment for long periods. Within eight years, the waiting list was
completely abolished. At the same time, eighty per cent of the

adult population of Edinburgh was screened by mass miniature X-rays, harvesting many more undiagnosed cases that might have acted as sources for new infection within the population. It was a marathon effort but they had demonstrated the seemingly impossible. Tuberculosis, which had previously been the commonest cause of death in young people in Edinburgh, had been brought under control, the death rate virtually abolished. They had proved their case.

One can imagine the effect when they tried to convince their colleagues. "For a number of years no-one, not even the MRC, believed our results. They thought we had fiddled our figures."[24]

Undeterred by this, in 1957, at the suggestion of Noel Rist, who was the chairman of the Bacteriological Committee of the International Union against Tuberculosis, Crofton instituted a huge international trial with the express purpose of persuading the world that tuberculosis really was one hundred per cent curable. "In order to persuade our colleagues, we dressed it up as 'A Study of the Causes of Failure'." Choosing a leading and influential centre in each of twenty-two countries, whose results might have a national influence, this ambitious trial deliberately focused on people with the most advanced forms of the disease. It needed all of the organizational ability of Reg Bignall at the Brompton Hospital in London. But when the results came in, it proved to be a magnificent success. The only deaths occurred in patients who had been moribund at the start or where doctors broke the protocols and failed to give standard treatment. "As people had seen the results in their own units, at last they believed them."[25]

In pointing to the real meaning of these experiences during his 1960 lecture, this humane and unassuming doctor told the world what would have to be done if it seriously intended to conquer the disease. It implied nothing less than an all-out war. The necessary action included pasteurization of milk, tuberculin testing of cattle and BCG vaccination of whole populations, mass radiography to find the disease early followed by adequate triple drug therapy in every infected patient, isolation of the infectious until they were no longer so, and such general population measures as reduction of overcrowding, all hopefully accompanied by general improvement in the standards of living.

In the United States, in 1960 and 1961, meetings with that same evangelical spirit were convened at Arden House, Harriman, New York, when a new and all-embracing campaign against tuberculosis was proposed to the US Public Health Service by the National Tuberculosis Association. The new spirit of optimism was enshrined in their stated aim, which was to "approach zero" level of infection in the United States. America had also discovered the effectiveness of triple therapy in pulmonary tuberculosis. Where in Europe, BCG vaccination was used to immunize contacts of newly diagnosed open cases, America had found an alternative in short-term isoniazid therapy which appeared every bit as effective in preventing the spread of the disease.[26] These two measures were now adopted as the foundation stones for National Tuberculosis Association policy throughout the United States. But for these policies to work they would need to be put into effect with the utmost diligence and at enormous cost. Soon the rest of the world would follow the British and American lead: organizations such as the World Health Organization, the International Union against Tuberculosis and the United Nations, would raise the banner for the complete eradication of the disease from the face of the earth.

vi

NOBODY UNDERESTIMATED THE difficulties of implementing this aim. In every country throughout the world, infected patients would have to be hunted down; like twenty million or more Typhoid Marys, they would have to be treated in isolation until no longer infected, every single close contact would have to be screened for the disease, treated if already infected, if not infected given the protection of BCG vaccination or short-term isoniazid therapy. If the world really did undertake to eradicate tuberculosis, the cost would be astonomical, the manpower needed would be legionary. Nevertheless, the aim was heroic and the opportunity was certainly a golden one. It simply had to work. In America, the Tuberculosis Association spelled out the price of failure: "If the opportunity to end tuberculosis is not seized now, it may be lost indefinitely."[27,28]

But was such a laudable aim no more than a Utopian ideal, certain to fail in the sad dystopias of the Third World?

In the poorer countries the problems had always promised to be awesome. The cost of admitting a patient to hospital, of intensive nursing for six months or so, with twice daily injections of streptomycin for the first two or three months, and subsequently two full years of drug therapy, were admittedly vast. Even during that early spirit of optimism, the British doctor, Wallace Fox, a pioneer in the global application of the cure, put the real problems of the Third World into perspective: "The actual cost of the drugs in anti-tuberculosis regimens is an important consideration in developing countries, where the total expenditure on all the health services is often of the order of four shillings per head of population per year."[29] There was, for example, no possibility of admitting millions of sufferers to sanitoria. If the cure were to work here, a totally different concept of therapy would have to be envisaged.

Fox now put this concept to the test in what would be called "The Madras Experiment". In 1956 a Tuberculosis Chemotherapy Centre was opened in Madras, India, under the joint auspices of the Indian Council of Medical Research, the Madras State Government, the World Health Organization and the British Medical Research Council. At this time there were just 23,000 beds for tuberculosis sufferers throughout India when an estimated 1.5 million people were suffering from the disease. From its outset this experiment tested the ability of the drugs to cure tuberculosis without the need for sanitoria, with their advantages of isolation of the infected, their ideals of rest and improved nutrition.

Two groups of patients were tested: one treated in a sanitorium while the other was treated at home – "home," in the words of R.Y. Keers, "in this context usually meaning an overcrowded hovel in the poorest quarter of Madras".[30] Injection with streptomycin was impossible in these circumstances, and instead each group was treated with daily PAS and isoniazid for a year. The patients were then followed up for five years to see if they had been cured. After this lengthy period of follow-up, 90 per cent of those treated in their hovels were clear of disease compared with 89 per cent of those treated in the sanitoria. The inference was not only clear – it was cast-iron proof that Crofton's and the Arden House ideal could now be applied to the poorest quarters of the world.

Suddenly even the pipe dream appeared to become possible. In the early 1960s, a wonderful new spirit of optimism inspired the international effort, which could only be encouraged by the discovery of a series of new anti-tuberculous drugs.

In 1963, twenty years after Albert Schatz found the streptomyces that produced streptomycin, the drug company, Lepetit, discovered that a mould with the delightful name *Streptomyces mediterranei* produced a new antibiotic, Rifamycin B. Chemical manipulation of its molecule by the pharmaceutical giant, CIBA, resulted in a new drug of remarkable potency against tuberculosis, rifampicin. Less toxic than streptomycin and as powerful as isoniazid, it could also be taken in tablet form. To this would be added pyrazinamide, discovered by Kushner and his colleagues, as a result of their continuing researches into the pyridine ring, and in 1967, ethambutol, discovered by Lederle laboratories in the United States. Rifampicin replaced streptomycin and ethambutol replaced PAS in the modern therapy, while isoniazid remains to this day one of the three front line drugs. To these six, were added others of less potency or greater toxicity, such as cycloserine and ethionamide. It seemed that even those very worrying problems of drug resistant germs could be relegated to history.

Throughout the developed world, with the successful application of triple therapy and the enthusiastic promotion of prevention, the death rate from tuberculosis came tumbling down. One by one the great sanitoria became redundant. Trudeau's famous sanitorium at Saranac closed in 1954. In Sweden every other sanitorium except the Renström, close to Gothenburg, closed their doors. Even in Davos, the sanitorium capital of the world, the famous old hospitals, with their fairytale architecture, were razed to make way for concrete blocks that would accommodate the modern fashion for winter sports.

The success of the great campaign resulted in a progressive

and massive reduction in both the infection rates and death rates from tuberculosis in every country throughout the developed world. Tuberculosis doctors found their expertise no longer needed and they became chest physicians with other interests. The thoracic surgeons could concentrate their efforts on heart disease and lung cancer.

This revolution did not happen quickly. The change came about slowly, steadily, over two decades, from the mid-fifties to the mid-seventies. By degrees, for the ordinary man and woman in the street, tuberculosis began to fade from consciousness. After the mid-seventies, nobody seemed to die from it any more – or so it seemed. A new generation throughout the wealthy nations, in England, the United States, Germany, France, Ireland, Italy, Spain, the Netherlands, Denmark, Canada, Australia, Scandanavia, Japan, went about their lives hardly aware that the disease existed, except in the poorer quarters of the Third World. They never knew the terror that had been tuberculosis. But was the terror really over?

In reality, of course, although it had become greatly reduced, tuberculosis had never quite disappeared, not in so much as a single developed country. On the contrary, in the tragic arenas of the Third World, poverty, war, corruption and the lack of any effective medical infrastructure had allowed the disease to march on in horrifying proportion. Yet even here, by the late 1970s and early 1980s, there were signs at last that the dedicated efforts of doctors such as Karel Styblo, working for the World Health Organization, and Annik Rouillon for the International Union against Tuberculosis, were achieving their first limited successes. It seemed that it could only be a matter of time, coupled with a better allocation of financial and technical aid, before the success in the developed countries would be paralleled throughout the Third World.

But as ever, when we seemed so close, tuberculosis would surprise us. By 1986–87, African workers began to notice something very strange. Some patients, young patients, were dying under mysterious circumstances – patients who had been diagnosed as smear-positive tuberculosis, who had been treated with good triple therapy, whose sputum had converted to negative. Something was going disastrously wrong with the anti-tuberculosis programme, masterminded by the International Union Against Tuberculosis and the World Health Organisation. With all of his immense energy and talent, Dr Karel Styblo, assisted by colleagues throughout Africa, checked for errors in diagnosis. They found none. They checked for errors in recording, for every conceivable pitfall in what had so recently proved a very successful programme of treatment. But no such error was to be found.

There was no flaw in the programme, no explanatory human error. What they were noticing was the arrival of a new phantasmagoria of terror. In the United States of America that terror had already made its mark in an unforgettable year, 1978, a year when once again, as throughout history, the Russian doll that was tuberculosis would show the world another inscrutable face. What could be so unusual about that otherwise unprepossessing year, 1978?

Two years earlier, New York had been the setting for a spectacular event, when, on 4 July, in the words of Randy Shilts, "Ships from fifty-five nations had poured sailors into Manhattan to join the throngs, counted in the millions, who watched the greatest pyrotechnic extravaganza ever mounted, all for America's 200th birthday party."[31] In time epidemiologists would look upon that eventful year of 1976 and those ships as the harbingers of a new plague, a virus the like of which the world had never known, yet which would bring a wasting and lingering death to the young in a manner that was all too reminiscent of a much older pestilence and one it now sought to emulate: this new plague would soon become familiar worldwide under its frightening acronym, AIDS. How curious it seemed that it was in 1978, the year when the first few cases of this previously unknown contagion were reported, that the infection rate for tuberculosis began to rise again in New York.

PART IV

THE TIME BOMB

22

An Alliance of Terror

I have taken my drop of water from the immensity of creation, and I have taken it full of the elements appropriate to the development of inferior beings. And I wait, I watch, I question it, begging it to recommence for me the beautiful spectacle of the first creation. But it is dumb, dumb since these experiments were begun several years ago; it is dumb because I have kept it from the only thing man cannot produce, from the germs which float in the air, from Life, for Life is a germ and a germ is Life.

Louis Pasteur

i

ON WEDNESDAY 17 October 1990, the *New York Post* carried a startling headline: "Highly contagious tuberculosis close to epidemic level in the city." "No matter where you are in New York today, you can be at risk."[1] This highlighted an investigation the newspaper had been conducting for many weeks into what appeared to be a modern epidemic of tuberculosis, a disease that its readers thought long dead and buried, in the foremost city of the Western world. That same year an expert from the World Health Organization made the extraordinary remark at a closed meeting on the world problem of tuberculosis: "Africa is lost". Thirty years after John Crofton had shown the world how tuberculosis could be eradicated, and after the experts in the United States had gathered to proclaim their "approach zero" declaration at Arden House, the optimism of three decades was faltering. What had gone wrong?

Although the disease had never been eliminated in America, no more than in any other country throughout the developed world, there had been a huge success in bringing down the numbers of infected people. Whereas in 1953 a total of 84,304 Americans had contracted it and 19,707 had died from it, by 1985 the new infection rate had fallen to 22,201, with 1,752 deaths that year.[2] Suddenly, poignantly, that decline had been halted. From 1985 onwards the United States would see a progressive rise in new cases. For example, in 1989, the increase would be 4 per cent on the previous year. By 1990 it would jump up a staggering 9.4 per cent in a year when no less than 25,701 Americans would once again contract tuberculosis.[3] Initial reaction was predictably visceral: Nobody would believe it.

Even as early as 1979, it was apparent to a small number of experts such as Lee Reichman, president of the American Lung Association, that tuberculosis was on the increase. But when he warned a succession of congressional committees throughout the 1980s of the coming epidemic, his words fell on deaf ears. Although it is easy in retrospect to criticise the official bodies, few would have been prepared to believe Dr Reichman at this time.

During the 1970s, the U.S. National Institute of Allergy and Infectious Diseases spent progressively less each year on tuberculosis research until, by 1979, only eight research grants were awarded, totalling a meagre $514,000.[4] Year by year, from 1981 to 1987, the Reagan administration opposed the very existence of a federal TB programme, calling on every occasion for its repeal.[5] For doctors such as Reichman, it was impossible to obtain adequate funding even for basic provision of anti-tuberculosis services, never mind new research. Like every city throughout the developed world, New York and New Jersey had closed down their TB hospitals and sanatoria in the late 60s and early 70s, placing the burden of tuberculosis care onto clinics and community care on an outpatient basis.

Ironically, it was the very success of drug therapy that had allowed the switch of emphasis from hospital inpatient treatment of tuberculosis to the poorly monitored community-based therapy. There was powerful motivation to accept any scheme for saving public money. By the mid-1970s New York

City was on the brink of its now famous bankruptcy. Even the funding of outpatient services was sharply reduced, worsening an already spiralling danger. The new generation of young doctors felt no awe of a disease that had been consigned to the limbo of history. Who could blame them if they were seduced by the *Vorsprung-durch-Technik* of molecular biology and genetic engineering? Any research and funding now devoted to the fight against infection was understandably earmarked for the struggle against AIDS. All the while, against this universal tendency for doctors, scientists and politicians to underestimate it, tuberculosis, the sinister chameleon, continued to change and to evolve.

Some fundamental questions had to be asked about the disease and its manner of treatment: Had we had taken a step too far in our zeal for community-based drug therapy? An important consideration in both hospital and community-based thinking was the conviction that after as little as a few days' therapy, tuberculosis patients were no longer infectious to others. In a seminal study, Luke Clancy, an Irish expert who had studied with Crofton, showed that even after several weeks of intensive drug therapy, guinea pigs inoculated with sputum from such patients were still infected by it. The implications were considerable, not only for staff looking after such patients but also for other patients they might encounter in the hospital setting. If such patients were discharged early into the community, the implications were a good deal more disturbing. In Clancy's own words, "We think this is important especially in the AIDS era. We feel that the notion that patients were no longer infectious after a few days' or even two weeks' chemotherapy has become elevated to the status of a dogma. We think that this is wrong and feel that . . . in low prevalence countries especially when we are considering immunosuppressed hospital patients, it represents a dangerous and unsustainable stance which must be revised."[6]

What was really happening to people after they had been discharged back into the community still taking multiple drug therapy for tuberculosis? This vitally important question was now brought into focus by Drs Karen Brudney and Jay Dobkin, working at Presbyterian Hospital in New York.[7]

The purpose in switching from hospital to community was undoubtedly to save money. But with tuberculosis – the long-term courses of treatment, the need for multiple drugs, often producing side-effects, the known tendency of people, no matter how intelligent or educated, to stop unpleasant medication as soon as they *felt* better – this carried obvious risks. When Brudney and Dobkin assessed the effectiveness of their impoverished community service, their conclusions were very disturbing indeed. After discharge from hospital, no less than 89 per cent of patients disappeared from community follow-up and never completed their treatment. The outcome was only too predictable: More than a quarter of them were back in hospital within a year, still suffering from tuberculosis. As the very first studies with the newly discovered streptomycin, PAS, and isoniazid had shown, precious as the cure undoubtedly was, poor supervision of its application could quickly turn to disaster.

Outside America, scepticism about the new threat posed by tuberculosis was even more deeply ingrained. In Britain, a country that had long since dissolved its anti-tuberculosis association, the media gave little coverage to what was happening in America. Those who warned about the new danger were dismissed as "panic-mongers," their message too "controversial" to be taken seriously.

Such scepticism in every developed country was compounded by another "misconception" concerning tuberculosis. For years, experts had reassured the public that a disease that had infected a third of humanity was not in fact highly contagious. It had been calculated that on average you had to share the same air with an openly infected patient for several hundred hours before you were at risk of being infected. If the myriad of mini-epidemics worldwide, often resulting from trivial or very brief contact, had not questioned this, a new outbreak in America surely would shake it to its roots. In 1989, a man working as a metal grinder in a shipyard in the town of Bath, Maine, developed a cough and a fever that would not go away. This was not a community downtrodden by poverty or homelessness. On the contrary, it was a prosperous town, spared the overwhelming problems of drug addiction or the

AIDS epidemic of the deprived inner city districts of New York. In Bath, tuberculosis was considered so unlikely that it did not even occur to the doctor when this man presented with his symptoms. The unfortunate man suffered from tuberculosis for eight months before the correct diagnosis was made, during which time no less than 417 of his workmates had become infected.[8]

Unimpressed by the warnings of the prescient few, and ignoring the rising tide of infection in the inner city ghettoes, most Americans continued about their business at home and at work, convinced that this forgotten plague did not threaten them. New York was the exception that proved the rule. Because the disease was, and always had been, more common amongst the poor, it was assumed that the more affluent were immune to it. Conditions in the less-privileged districts, such as central Harlem, were so miserable that middle-class America could readily believe anything could take fertile root there. An imaginary iron curtain, wondrously germ-repelling, was drawn about the ghettoes. What a shock it was when, in July 1992, all dealers working on the exchange floor of the New York World Trade Center were ordered to take a tuberculin test. Staff were forbidden entry to the trading floor unless they could demonstrate that they had proved negative on skin testing. This followed the discovery that two employees had developed tuberculosis. The plague had penetrated to the very heart and symbol of Western affluence.

Of course it did not stop there. In January 1992, four months after their twins were born, prosperous lawyers Andres Valdespino and his wife, Michelena Hallie, noticed that one of their babies had a cold that would not go away. The family lived in North Tarrytown, an attractive rural town north of New York. Their doctors had difficulty arriving at a diagnosis. It was not until his twin brother developed the same symptoms that tuberculosis was diagnosed. By this time it was also diagnosed in his father, his mother and another brother. Their unhappy experience was reported in *The New York Times* on December 6 that year. "I felt so immune," exclaimed an understandably worried mother. "We live in this tiny town in Westchester, in the middle of the forest." Although the new outbreaks of tuberculosis were initially based almost entirely in the big metropolitan areas, the disease was now spreading into the neighbouring rural counties. For example, in the 16 counties surrounding Houston, a city with one of the highest tuberculosis rates in America, new cases had risen by 80 per cent between 1989 and 1992. This was creating yet another problem for sufferers: initial incredulity was often leading to a delay in making the correct diagnosis.

The upsurge of the disease was so alarming that in October 1992 *The New York Times* printed a series of articles under the title "Tuberculosis: A Killer Returns," which drew urgent attention to the escalating danger. "The United States has stumbled into its first preventable epidemic, a wave of tuberculosis with strains so virulent they threaten to return pockets of American society to a time when antibiotics were unknown."[9] By December 1992, in spite of every effort at controlling the disease in New York and elsewhere, its rapid spread was so worrying that 34 scientists, ethicists and public health leaders came together to form a voluntary panel, which issued a report on "The Tuberculosis Revival," with some controversial and far-reaching recommendations on the social and ethical implications for American society. These included the suggestion that new legislation should be introduced to force every infected patient to agree to direct observation of their compliance with drug treatment. "It is absolutely essential that we never again draw lines in health care between the haves and have-nots," said Nancy Dubler, one of the panel.

America was waking up to a fact that would have been familiar to Hippocrates two and a half millennia earlier: when it comes to tuberculosis, everybody is at risk.

Elsewhere in the developed world, the forgotten plague would stage a similar comeback, as if America had cast the template for an incredible – indeed, rather mysterious – reincarnation.

In the United Kingdom, the numbers of new cases of tuberculosis continued to fall until 1988, after which they remained virtually stationary for two years before rising by 5 per cent in 1991. Figures available for the first half of 1992 predicted an even more dramatic rise. This was the first time the British authorities had seen any rise at all in forty years. It was so unexpected it caught Virginia Bottomley, the Health Minister in the British Parliament, unprepared, precipitating that same visceral reaction as a few years earlier in America. There was, she assured the country, no tuberculosis problem. However, just two weeks later, she was forced to concede the opposite in Parliament, when she provided figures for the Greater London area. It was now revealed that, since 1987, the disease had been steadily increasing in London. By 1991, there had been no less than 1,794 cases of tuberculosis in the city, giving it one of the largest tuberculosis burdens of any city in the developed world.

In Britain, where it had been planned to end the country-wide BCG vaccination of school children in 1990, and where fifteen local health authorities had already discontinued it, this became the subject of discussion and controversy in the media. Most of the British health authorities now thought it prudent to continue vaccination, a policy that met with the approval of Dr P. D'Arcy Hart, who had directed both the first British trial of streptomycin and the subsequent large-scale trial of BCG vaccination in school children, and who was still working with the British Medical Research Council.

In a manner that would shake the Olympian complacency of many a government and health ministry, the British pattern was repeating itself in most of the countries of Western Europe.

In a press release titled "Tuberculosis Is Rising in Industrialized Countries," dated 17 June 1992, the World Health Organization listed no less than ten countries in which tuberculosis was dramatically increasing. It surprised many to see Switzerland, Denmark, the Netherlands, Sweden, Norway and Austria included, in addition to Ireland, Finland, Italy and the United Kingdom. From country to country, different explanations were now proffered by ministries of health for this extraordinary reawakening of the forgotten plague. In London, for example, where the problem district of Camberwell was witnessing a tuberculosis rate five times the British national average – and already half the level of some of the worst areas in the developing world – one in three of the tuberculosis sufferers was homeless. Dr Peter Davies, on behalf of the British Thoracic Society, rightly stressed the link with poverty and the location of the new outbreaks in deprived inner city enclaves. Yet in prosperous Scandinavia, Holland and Austria there seemed a less obvious link to ghetto conditions. Here the increase was attributed to immigrants from war-torn central Europe and elsewhere, where it had long been endemic. And so it went, from country to country, alternative reasonable explanations would be advanced for the problem on their particular doorstep. Yet this very diversity of explanations could hardly account for the fact that the disease, which had been inexorably falling in every developed country for forty years, was suddenly and progressively increasing in ten countries simultaneously. Simple logic dictated there must be some common factor, or factors – indeed, there had to be a very powerful explanation the United States and Western Europe had in common.

In this evaluation, nothing could be more pertinent than the realization that this strange and frightening recrudescence of tuberculosis in the United States and Europe was only the tip of a global iceberg.

In 1991, Professor John Murray, of San Francisco General Hospital, drew attention to the fact that during the previous five years there had been an ominous worldwide resurgence of tuberculosis, with a veritable explosion in sub-Saharan Africa.[10] The problem was so urgent that on 26–27 October 1990, a meeting was convened at the World Health Organization in Geneva, when representatives of tuberculosis control programmes attended from all over the world. Their conclusions were as close to frightening as this conservative medical gathering would allow.

Eight million or more people worldwide would contract open tuberculosis this year alone. "It is estimated that tuberculosis caused 2.9 million deaths in 1990, making this disease the largest cause of death from a single pathogen in the world."[11]

While the largest numbers of deaths occurred in the developing world, a surprising 400,000 people were still contracting it in industrialised countries and 40,000 people were still dying from it. The global situation was so alarming that on 1 March 1990, Dr Christopher Murray, of the Harvard School of Public Health, and Karel Styblo and Annik Rouillon, of the International Union Against Tuberculosis, based in Paris, joined forces to warn that "the magnitude of the tuberculosis problem worldwide was now staggering."[12]

It was estimated that approximately 1.7 billion people, or one third of the world's population, were still infected with the disease on the basis of skin testing. This included 10 million Americans, 1 million of whom lived in New York. No country in the industrialised world was excepted from this vast reservoir of latent infection. But this was hardly a cause for alarm since, judging from previous experience, only a small proportion of these latent infections would ever mushroom into active tuberculosis. However, a new convergence of forces would give the vast numbers of people carrying latent infection ominous significance.

At last, doctors both in the United States and at the World Health Organization had arrived at a very important –indeed, a shocking – realization. Although there were additional factors involved, most notably homelessness and social deprivation, the most important trigger for this new global threat was now obvious: It was the AIDS virus.

The emerging threat so worried three eminent bacteriologists – Stanford and Grange of London, and Pozniak of the University of Zimbabwe – that they wrote a special article for the *Lancet* in which they spelled out what was likely to happen in words that nobody could fail to understand. In an article that took its title from the WHO expert's comment, "Is Africa Lost?," they explained how, with this congruence of AIDS and tuberculosis, the world was facing "the greatest public health disaster since the bubonic plague."[13]

ii

AIDS IS CAUSED by infection with a virus new to medicine, the human immunodeficiency virus. It belongs to a group of viruses, the lentiviruses, that remain dormant in an infected

person for a very long time before the disease begins to show.
There are in fact two related viruses, HIV-1, which is found
worldwide, and HIV-2, which occurs principally in West
Africa. The virus infects a certain type of human white cell,
the CD4 subset of T lymphocyte, which plays an important
part in the immune response of the human body to infection.
The HIV virus also damages monocytes, another key cell in
the human defences. If a writer of science fiction had racked
his brain to come up with the most sinister imbroglio of
doom, he could not have invented anything more threatening. Those very immune cells which are destroyed by the
HIV virus are also the cells that enable the body to fight tuberculosis.

In those 1.7 billion people worldwide who, often without
being aware of it, are still harbouring the tuberculosis germ in
those little "healed" cicatrices in their lungs, these are the very
cells that are keeping the tuberculosis germs under control.

A person who is infected with the AIDS virus but has not
yet developed any obvious symptoms or signs of disease is
said to be HIV positive. When the disease becomes manifest,
the person is said to have full-blown AIDS. Although the first
clinical cases of AIDS were reported as recently as 1981, doctors soon noticed that the two diseases have a surprising number of features in common. In the words of Festenstein and
Grange: "In both cases it is possible to be infected but clinically
healthy – overt disease may not commence until many years
after the initial infection. During the interval before illness
commences, the only signs of infection are, respectively, a
positive tuberculin test and circulating antibodies (HIV posi-
tivity)."[14] There are other, rather more worrying, habits the
two diseases share.

The city of New York, in common with every other city
throughout the industrialized world, saw an unrelenting fall
in the numbers of its citizens contracting tuberculosis from the
1950s onwards. Where in 1960 a total of 4,699 cases were reported, this number had dwindled to an all-time low of 1,307
in that auspicious year, 1978, when the fall in the disease rate
had stopped. Ever since 1978, the numbers of new cases diagnosed per year had gradually risen again. In 1989, Dr Jack

Adler, then Medical Director of the New York Bureau of Tuberculosis, in analysing this strange reversal of trends, reported that "Tuberculosis cases in New York City increased again in 1989. This incidence represents a 9.8 per cent increase over 1988's and a 68 per cent increase over 1980's. The 1989 case rate is the highest in two decades."[15]

He went on to emphasize that the disease continued to climb upward among 25–44-year-olds in all racial and ethnic groups, but particularly in black and Hispanic males. The high incidence of disease in this age group was particularly distressing because these were the individuals of child-bearing age. Where in 1987 there had been forty-eight cases of tuberculosis affecting children under fifteen years old, by 1988 these numbers had almost doubled, to ninety-one.

Since then this pattern in New York has not improved: It has progressively worsened. In the year ending November 1991 roughly 4,000 new cases of tuberculosis were reported. People are not just contracting the disease, many are also dying from it. In 1989, for example, of approximately 2,500 cases in New York alone, 233 died from tuberculosis. When asked for a simple explanation of this phenomenon, Dr Adler, while acknowledging there were other factors, notably poverty, drug addiction, and immigration from the developing countries, had no doubt in pointing to the main causative factor: "I can give it to you in a word of four letters – AIDS."[16]

New York was far from alone in the United States in witnessing this triggering of tuberculosis by the AIDS virus. On 27 September 1991, Dr Gisela Schecter, director of the Tuberculosis Clinic at San Francisco General Hospital, reported an outbreak of the disease among the residents of a home for HIV-infected persons in the city, which graphically illustrated the difficulties the health care workers were now facing.[17]

On 19 December 1990, a resident who had lived in the home since November was admitted to hospital with a history of several weeks' productive cough, fever, and night sweats. Soon diagnosed as suffering from active pulmonary tuberculosis, he received anti-tuberculous drug treatment and did not return to the home. On 19 January 1991, another resident was admitted to a local hospital with a history of seven days' productive cough, fever, chills, and shortness of breath. Tuberculosis germs were shown in the sputum and were subsequently cultured from his blood and pleural fluid (from the cavity surrounding the lung). He was given appropriate treatment and then discharged back to the residential home. But, following a pattern that would become worryingly commonplace, he did not take his treatment as prescribed. When readmitted to hospital on 15 February, his sputum was again positive for the germs. His lungs were now infected with *Pneumocystis*, a protozoal parasite that commonly infects AIDS patients. In spite of drug treatment for both infections, he died on 10 March from overwhelming destruction of his lungs.

From 21 February to 4 March, four additional residents of the HIV home were admitted to hospital, suffering from pulmonary tuberculosis. On 6 March, the Tuberculosis Control Division for the city visited the two-and-a-half-storey residential home and screened the remaining seventeen residents and fourteen members of the staff. Seven of the residents and four of the staff now had positive skin tests. Three of the seven residents had the typical appearance of the disease on chest X-rays, two of whom grew the germs from sputum cultures. It was concluded that twelve of the residents had contracted pulmonary tuberculosis from a single infected patient. The outbreak was remarkable not only for the large percentage of residents who had contracted active disease within the residential home but also for the ferocious speed with which the disease had seemed to explode in the infected patients. In the AIDS patients, tuberculosis had undergone a dramatic metamorphosis of its normal character, proliferating and invading with the fulminant speed of an acute bacterial infection.

San Francisco General Hospital, a pioneer in the study and treatment of AIDS, had been one of the first institutions in America to recognize the resurgence of the more ancient enemy. By 1991 the hospital was fighting a battle against the disease that would have been familiar to the campaigners of the 1930s and 1940s. All health care workers within the city were subjected to twice yearly tuberculin skin tests. There was a stepped-up tuberculosis awareness campaign for all doctors working within the city. They went so far as to invent a new mask, called a particulate respirator, designed to prevent their staff from contracting the disease from their patients.

It was now established that AIDS patients were highly vulnerable to picking up tuberculosis, whether from the infected cough of an open sufferer or from activation of latent or apparently healed infection from years previously. But the habit-sharing of the two plagues was even more insidious and vital than anybody had first realised. The American doctors were observing an equally malign cooperation in reverse.

A new study showed that not only was infection with HIV triggering a latent infection with tuberculosis, but that, within two and a half months, the tuberculosis itself had the capacity to activate the HIV infection, causing it to blossom into full-blown AIDS.[18] In effect, each disease was triggering the other, so that, within just months of becoming HIV positive – and often completely unaware he or she was harbouring the tuberculosis germ from childhood – the unfortunate man or woman now went into a devastating decline, with overwhelming infection from both diseases at the same time.

This horrific picture was all too typical of the pattern now emerging worldwide, in which the twin plagues of AIDS and tuberculosis had come together in a synergy of terror never seen before in medical history.

iii

SOME DEVELOPED COUNTRIES, such as Britain, have so far escaped major outbreaks of the new TB-AIDS epidemic, partly because AIDS is much less common and also because, by chance, HIV infects predominantly young white or black males while latent tuberculosis is commonest in the elderly white population or in immigrants from the Asian continent, in whom HIV infection is, as yet, uncommon. But clusters of tuberculosis in AIDS patients are now being reported in Britain, and AIDS is part of the explanation of the new rise of tuberculosis in Dublin. In at least one major Spanish city, the relationship between the two plagues is rather more established.

In 1988 alone, 1,012 new cases of tuberculosis were diagnosed in the city of Barcelona, an increase of 36.7 per cent compared to the previous year. Many of the sufferers were young men aged 20–29, who were concomitantly infected with HIV, secondary to intravenous drug abuse.[19] This arrival of the AIDS-tuberculosis syndrome is now being reported, although as yet on a small scale, from many other developed countries in addition to the United States and Spain, including Italy and Australia. In Paris, particularly in the Île de France district, a new and unexpected increase in tuberculosis is almost certainly AIDS-related. In another Spanish city, San Sebastian, in the Italian cities of Bari, Florence and Pisa, in the German cities of Frankfurt and Berlin, AIDS is triggering a significant percentage of the recent increase in tuberculosis.[20] Meanwhile, in a report published in late 1992 by the British Health Ministry's *Weekly Epidemiological Bulletin*, medical authorities reported that AIDS was now the principal cause of death in Parisian men between the ages of 24 and 44 years, bringing the capital of France on a par with New York and San Francisco. How worrying that there are now an estimated 1 million people infected with HIV in the United States and 500,000 in Europe, including Russia.[21]

In Japan, where the epidemic wave of tuberculosis peaked much later than in America or Western Europe, a high proportion of the population are latently infected and reactivation tuberculosis is still relatively common; given its proximity to South-East Asia, where HIV infection is now epidemic, the danger must be considerable. Thailand, with its huge sex industry, is desperately vulnerable. In 1992, a total of 400,000 Thais were already HIV positive, with health workers estimating that 500 more Thai citizens were being infected with the AIDS virus every day. Yet even this alarming figure is dwarfed by the prediction that by the end of the century, as many as 4 million Thais will be HIV positive. The fact that such "sex-tourism" is now being diverted to Vietnam and Laos, where the bars advertise themselves as "AIDS-free with guaranteed virgins," can only be sowing the seeds of catastrophe. Today more than 3 million people in South-East Asia are already estimated to be HIV positive. In this light it is tragic that the

World Health Organization now deems it too late to prevent an explosion of HIV infection in India, where hundreds of millions are harbouring tuberculosis and where more than 1 million are already infected with the AIDS virus. Indeed, the WHO is now predicting that by the end of the century, South-East Asia will have overtaken Africa, when it is anticipated that no less than 40 million Asians will be HIV positive. Many other Asian countries, particularly China, with its gigantic tuberculosis problem, are vulnerable.

Saddest of all, in sub-Saharan Africa, where 171 million people are infected with latent tuberculosis, the catastrophe has already happened. In 1992, an estimated 6.5 million Africans were infected with the HIV virus, of whom 3.12 million were additionally infected with life-threatening tuberculosis. Little wonder that the expert at the World Health Organization meeting was heard despairingly to confess that "Africa is lost."[22] Perhaps as revealing was the fact that at the meeting of the World Health Organization where this remark was made, nobody questioned this melancholy conclusion.

It seems almost insane that in these days of global travel, when somebody can fly from continent to continent in hours, the affluent countries perceive so little threat to themselves in such unmitigated suffering throughout the developing world. In the blunt summation of the International Union: "Tuberculosis has been a neglected international and national health priority for nearly two decades."[23] How easily we forget the great terror.

A remarkable little band of dedicated doctors and scientists gave us the cure for tuberculosis. But their brave and inspired struggle had been fought out at considerable personal cost. The marriages of Koch, Lehmann and Domagk would all break down. Dubos' first wife died from the disease, and his second wife, Jean, and his colleague Bernard Davis, like William Feldman, contracted it from their work and were lucky that their lives could be saved by the very cure they had helped to discover. Dubos and the young German doctor Karl Jahnke were also infected from their work but recovered at the whim of the disease. The chemists Rosdahl, Klarer and Mietzsch believed for the rest of their lives that their contribution towards the cure had been neglected, just as the streptomycin controversy blighted the future life and career of Albert Schatz. How poignant it seems, some forty years after the cure was discovered, that the world failed to extend their wonderful achievement to its full global potential.

In 1960, when in the euphoria of that new spirit of optimism, the World Health Organization held its seventh meeting, it stressed that "tuberculosis is the most important specific communicable disease in the world as a whole, and its control should receive priority and emphasis both by the WHO and by governments."[24] Sadly, just four years after its conception, the Utopian ideal of global conquest of the disease was already acknowledged by that same expert body to be failing. Thirty years later the experts would not only confirm that lamentable trend of earlier reports but also issue warning after warning on the alarming new global threat from the disease. In 1991, in the opinion of Styblo and Enarson, "infection with the human immunodeficiency virus (HIV) is now the greatest risk factor for tuberculosis, having caused the greatest deterioration in the epidemiological situation in the last 100 years."[25] In an important global overview, in 1991, the World Health Organization experts Sudre, ten Dam and Kochi would hammer the message home: "This report confirms the staggering global magnitude of the tuberculosis problem and the urgent need to revive anti-tuberculosis control programmes throughout the world."[26]

Why had all those fine efforts of so many highly motivated and dedicated experts failed?

C.J.L. Murray, dissecting out the cause of that failure in 1991, would be blunt: "The neglect of tuberculosis as a major public health priority over the last two decades is simply extraordinary. Perhaps the most important contributor to this state of ignorance was the greatly reduced clinical and epidemiological importance of tuberculosis in the wealthy nations."[27]

It was all very well for highly motivated groups to lay down the ground rules for the impoverished health authorities of developing countries – they could perform superbly efficient controlled trials, imbued with laudable missionary spirit – but it was another matter entirely for those hard-pressed countries, racked by wars, famine, extreme poverty and ignorance, to accomplish miracles year after year, with virtually no money or resources.

All the time the disease was being battened down to controllable levels in the developed countries, it remained a fearsome killer in the poorer countries of the world. In many areas of sub-Saharan Africa, it could be assumed that virtually everybody had contracted it. Throughout Asia, with its teeming populations, and Oceania, with its poorly equipped medical services, the disease had swarmed in epidemic proportion. These facts can only imply an appalling neglect of such unfortunate people by our more fortunate selves in the developed world. In these days, with such ease of movement from one country and even one continent to another, this was not only morally indefensible, it was also reckless. Nothing was more predictable than that soon the problem would turn up in our own backyard.

iv

IN 1985, a twenty-four-year-old immigrant woman suffering from tuberculosis arrived in the United States.[28] Her disease had been treated in her native Korea but nobody knew what drugs she had taken. When she arrived in America, her chest X-ray showed early involvement of the apices of both lungs. She was treated with isoniazid, rifampicin and ethambutol in combination. Four months later she had deteriorated, with a productive cough, chills, fever, sweats and weight loss. Her chest X-ray showed a considerable worsening, with cavities at both apices. She was now admitted to hospital, ethambutol was stopped and pyrazinamide, ethionamide, cycloserine and streptomycin were added to the isoniazid and rifampicin. In spite of this, she continued to worsen, her chest X-ray became more alarming, her cough remained productive and every sputum sample that was examined showed an abundance of tuberculosis germs.

At this stage she was transferred to the care of Dr Michael D. Iseman, Chief of Clinical Mycobacteriology at the Division of Infectious Disease in the National Jewish Center for Immunology and Respiratory Medicine, at Denver, Colorado.

Dr Iseman, a world expert on multi-drug–resistant (MDR) tuberculosis, cultured her germs and confirmed that they were resistant to isoniazid, streptomycin, ethionamide, rifampicin, pyrazinamide, cycloserine and rifabutin, with only partial sensitivity to ethambutol. By now the left upper lobe was totally destroyed and the remainder of the left lung was extensively diseased. There was a less severe infection in the right lung. In desperation, a new course of treatment was attempted, using PAS, ethambutol and the rather more speculative capreomycin, kanamycin and ofloxacin. "Owing to the extensive drug resistance, therapeutic pneumoperitoneum (an old 'collapse' technique) was begun." As in the earliest days of streptomycin and PAS, this treatment allowed sufficient improvement for her left lung to be removed. The surgery saved her life and she remained well three years after the operation.

Dr Iseman, who was now treating hundreds of similar cases, saw it as a matter of urgency to find out how her tuberculosis had developed this terrifying degree of resistance to every known anti-tuberculous drug.

From the very first days of streptomycin and PAS, resistant germs had been encountered. The doctors at that time had not understood the mechanism by which this happened. But science had progressed in the intervening forty years. In the 1950s, Oswald Avery had discovered DNA as the wonder molecule of life and heredity, which was soon followed by the Nobel Prize-winning elucidation, by Watson and Crick, of its three-dimensional chemical structure. Now we understood how, during cell division, the DNA code of any living cell could randomly alter. This is what we really mean when we refer to the process of mutation. Germs can also mutate. It is the principal means by which they develop resistance to antibiotics. A mutated germ then passes on the new DNA coding for that resistance to all its offspring. At last we had an explanation for that dangerous development of resistance in the early tuberculosis trials. Now we know that the tuberculosis germ has a terrifying capacity to mutate.

How it does so can be explained very simply. Let us say that we start with a single germ that is sensitive to any of the anti-tuberculous drugs. If that germ then divides and its progeny continue to proliferate until there is a pool containing 1 million germs (a fairly average number in a newly infected patient), some of the myriad mutations that have taken place will have resulted in germs that are resistant to each of the anti-tuberculous drugs in turn. Fortunately, a single germ does not evolve all of these resistant mutations at the same time – this would be the formula for Armageddon. In practice, while one germ mutates the resistance to streptomycin, a different germ mutates the resistance to isoniazid, and so on. Not a single drug is exempt from this terrifying mutation capacity. Indeed, there will be germs present that are already resistant to drugs that have not yet been invented. The potential is obvious and awesome.

During the 1950s and 1960s, doctors such as Crofton had discovered by direct observation of the germ's behaviour that triple therapy prevented drug resistance from developing. In 1985, Michael Iseman could now put forward a theory why this worked.

Naturally occurring tuberculous bacteria are rarely resistant to more than one drug. Some bacteria may be resistant to drug A, others to drug B. If you give the patient both drugs A and B, drug A will kill the bacteria resistant to B, and B will kill the bacteria resistant to A. This then was the rationale behind combined therapy. To this equation of perfection, Iseman now added the factor of human fallibility. A patient harbouring a billion germs is started on two drugs together – say, isoniazid and rifampicin. After a few weeks of therapy, the patient – who is not a supervised inpatient but a sick and poor outpatient, harassed by personal stresses and worries, and perhaps struggling with the additional burden of taking concomitant multiple-drug therapy for AIDS – decides that rifampicin is producing intolerable side effects. Without telling the prescribing doctor, the patient now stops rifampicin and continues to take isoniazid alone. Because the

majority of germs are initially killed off, the patient feels temporarily better but, after several months, germs resistant to
isoniazid grow and multiply. The doctor now makes the error of assuming the patient is taking both drugs. Tests on the
resistant germ reveal that it is only resistant to isoniazid, so
the rifampicin is continued and another drug, such as ethambutol, is added. In effect the patient continues to take only
one drug, and his germs, already resistant to isoniazid, now
develop a resistance to ethambutol as well. Spread of his
germs to other contacts now infects them with germs that are
already resistant to two drugs. The contact is given triple
therapy, containing two of the drugs to which the germ is
resistant. In time the contact is growing germs resistant to
three drugs. And so the cycle expands and spreads.

Through this mechanism, as early as 1985, Dr Iseman predicted the emergence of a superbug, resistant to all effective
drugs. This "truly chilling" possibility was aptly summed up
in the title of his editorial: "Tailoring a Time Bomb."[29]

Just seven years later there would be evidence from four
continents that Iseman's hypothesis was now fact.

On 25–26 January 1992, the *International Herald Tribune*, published in Paris, carried a banner headline: "Drug-Resistant
Strains of Tuberculosis Are 'Out of Control,' U.S. Says." Multi-
drug–resistant tuberculosis germs had now appeared in seventeen American states, with mini-epidemics in Florida,
Michigan, New York, California, Massachusetts, Texas and
Pennsylvania. The pattern in Miami, Florida, and in New York
was typical of what was happening in the other states.

In 1990, a new tuberculosis outbreak took place in a large
municipal hospital, starting in a ward dealing with AIDS patients. What worried the Miami doctors was the fact that these
patients were infected with germs resistant to all of the first-
line and most of the second-line anti-tuberculous drugs.[30] In
that same year, in New York, similar outbreaks of antibiotic-
resistant tuberculosis broke out in three of the city's hospitals,
from where it spread to at least one of the city's prisons. Within
the hospitals, infection was spreading in a nosocomial
manner – from patient to patient and from patients to staff. As
in Florida, the resistance to antibiotics made these outbreaks

almost impossible to treat. Inevitably the majority of sufferers died, many within just weeks of diagnosis.[31]

The article in the *Herald Tribune* quoted Dr Dixie Snider, a senior expert from the Centers for Disease Control, in Atlanta: "At no time in recent history has tuberculosis been of such great concern as it is now, and legitimately so, because tuberculosis is out of control in this country."

Bacterial strains resistant to the standard antibiotic treatment were already emerging in many other countries. In 1991, when Dr John Stanford, an eminent bacteriologist working at Middlesex Hospital, London, visited the Chest Hospital of Mashad, in the North of Iran, he discovered, to his shock, that whole wards were full of patients suffering from tuberculosis resistant to all of the first- and second-line anti-tuberculous drugs.[32] Dr Tony Jenkins, the director of British public health services, based in Cardiff, Wales, has for some years been receiving sputum samples from tuberculosis patients attending the Tibetan Welfare Delek Hospital, a charitable institution in the little town of Dharmsala in northern India and which ministers to Tibetan refugees. Approximately 50 per cent of the sputum samples tested over the past two years have grown germs resistant to the first- and second-line anti-tuberculous drugs.[33] The emergence of multi-drug–resistant tuberculosis is being increasingly reported from other centres, in Asia, South America, Europe, Africa and the Middle East.

On 21 January 1992, the first banner headline covering the new threat appeared in a British newspaper when the *Evening Standard* of London carried a headline, "Hospital warning as lethal TB supergerm spreads." Even in Britain, where the authorities had long prided themselves on their vigorous control of the disease, it appears that perhaps as many as a dozen people, mostly vagrants, are wandering the streets of London and other cities while coughing up tuberculosis germs resistant to all effective antibiotics.[34] In late 1992 the inevitable happened. The first British case of multi-drug-resistant tuberculosis complicating HIV infection was diagnosed by Dr Anton Pozniak in a 30-year-old Ethiopian woman who had been admitted to a London hospital.[35]

Paradoxically, this most dangerous development of all, the

emergence of a superbug, seems of least importance in Africa, where the disease is at its most vicious, because people are dying often without receiving any drugs at all. But in Asia, Oceania, Mexico and South America, where, in an ignorant abuse of the cure, people can buy drugs without prescription over the rural shop counter, the emergence of bacterial resistance on a large scale is likely to accelerate. And with this a nightmare of old has come back to haunt the health workers themselves.

Unlike AIDS, which poses a very small risk to staff, even if they are in close daily contact with infected patients, tuberculosis, transmitted by inhalation, poses a very real risk. In a recent survey at Cook County Hospital in Chicago, almost half of a sample group of doctors in training to become internists were found to be skin-test positive, indicating that they had become infected with tuberculosis during their work.[36] Previously, any such doctor, nurse or health care assistant who contracted the disease in this way had the ultimate consolation that they could be cured; now with the advent of MDR tuberculosis, such reassurances were no longer possible. To date an unknown but considerable number of health care workers have converted to skin-test positive, indicating latent infection, from their work. At least sixteen health care workers in the United States have become clinically infected with MDR tuberculosis, and five have died from it. Although some who died were themselves immuno-compromised and thence more vulnerable, this was the signal for many hospitals, clinics and institutions to take a long, hard look at how they could make the workplace safer. Ultra-violet lamps were introduced in air-ducts ventilating high-risk areas, as were negative pressure to isolation rooms and rigorous insistence on infection control techniques, including special masks. Better-equipped isolation units were installed in affected prison hospitals. It went so far that the U.S. National Institute for Occupational Safety and Health shocked the medical profession by recommending that those treating tuberculosis patients should wear "scuba-like masks of thick rubber connected to a motorized air pump."

While caring doctors such as Iseman and Reichman refused such intrusion into the doctor-patient relationship, other staff in many hospitals had become sufficiently frightened to move out of the tuberculosis wards and choose alternative careers.[37] Some patients known to be coughing up MDR germs refused to be hospitalised for treatment, causing restrictive legal powers from earlier years to be resurrected so that public health officials could detain them in hospital for compulsory treatment in isolation. In New York City, between 1988 and 1991, seventy-seven such detention orders were signed.[38] Perhaps most worrying of all, in a recent study of 466 patients with MDR tuberculosis in New York City, 70 per cent of them had picked up the multi-resistant germ as their initial infection.[39] This came as a shock to many doctors who thought that with the evolution of multi-drug resistance, the germ automatically lost its virulence. There was no denying that these germs were highly contagious.

Could the inconceivable happen? Could a multi-drug-resistant germ arrive in epidemic form onto the streets of our modern cities? In our affluent cultures and societies, an entire generation of young people have grown to maturity with little contact with tuberculosis or its sufferers. Where in previous decades, families throughout the industrialized world had many children, anticipating considerable losses, our nuclear families of one or two children assume a long life, free of the threat of killer epidemics. Given the advances of modern medicine, such a terrible scenario would seem unlikely. Yet there must be an element of uncertainty. The germ that causes tuberculosis is not only one of the most awesome of enemies that humanity has ever faced, it is also one of the most unpredictable.

V

STEP ONE IN the strategy of battle is to know your enemy. We need to understand the unique nature of the germ that causes tuberculosis and from this knowledge evaluate the very real threat it poses. Useful new information is already emerging from studies of the cellular biology of the germ. For example, Ying Zhang and colleagues, working at the MRC Tuberculosis

Unit at Hammersmith Hospital in London, have clarified the genetics involved in the mechanism of isoniazid resistance;[40] in time such understanding may speed up the recognition of multi-drug–resistant germs in newly diagnosed sufferers and it may facilitate the design of new anti-tuberculous drugs.

It is possible that BCG vaccination, which never found favour in the United States or the Netherlands, has given the remaining countries of Western Europe an additional degree of protection. But vaccination of 70 per cent of the world's children in the high-risk countries has not prevented the modern explosion of the disease, and even the committed authorities in Britain, France, Germany and Scandinavia claim no more than partial protection; indeed, no less a world authority than Karel Styblo believes that its protection is of limited duration, mainly effective in reducing the risk of meningitis and blood-borne tuberculosis in children.[41] BCG vaccination will not prevent the new global epidemic, though it may be worth considering for exposed health-care workers and children in high-risk inner city areas. In the presence of AIDS, there are additional difficulties.

It is the common experience of doctors treating AIDS patients that many who were previously vaccinated have readily gone on to develop tuberculosis. BCG is, of course, only given to people who are shown to be skin-test negative. This is a problem with AIDS patients, in whom the skin test for tuberculosis (Mantoux or Heaf) often becomes negative, even in the presence of tuberculosis, both latent and clinical. This, taken with the fact that the living BCG germ may also become invasive in people already suffering from AIDS, will severely limit its use wherever AIDS is common.

Every affected city or district must have at the very least isolation wards equipped with the necessary facilities to prevent spread both in the community and, within hospitals, to staff and other patients. The key, as always, is adequate funding. Although the situation in New York remains very serious, with a documented progressive increase in MDR tuberculosis, Dr Thomas R. Frieden, the current Medical Director of the U.S. Bureau of Tuberculosis Control, has received funding for a major improvement of clinics and X-ray screening facilities.

Most vital of all, money has been made available for closer monitoring of drug compliance in the community. Time will tell if, as Dr Frieden believes, such measures will meet with deserved success. Outbreaks in prisons and similarly vulnerable institutions can be anticipated and measures taken to prevent them. Most difficult of all, the HIV epidemic will need to be brought under control. Other vital factors in the deprived inner cities, particularly homelessness, alcoholism, drug addiction, and the shoddy medical services that accompany poverty, will require sympathetic attention. Even these measures, expensive as they will prove, are no more than a beginning, and they will eventually fail if the wealthy countries simply look to themselves.

The world must come to terms with the fact that the concurrence of AIDS and MDR tuberculosis has primed a time bomb that, in the tragic social conditions of the Third World, has already exploded. Yet, perhaps for less time than we realize, the opportunity to conquer tuberculosis is still within our grasp. Never in history has there been a more cogent need for a global strategy that can only be funded by the more wealthy nations. The dedicated organizations such as the WHO, the International Union, and UNICEF will need all the help they can get.

A comprehensive new study has calculated that the present epidemic of AIDS-tuberculosis in Africa is likely to escalate in the next ten years.[42] When one considers that the level today is twice that of five years ago, the projected figures in this study can only be described as apocalyptic. No sentient human being can ignore this tragedy. In 1992, the World Health Organization, in association with the International Union Against Tuberculosis, initiated a new strategy, partially funded by the World Bank, that is aimed at controlling tuberculosis throughout the world. Whatever the outcome, we should not delude ourselves that the disease will be eradicated in the twentieth century. With 1.7 billion people carrying the germ, this cannot happen. The experts are aiming for something rather more realistic – a much tighter control of the disease. Most important of all, millions of lives might still be saved.

New ideas and new heroes are desperately needed. One such novelty, currently being tested in Africa by Stanford and his colleagues, involves vaccinating sufferers with a killed germ, *Mycobacterium vacae*, in tandem with intensive short-term antibiotic therapy.[43] This has the advantage that it could be used in areas with a high incidence of HIV infection. But whatever the eventual role of such innovations, we already possess a reliable way forward, one that has already proven itself in the arena of battle. In a review soon to be published under the title *Tuberculosis: Where Are We Now?*, Karel Styblo and Annik Rouillon have made it clear where the answer lies: "There is no doubt that case-finding of infectious (particularly smear-positive) cases of pulmonary tuberculosis and their cure are the key to any effective control of the disease, both in developed and developing countries."[44] By "cure" these authorities mean the use of multiple drug therapy. Such is the debt owed to a tiny handful of unsung heroes, that even when faced with this new and very dangerous threat, their cure, so hard-won and so brilliant, remains the mainstay of the global effort.

But faced with the spectre of multi-drug-resistant tuberculosis, the application of the cure is not as straightforward as it might have been when that cure was first discovered. The discovery of effective new anti-tuberculous drugs must surely be the most urgent priority in the new initiative.

vi

IN AN INTERESTING new development, the molecular structure of the streptomyces-derived drug rifampicin has been modified in the research laboratories of the Italian pharmaceutical company Farmitalia Carlo Erba (Adria Laboratories in the United States) to produce a new drug, rifabutin. Although rifabutin has similarities to rifampicin, there are significant differences. In particular it is more soluble in fat, giving it enhanced penetration into diseased tissues, where it also remains active much longer. Because of the waxy coat of tuberculosis germs, this enables the drug to kill germs at much smaller doses, and trials of rifabutin, administered as part of a multiple therapy, have recently shown that it benefits 60 per cent of AIDS patients infected with MDR tuberculosis.[45] Recent research has shown a second and equally exciting role for rifabutin.

AIDS is triggering more than one form of tuberculosis. In the very early stages of infection with HIV, often when they have no symptoms of AIDS, patients are vulnerable to infection with the human tuberculosis germ, a disease familiar to humanity since the Stone Age. Only recently have we come to realise that as AIDS manifests with symptoms and the virus begins to damage the immune system of the infected person, they are vulnerable to a very different form of tuberculosis, a life-threatening infection with the avian or bird strain of the disease, called *Mycobacterium Avium Complex*. Better known by its acronym, MAC, this bizarre infection was virtually unknown before the arrival of the AIDS virus, yet there is gathering evidence that it may be responsible for much of the wasting, exhaustion and fever that torment the final days of AIDS patients, symptoms that had long given AIDS a curious resemblance to the age-old consumption.

Although there is a widespread impression amongst the public that little progress has been made in the medical battle against AIDS, this is far from the case. Significant and ongoing progress has been made in the development of antiviral drugs, such as zidovudine (ZDV, AZT), interferon-alpha, didanosine (ddI) and zalcitabine (ddC). Advances such as these have helped people with AIDS to live longer, but as the immune depression caused by the virus deepens, a number of unusual microbes that rarely infect those with normal immunity threaten the life and health of AIDS patients. Thanks to advances in therapy, two such opportunistic invaders, *Pneumocystis* and *Toxoplasma*, are largely preventable. The most common secondary infection that still threatens the life of the AIDS patient is MAC infection. Indeed, there is gathering evidence that if people with AIDS live long enough, almost all of them become infected with this very unpleasant germ.

Perhaps this is not so surprising, since MAC germs are common in nature, being found in soil and ordinary tap water.

Harmless to people with an intact immune system, they attack the immuno-compromised AIDS patients, invading the bloodstream and proliferating in the internal organs, including the bone marrow. The unfortunate patient suffers night sweats, fevers, chills, profound weight loss, and diarrhoea. With the bacteria swarming in ever-increasing masses throughout the tissues of the body, the stricken man or woman goes into a terminal decline of wasting and exhaustion. Until now, this infection has been extremely difficult to treat, even with barely tolerable cocktails of four or five of the most powerful anti-tuberculous drugs. Recent research has suggested that rifabutin might have an important role in the treatment and prevention of this remorseless infection.

Two large controlled trials of rifabutin in MAC infection have now been conducted in the United States and Canada, involving more than a thousand patients from seventy-three different medical centres. The purpose of the trials was to assess if the administration of rifabutin in AIDS patients before they developed MAC infection would prevent the MAC infection from developing. The results, presented in July 1992 by two of the investigators, Dr FM Gordin and Dr W Cameron, to the VIII International Conference on AIDS/STD in Amsterdam, showed that in approximately 50 per cent of patients given rifabutin, MAC infection was indeed prevented. In the words of Dr Gordin, "The use of rifabutin represents a major breakthrough in our ability to prevent one of the most devastating opportunistic infections in persons with HIV disease."[46]

vii

WHEN, IN THE 50s and 60s, the pioneers placed the ball of tuberculosis eradication into our hands, we ran with it for a time and then we dropped it. The time has come to pick up the ball again, and this time we must run with it all the way to victory. The hard lessons of past failure must be learnt so that we do not make the same mistakes again. But let us not fool ourselves that the task will be easier. The burden of infection may be much smaller in the developed world than it was in

1960, but it is newly complicated by AIDS and the emergence of multi-drug–resistant germs, and it is rapidly growing. In the developing world, with 1.7 billion latently infected, and racked by wars, famine, overpopulation, poverty and the spiralling AIDS epidemic, the task is truly leviathan. It is not, however, impossible. In December 1992, a panel of 34 American scientists, ethicists and public health leaders came together in a determined effort to introduce broad new measures to stem the rampant spread of tuberculosis nationwide. One important recommendation is that all patients discharged into the community should be closely monitored to make sure they take their treatment until they are completely cured.

On the international front, a highly original extension of the Mutual Assistance Programme of the International Union has been put forward by Dr Annik Rouillon, which is given here in modified form. This is the suggestion that individual wealthy nations might adopt one stricken developing country with regard to famine, AIDS and tuberculosis. This would reduce the perceived problems in the donor country to manageable size, and it would be relatively easy to monitor the effectiveness of its efforts, to ensure that those efforts were put to good effect.

So, as the world enters the last decade of the twentieth century, a new battle begins against one of the oldest and most formidable scourges of humanity. Eventually success or failure will boil down to whether there is the will in the developed world to spend sufficient money to win the battle. It is likely to depend more on compassion than on molecular biology.

Postscript

Josef Klarer died at the age of fifty-five years, in 1953. His colleague, Fritz Mietzsch died at the age of sixty-two, in 1958. Gerhard Domagk died of an infection in his bile ducts on 24 April 1964 at Burgberg in Germany, when he was sixty-eight years old. Selman Waksman died on Cape Cod in the United States, of a cerebral haemorrhage in 1973, aged eighty-five. William Feldman died on 15 January 1974, aged eighty-one. René Dubos died from pancreatic cancer in New York City on his 81st birthday, 20 February 1982. Jorgen Lehmann died while this book was being written in Gothenburg, Sweden, of pneumonia complicating Parkinson's disease, on 26 December 1989, three weeks before his 92nd birthday.

Albert Schatz, H. Corwin Hinshaw, Karl-Gustav Rosdahl, Professor Åke Hanngren, Wallace Fox, Betty Bugie (now Gregory) and Doris Jones (now Ralston) are alive and enjoying their respective retirements. Sir John Crofton lives in Edinburgh, where he is still very active in the global struggle against tuberculosis. At the time of writing, Frederick Bernheim and Robert Behnisch are both alive but in poor health.

After Jorgen Lehmann had retired for the second time at the age of eighty-five years, a colleague met him walking through the Sahlgren's Hospital. When asked what he was doing there, Lehmann smiled and explained: "The air in these corridors is life to me!"

Sources and References

At the start of each chapter section, I have given some idea of where the bulk of the reference material originated. Much is of course new and is therefore not available from other published sources.

Introduction

1. Clinical Pharmacology, by D.R. Lawrence. J. & A. Churchill Ltd, 3rd ed 1966; 79.
2. Waksman's autobiography was, *My Life with the Microbes*, published in the UK by Robert Hale, 1958. He subsequently wrote *The Conquest of Tuberculosis*, published in the UK by Cambridge University Press and in the US by the University of California Press, 1964.

1 The Reign of Terror

I must express my gratitude to Dr Keith Manchester and Dr Charlotte Roberts, who helped me with the palaeopathology in this chapter. I would also like to thank my surgical colleague, Mr John Rowling, for his kindness in allowing me to read his thesis on disease in ancient Egypt and for his charming conversation on the papyri and sources of reference for disease in the old world. I would also like to thank Professor Brock and Springer Verlag for their kind permission to allow me to refer to Brock's excellent biography of Robert Koch. Not least, though it no longer features in the text, my grateful thanks to Dr Stephen Webb, Assistant Professor of Australian Studies, Bond University, Queensland, for his fascinating information on the bones of Australian Aborigines.

1. Dubovsky (1983) Tuberculosis and art. *S A Mediese Tydskrif Deel*; **64**: 823–826.
2. This information was kindly offered to me by Dr Keith Manchester, of Bradford University and confirmed by Angela Milner of the Natural History Museum, London. The infection was "avian osteopetrosis".

3. Personal communication, Keith Manchester.

4. Wells C (1964). *Bones, Bodies and Disease.* Thames and Hudson. The skull is in the Natural History section of the British Museum (spec no 686).

5. Cave AJE (1939). The evidence for the incidence of tuberculosis in ancient Egypt. *Br J Tuberc*; **33**: 142–152.

6. Bartels P (1907). Tuberkulose (Wirbelkaries) in der jung̈eren Steinzeit. *Arch Anthropol*; **6**: 243–255.

7. Formicola V, Milanesi Q, and Scarsini C (1987). Evidence of spinal tuberculosis at the beginning of the fourth millenium BC from Arene Candide Cave (Liguria, Italy). *Am J Phys Anthropol*; **72**: 1–6.

8. Sagar Ph, Schalimtzek M, and Moller-Christensen V (1972) A case of spondylitis tuberculosa in the Danish neolithic age. *Dan Med Bull*; **19**: 176–180

9. Ortner DJ (1979). Disease and mortality in the early bronze age people of Bab edh-Dhra, Jordon. *Am J Phys Anthrop*; **51**: 589–598.

10. Personal communication.

11. Manchester K (1984). Tuberculosis and leprosy in antiquity: an interpretation. *Medical History*; **28**: 162–173.

12. Bony changes suggestive of tuberculosis have also been found in two skeletons from Ashton, Northamptonshire and one from Dorchester. These all date from the Roman period prior to the late 4th century – see Stirland A and Waldron T (1990). The earliest cases of tuberculosis in Britain. *J Arch Sc*; **17**: 221–230.

13. Tuberculosis in America pre-dating Columbus is now generally accepted. Pfeiffer S (1984). Paleopathology in an Iroquoian ossuary, with special reference to tuberculosis. *Am J Phys Anthrop*; **65**: 181–189. Ritchie WA (1952). Palaeopathological evidence suggesting pre-Columbian tuberculosis in New York State. *Am J Phys Anthrop*; **10**: 305–317. Also see – Palaeopathology in an Iroquoian ossuary, with special reference to tuberculosis. *Am J Phys Anthropol*; **65**: 181–189.

14. Clark GA, Kelley MA, Grange JM and Hill M C (1987). The evolution of mycobacterial disease in human populations. *Current Anthropology*; **28**: 45–62.

15. Suzuki T (1985). Palaeopathological diagnosis of bone tuberculosis in the lumbosacral region. *J Anthrop Soc Japan*; **93**: 381–390.

16. Krishnaswami I A (1937). Veterinary science in India, ancient and modern, with special reference to tuberculosis. *Agriculture and Livestock in India*; **7**: 718–24.

17. For a comprehensive dissection of Koch's speech, see, Professor Thomas B Brock (1988). Robert Koch, a Life in Medicine and Bacteriology. Published (in Europe) by Springer Verlag.

18. I have taken this quote from Brock, p 128. Brock's original reference is: Loeffleur F (1907). Zum 25 jahrigen Gedenktage der Entdeckung des Tuberkelbacillus. *Deutsche Medizinishe Wochenschrift*; **33**: 449–451.

19. Ibid.

20. Brock; 129.

21. Koch R (1882). Die aetiologie der Tuberculose. *Berliner Klinische Wochenschrift*; **19**: 221–230. An English translation was published in 1982, *Rev inf dis*; **4**: 1270–1274.

22. Brock; 128.

23. London *Times*, 22 April 1882.
24. *New York Times*, 3 May 1882.

2 The Lines of Battle

1. Wales JM, Buchan AR, Cookson JB, Jones DA and Marshall BSM (1985). Tuberculosis in a primary school: the Uppingham outbreak. *Br Med J*; **291**: 1039–40.
2. Frew AJ, Mayon-White RT and Benson MK (1987). An outbreak of tuberculosis in an Oxfordshire school. *Br J Dis Chest*; **81**: 293–5.
3. Bosley ARJ, George G and George M (1986). Outbreak of pulmonary tuberculosis in children. *Lancet*; i: 1141–1143.
4. A useful world review of modern epidemics, although now well out of date is – Lincoln EM (1965). Epidemics of tuberculosis. *Adv Tuberc Res*; **14**: 157–201.
5. MacDonald B (1948). *The Plague and I.* Published by Hammond, London: 27–28.
6. Shirer WL (1960). *The Rise and Fall of the Third Reich.* Pan, London, 3rd edition 1964; 28.
7. Private communication from my colleague, Dr J. Moroney.
8. Williams H (1973). *Requiem for a Great Killer.* Health Horizon, London; 33.
9. When streptomycin was first assessed by the MRC in the United Kingdom, the sanitorium regime was used as the "control". Admittedly the patients selected for therapy were suffering from rapidly advancing acute pulmonary tuberculosis. Two thirds of those treated by the conventional sanitorium regime were dead within five years.
10. I am very grateful to Professor Hinshaw for his very generous permission to quote from a preliminary chapter to a book, written by him, though not published.
11. I would prefer to keep my source of this account confidential.
12. Ellis AE (1958). *The Rack.* William Heinemann Ltd, London. Although not such a literary prodigy as Mann's *The Magic Mountain*, this book reads so factually that it seems likely that its harrowing content was based upon real personal experience.
13. I watched the demolition of one of the old sanitoria in Davos in 1975.
14. Hinshaw HC, see reference 10.
15. Williams H; 41.
16. Ibid; 49.
17. For a very comprehensive history of a single sanitorium read, Bignall JR (1979). *Frimley: The Biography of a Sanitorium.* Published by the Board of Governors, National Heart and Chest Hospitals, Bromptom Hospital, Fulham Road, London SW3 6HP.

3 New Jersey

I am extremely grateful to Byron Waksman for both allowing me to interview him and for the courtesy of allowing me unlimited access to his father's published books.

Since Selman Waksman wrote his autobiography – and a very eloquent and fascinating one at that – I have relied heavily on this for details of his life.

1. Byron Waksman interview.
2. Waksman SA (1958). *My Life with the Microbes*. Robert Hale Ltd; 22.
3. Ibid; 31.
4. Ibid; 32–33.
5. Ibid; 37.
6. Ibid; 50–51.
7. Ibid; 50–51.
8. Ibid; 40.
9. Ibid; 43.
10. Ibid; 48
11. Ibid; 55
12. Ibid; 55
13. Waksman SA (1964). *The Conquest of Tuberculosis*. University of California Press; 103.
14. My Life With the Microbes; 65
15. Ibid; 70.
16. Ibid; 157.
17. Ibid; 157.
18. Ibid; 131.
19. Ibid; 132–133.
20. Oral History, University of Columbia, New York. René Dubos; 33.
21. Waksman SA (1960). Dr René J Dubos – A Tribute. *J Am Med Assoc*; **174**; 503–507.
22. Ibid.

4   The Philosopher-scientist

I am deeply grateful to the Rockefeller University for help in researching the life and work of René Dubos. Carol Moberg in particular was both kind and generous to me. This aspect of the story could not have been written without the assistance of the Rockefeller Archives, based at Tarrytown, where Renee D. Mastrocco was very helpful. I must also thank the Rockefeller University Press for their generosity in allowing me to quote from their book, *Launching the Antibiotic Era*, publ 1990, ed Carol L Moberg and Zanvil A Cohn. My grateful thanks are also due to Rollin Hotchkiss, who, despite his busy retirement schedule, gave time to fill me in on some vital details that only he knew about. The Oral History Department of the University of Columbia were very patient and helpful – I owe them a major debt of thanks. I am also deeply grateful to Harcourt Brace Jovanovich for their kind permission to quote from *Quest: Reflections on Medicine, Science and Humanity*, a wonderful little book which takes the form of a question and answer interview of Dubos by Jean Paul Escande, translated by Patricia Ranum.

1. At one time, Professor Hinshaw had planned to write his own book, with the title, *Conquest of a Plague*. This quote is from the introduction to that unfinished journal.
2. Oral history archives, University of Columbia; René Dubos mentions this same incident in almost every biographical interview.
3. *Quest: Reflections on Medicine, Science and Humanity*. Harcourt Brace Jovanovich. Translated by Patricia Ranum; 5–6.
4. Ibid.
5. Oral history; 14–16.
6. Ibid; 16–17.
7. Ibid; 16–17.
8. Ibid; 16–17.
9. Ibid; 16–17.
10. Ibid; 17.
11. Ibid; 29.
12. Ibid; 30.
13. Ibid; 34.
14. Ibid; 37.
15. Ibid; 38.
16. Ibid; 38.
17. Ibid; 38–39.
18. Benison (1976). See reference 2, Chapter 5; 463.
19. Dubos RJ (1976). *The Professor, the Institute and DNA*. The Rockefeller Press; 10.
20. Avery discovered that DNA was the molecule of heredity. Crick and Watson discovered its chemical structure.
21. As 18; 463.
22. As 18; 463.
23. Oral history; 39
24. Ibid; 40.
25. Ibid; 40.
26. As 19; 77–78.
27. Quest; 7.
28. This letter is in the Rockefeller archives.
29. *Medical World News*, 5 May 1975. Medicine's Living History: Dr René Dubos recalls his discovery of the first antibiotic; 78.

5 The Cranberry Bog Bacillus

See introduction to Chapter 4.

1. Oral History of René Dubos. This is a transcript from a series of tape-recorded interviews, in which Saul Benison recorded Dubos' life and career. It is the copyright of the Oral History Research Office, Columbia University, New York.
2. Ibid. This is taken from a published excerpt of the oral history as detailed in 1,

published as follows: Benison S (1976). René Dubos and the capsular polysaccharide of pneumococcus. *Bull History Med*; **50**: 465–466.

3. Dubos researched the mysterious life of Oswald Avery after his death. This was published as a biography: Dubos RJ (1976). *The Professor, the Institute, and DNA*. The Rockefeller Press, New York.

4. Ibid; 50–51.

5. Ibid; 53.

6. As 2; 466.

7. Ibid; 467.

8. Ibid; 471.

9. Ibid.

10. Avery OT and Dubos RJ (1930). The specific action of a bacterial enzyme on pneumococci of type III. *Science*; **LXXIIB**: 151–152.

11. As 2; 474.

12. Carol Moberg interview.

13. Medicine's living history. Dr René Dubos recalls his discovery of the first antibiotic. *Medical World News*, May 5, 1975: 79. Note: Drs Jacques Monod, Francois Jacob and Andrew Lwoff, of the Pasteur Institute, would later take the adaptive enzyme work further with the advantages of a more advanced scientific technology and would win the Nobel Prize in 1965 for it.

14. Waksman SA (1960). Dr. René J Dubos – A Tribute. *J Am Med Assocn*; **174**: 111–113.

6 One of Three Survivors

It would have been impossible to research the life of Gerhard Domagk without the assistance of the Bayer Pharmaceutical Company. In particular, the diary of Gerhard Domagk, which I discovered in the archives at Leverkusen, was invaluable to me and many quotations in the following derive from this. I am extremely grateful to them for permission to quote freely from material in their archives. I am also very grateful to Götz Domagk, who allowed me free access to his father's diary and even translated Hoff's paper for me. Virtually all of the original reference material is in German, so that I have relied on translations by five separate linguists. Since the diary pagination is irregular and I am working from multiple translations, I have not attempted to provide page numbers. I was also assisted by several of Bayer's own publications, including the following three. 50 YEARS OF ANTIBACTERIAL CHEMOTHERAPY, 1935–85. A PIONEER WHO MADE MEDICAL HISTORY. FROM GERMANIN TO ACYLUREIDOPENICILLIN. I owe much thanks also to Professor Hans Schadewaldt, Hinrich Otten, Professor J. Köbberling, who furnished me with the details of the Wuppertal-Elberfeld Hospital, and Klee's assistant, Professor Karl Jahnke, who permitted me to interview him and helped clarify many details.

1. This is the title of Domagk's diary. It underlines the importance he himself attached to his experiences during the first world war, when he was one of just three who survived from his class at school. The document is typewritten and corrected in his own hand. Götz explained that his father would dictate part of

this at regular intervals to his secretary and then correct the typescript after she had typed it.

2. Domagk's diary.
3. This is from a booklet, which transcribed Hoff's memorial speech to Gerhard Domagk after his death on 24 April 1964. *Gerhard Domagk – Gedenkrede*. A photocopy of the original was sent to me by his son, Götz, who is Professor of pathology (Abteilung Enzymchemie) at the Georg-August Universität Göttingen. Professor Domagk kindly translated the Hoff booklet into English for me.
4. Domagk's diary.
5. Ibid.
6. Ibid.
7. Ibid.
8. Ibid.
9. Ibid.
10. Ibid.
11. Ibid. This is clearly where he obtained the title for his diary.
12. Ibid.
13. As 3.
14. Domagk's diary.
15. Domagk G (1924). Untersuchungen über die Bedeutung des reticuloen-dothelialen Systems für die Vernichtung von Infektionserregern und für die Entstehung des Amyloids. *Virchows Arch Path Anat*; 253: 594.
16. Domagk's diary.
17. Ibid.
18. Rolleston JD. The Folklore of Tuberculosis. *Tubercle*; **22:** 55–65.
19. Domagk's diary.
20. Behnisch R (1986). *From dyes to drugs. Discoveries in Pharmacology, Volume* 3: Pharmacological Methods, Receptors & Chemotherapy. M J Farnham & J Bruinvels eds. Elsevier Science Publishers B V (biomedical division): 240–242.
21. Domagk's diary.

7 **The Prontosil Miracle**

(See introduction to Chapter 6).

1. Hitler's illness is believed to have been tuberculosis, which he contracted at the age of 14. His father died from a pulmonary haemorrhage thought to be due to chronic tuberculosis.
2. I have based this case report partly on Klee's paper (reference 4) and on my conversations with Professor Karl Jahnke.
3. Domagk G (1935) Ein Beitrag zur Chemotherapie der bakteriellen Infectionen. *Deutsche Medizinische Wochenschrift*; **61:** 250–253.
4. Klee Ph and Römer H (1935). Prontosil bei Streptokokkenerkrankungen. *Deutsche Medizinishe Wochenschrift*; **61:** 253–256.

5. McDermott W (1969). The story of INH. *J Inf Dis*; **119**: 678–683.
6. Colebrook L (1928). A study of some organic arsenical compounds with a view to their use in certain streptococcal infections. MRC Special Report Series, No. 119. HMSO, London. Also, Colebrook L and Hare R (1934). Treatment of puerperal infection due to Streptococcus Pyogenes by organic arsenical compounds. *Lancet*; **i**: 1279.
7. Colebrook L and Hare R (1927). On the bactericidal action of mercurochrome. *Br J Experimental Path*; **8**: 109.
8. Colebrook L (1935). Treatment of puerperal fever by antistreptococcal serum. Lancet; **i**: 1085.
9. Colebrook L and Kenny M (1936). Treatment of human puerperal infections, and of experimental infections due to haemolytic streptococci in mice, with Prontosil. *Lancet*; **i**: 1279.
10. Colebrook L and Kenny M (1936). Treatment with Prontosil of puerperal infections due to haemolytic streptococci. *Lancet*; **ii**: 1319.
11. Domagk's diary. This incident was also described to me in detail by his son, Professor Götz Domagk.
12. Domagk's diary.
13. Tréfouël, Mme J, Tréfouël FN and Boet D (1935). Activité du p-aminophenyl sulfamide sur les infections streptococciques expérimentales de la souris et du lapin. *Comptes rendus des séances de la Société de biologie et des ses filiales*; **120**: 756–758.
14. Rich AR and Follis RH (1938). The inhibitory effect of sulfanilamide on the development of experimental tuberculosis of the guinea pig. *Bull Johns Hopkins Hosp*; **62**, 77–84.
15-33. All these references are taken from Domagk's diary.

8 Visionaries

1. Waksman was an admirer of Haffkine, who, like himself, was Jewish and had been forced to leave Russia to achieve intellectual liberty. Waksman in fact wrote a biography of Haffkine. Waksman SA (1964). *The brilliant and tragic life of W M W Haffkine*. Rutgers Univ Press.
2. Allison VD (1974). Personal recollections of Sir Almroth Wright and Sir Alexander Fleming. *Ulster Med J*; **43**: 89–98.
3. Maurois A (1959). *The Life of Alexander Fleming*. Penguin Books; 137.
4. Ibid; 138.
5. Comroe J H Jr (1977). *Retrospectoscope. Insights into Medical Discovery*. Von Gehr Press (California); 3.
6. As 3; 161.
7. *A Pioneer who made History*. Booklet on the life of Domagk published by Bayer.
8. Woodruff HB (1981) A soil microbiologist's odyssey. *Ann Rev Microbiol*; **35**: 1–28.
9. These experiments are reviewed by Long in his scholarly text. Long ER (1958). *The Chemistry and Chemotherapy of Tuberculosis*. The Williams & Wilkins Co, Baltimore.

10. Bernheim is a very much underestimated man. It is virtually impossible now to get any biographical details. At the time of writing, he was suffering from an illness which prevented his speaking.

11. The same author as 5 above, who was a Californian Professor of Respiratory Medicine and a friend of H. Corwin Hinshaw. These articles were taken from the book in reference 5 and printed as papers. Comroe J H Jr (1978). Pay dirt: the story of streptomycin. *Am Rev Resp Dis*; **117**: 957–968.

12. Bernheim F (1940). The effect of salicylate on the oxygen uptake of the tubercle bacillus. *Science*; **92**: 204–205.

9 One Small Candle

I am particularly grateful to the Ferrosan drug company for their assistance and courtesy when I travelled to Sweden. It was very fortunate that Jarl Ingelf, the promotion and literary editor to Ferrosan, had conducted a series of biographical interviews with Jorgen Lehmann. These were published in the company magazine, *Observanda Medica Ferrosan*, over a series of editions from 1979 to 1981 under the title, "From Salicylate to Para-Aminosalicylate, PAS: a dreamlike idea which became reality". Lehmann also spoke at length about the various adventures of his life in two interviews, which he gave to a Swedish radio programme called *Vetandets Värld* in February 1979. The tapes of these, which were kindly provided to me by Professor Sven Lindstedt, reveal his characteristic bubbling humour and quick wit, even in old age. Both are important biographical sources on Lehmann's life and thinking. Ferrosan has now been incorporated into Kabi Pharmacia and most of the archives transferred. I would like to thank Jarl Ingelf, the two chemists Sven Carlsten and Hans Larsson, and Stig Nylen, formerly the director of Ferrosan, for their kindness and courtesy in allowing me to interview them and in providing me with much invaluable information and illustrations. I would also like to thank Dr Bernard Deane, and his company, Kabi Pharmacia, for their courtesy and help.

My researches in Sweden were made a delight by the friendship and assistance of many people. Karl-Gustav Rosdahl provided me with much original information about his role in the PAS story. In Stockholm, Orla Lehmann and Professor Åke Hanngren became my friends. In Gothenburg, Maja Lehmann, recently bereaved, was kind beyond words. Professor Sven Lindstedt at the Sahlgren's Hospital was very entertaining and informative and his secretary, Agneta Magnusson, was tireless in translating the *Observanda* articles and the *Vetandets Värld* radio interviews into English. There were many others, whom I have not room to mention, all of whom made my Swedish research a genuine pleasure.

Much of the more personal and intimate information in this chapter comes from my interviews with Orla and Maja Lehmann. Their frankness and honesty in answering my many queries was admirable.

1. *Vetandats Värld*.
2. Åke Hanngren interview.
3. Lehmann, who found it highly amusing, told this story to Åke Hanngren. Personal communication.

4. *Vetandats Värld*.
5. Orla Lehmann interview.
6. Maja Lehmann interview.
7. Ibid.
8. Orla Lehmann interview.
9. Ibid.
10. This patient's story is told in both the *Vetandats Värld* and the *Observanda* articles.
11. *Observanda* articles.
12. As 1.
13. Ibid.
14. Ibid.
15. *Observanda* articles.
16. As 1.
17. Lehmann would, in his inimitable way, describe this interesting development. "Professor Link is an extraordinary personality with radical views. He rarely answers letters and he hates doctors. The reason for this is that when he developed tuberculosis and, while in a sanitorium for treatment, he heard about the existence of PAS. His American physician knew nothing of it and regarded it with complete mistrust. Link was desperate to get it yet could not obtain it. He finally did succeed in obtaining a supply of PAS and was successfully treated with it. In this way, dicoumarol and PAS shook each other by the hand in the personality of Professor Link." – *Observanda* articles.
18. Both *Observanda* articles and the *Vetandats Värld* interviews.
19. Bernheim F (1940). The effect of salicylate on the oxygen uptake of the tubercle bacillus. *Science*: **92**; 204.
20. *Observanda* articles.
21. The background information on tuberculosis in Sweden was provided to me by Åke Hanngren. A review of the history of the economic implications of tuberculosis in Sweden from 1750–1980 was conducted by Puranen. Puranen Britt-Inger (1987). *Tuberculosis, the occurrence and causes in Sweden from 1750–1980*. Umeå studies in economic history, number 7. Department of Economic History, Umeå University, Umeå. The quote with regard to Stockholm comes from her summary: *Aims, Sources and Areas of Study*.
22. *Vetandats Värld*.
23. Saz AK and Bernheim F. The effect of 2,3,5, tri-iodobenzoate on the growth of tubercle bacilli. *Science*, 1941: **93**; 622–623.
24. Fildes P (1940). A rational approach to research in chemotherapy. *Lancet*; 955–957.

10 Triumph and Tragedy

1. Escande J-P (1979). *Quest: Reflections on Medicine, Science, and Humanity*. Harcourt Brace Jovanovich (New York and London); 62.

2. Dubos RJ (1976). *The Professor, the Institute and DNA*. The Rockefeller Press; 164.

3. Ibid.

4. Ibid.

5. Carol Moberg, personal communication.

6. Rollin Hotchkiss, personal communication.

7. I based this on the personality which is clearly evident in her writings in the Rockefeller archives, upon the opinion of Carol Moberg and Rollin Hotchkiss, and Dubos' own writings about her.

8. Carol Moberg, personal communication; also Dubos RJ (1975). *Medical World News* (McGraw-Hill) May 5; 77-87. The latter carried an article written by Dubos about his life under the title, *Medicine's Living History*.

9. Oral history; 353.

10. Ibid; 353.

11. The story of the DNA discovery is told in reference 2.

12. Dubos RJ (1975). *Medical World News* (see ref 8); 81.

13. Dubos RJ (1939) Bactericidal Effect of an Extract of a Soil Bacillus on Gram Positive Cocci. *Proc Soc Exp Biol Med*; **40**: 311-2.

14. Oral History; 448.

15. Proceedings of the Third International Congress of Microbiology, Sept 2-9, 1939. Abstracts of communications, publ 1940: 261-262.

16. *Quest*: 8-9. Also André Maurois (1959). *The Life of Alexander Fleming*. Published in translation by Penguin in association with Jonathan Cape; 175.

17. *Quest*; 9.

18. As 12; 82.

19. *L'Express* (Paris). Nov 3, 1979. Interview with René Dubos. Translated by the author.

20. Carol Moberg interview.

21. Oral History; 448.

22. Rollin Hotchkiss (1990). *Launching the Antibiotic Era*. The Rockefeller Press. Chapter headed, *From Microbes to Medicine: Gramicidin, René Dubos and the Rockefeller*.

23. Ibid.

24. Ibid.

25. Ibid.

26. This poem is in the Rockefeller archives, who kindly gave me permission to quote it.

27. Rhines C (1935). The persistence of avian tuberculosis bacilli in soil and in association with soil micro-organisms. *J Bact*; **29**: 299-311.

28. René Dubos subsequently told Carol Moberg that Marie Louise had responded well to the prolonged rest at the sanitorium. This is confirmed by her appearance on photographs at this time, when she looks to have gained weight and appears relatively well.

29. See reference 19. Also based upon Carol Moberg interview.

30. Personal conversation with Rollin Hotchkiss.

31. The handwritten letter, together with a typed version, is in the Rockefeller archives.
32. As 12.
33. *Launching the Antibiotic Era*; see reference 22: 94.
34. Ibid.
35. Dubos RJ and Dubos J (1953). *The White Plague: Tuberculosis, Man and Society*. Victor Gollancz Ltd, London.
36. Some details of their tuberculous infections and how they were managed are contained in the Rockefeller archives. Dubos himself contracted tuberculosis in a finger. Jean and Dr Davis contracted pulmonary tuberculosis and were treated with triple therapy.
37. These are just some of his many books. *The Bacterial Cell. Louis Pasteur: Free Lance of Science. The White Plague. Bacterial and Mycotic Infections of Man. Mirage of Health. Pasteur and Modern Science. Dreams of Reason. Torch of Life. The Unseen World. Health and Disease. Man Adapting. Man, Medicine and Environment. Reason Awake! Science for Man.*
38. There is a copy of this moving document, which was not written for publication, in the Rockefeller archives. This was kindly translated for me by Claudine Murrell.

11 New Beginnings

1. Harley Williams (1973). *Requiem for a Great Killer*. Health Horizon, London; 91–92.
2. George Bankoff (1946). *Tuberculosis*. MacDonald & Co, London; 153–154.
3. Ibid.
4. Ibid.
5. As 1.
6. As 2; 153.
7. Waksman SA (1964). *The Conquest of Tuberculosis*. Univ of California Press; 3.
8. Ibid.
9. Waksman SA (1958). *My Life with the Microbes*. Robert Hale, London; 16.
10. Ibid; 205.
11. Woodruff HB (1981). A Soil Microbiologist's Odyssey. *Ann Rev Microbiol*; **35:** 1–28
12. Ibid.
13. Ibid.
14. Waksman SA (1962). *By Their Fruits*. Publ Merck, Sharpe & Dohme; 10.
15. It would subsequently be tested, when it would prove to have definite antituberculous properties. See refs 7 and 11.
16. As 11.
17. Ibid.
18. As 9; 207.
19. Ibid; 210.
20. Ibid; 211.

21. In *The Conquest of Tuberculosis*, Waksman gave the year as 1943, whereas in *My Life with the Microbes*, he gave it as 1941. I have taken it as the former since it only makes sense in this context.
22. As 7; 105–106.
23. As 9; 211–212.
24. Ibid.

12 A Phoenix from the Ashes of Elberfeld

1. Domagk's diary.
2. Ibid.
3. Ibid.
4. Ibid.
5. Ibid.
6. Robert Behnisch (1986). *Discoveries in Pharmacology, Volume 3*: Pharmacological Methods, Receptors and Chemotherapy. Ed M J Farnham & J Bruinvels. Chapter 5: From dyes to drugs; 256. This Chapter is an interesting compilation of the Bayer researches as seen through the eyes of one of the participating chemists.
7. Domagk's diary.
8. Domagk's diary.
9. Ibid.
10. As 7; 250.
11. As 7; 276.
12. Behnisch R (1986). *Die Geschichte der Sulphonamidforschung.* Medizisch Pharm Studiengesellschaft. Mainz.
13. Domagk's diary.
14. As 7; 245.
15. Domagk's diary.
16. Ibid.
17. Ibid.
18. This is based partly on a series of personal communications with Professor Karl Jahnke, who was Klee's assistant in the 1940s. It is also based on Professor Jahnke's biography of Philipp Klee in *Wuppertaler Biographien* (1987); 49–59.
19. Domagk's diary.
20. Ibid.
21. As 18.

13 Streptomycin

Professor Albert Schatz and his wife, Vivian, were kind enough to allow me to interview them at length at their home in Philadelphia. These interviews were invaluable in painting the precise picture of the day to day researches at Rutgers that led to streptomycin. A large volume of new information arose from these interviews, which will be referred to simply as "Schatz interviews". I also had the good fortune to be able to discuss the streptomycin discovery and the scene at Rutgers with Betty Bugie (married name Gregory). I have referred earlier to the invaluable help I obtained from Selman Waksman's son, Byron. I must also thank Professor Hubert Lechevalier, until recently Professor of Microbiology at Rutgers, and his wife, Midge (Mary) who were so informative and courteous. The Rutgers Special Archive should also be mentioned for their very generous and prompt assistance, particularly with the illustrations.

1. Eva, Picasso's second mistress, with whom he eloped from his first in 1912, first developed symptoms of pulmonary tuberculosis in 1913. She died from it on 14 December 1915.
2. Schatz interviews.
3. Ibid. One only has to listen to the emotion with which Professor Schatz still recounts these memories to realise how deeply the terror of tuberculosis, and infectious disease in general, influenced the world prior to the antibiotic era. I can remember exactly the same regard for tuberculosis from my childhood in Clonmel, in the south of Ireland.
4. Ibid.
5. The thesis is lodged with the Rutgers State University of New Jersey.
6. Schatz interviews.
7. For this vivid portrayal of the working atmosphere during research that would shake the world, I am indebted to Doris Jones (married name Ralston). The quotes are taken from a lecture she delivered on this subject, which should surely be captured for posterity in a journal of medical or scientific history.
8. Ibid.
9. Ibid.
10. Schatz interviews.
11. Ibid.
12. Ibid.
13. Ibid.
14. Ibid.
15. Ibid.
16. See reference 7.
17. Ibid.
18. Schatz interviews.
19. Ibid.
20. Ibid.
21. See reference 7.
22. Schatz interviews.
23. A totally new antituberculous drug, Rifampicin, derived from the rifamycins, would be discovered almost twenty years later, in 1963; though not at Rutgers but in the laboratories of the drug firm, Lapetit. Interestingly, this too derived from a streptomyces and would in its turn permit the pharmaceutical company, Farmitalia, to derive yet another useful drug, from it rifabutin, in 1982.
24. Schatz interview.
25. Ibid.

14 First Cures

Professor H. Corwin Hinshaw afforded me both a taped interview by post and, when I visited him in California, a detailed oral interview. He also provided me with a wealth of written information, including the first chapter of a book he had intended to write but had never completed. I am indebted to him for the courtesy with which he treated me and for this intimate record which would otherwise have been unavailable for posterity. I shall refer to this taped and oral information as "Hinshaw interviews" in this and subsequent chapters.

1. Myers, JA (April 1961). William Hugh Feldman. *The Journal-Lancet*;173–181.
2. Ibid.
3. Hinshaw interviews.
4. Feldman WH, Hinshaw HC and Moses HE (1940). The Effect of Promin (Sodium Salt of P.P'-Diamino-Diphenyl-Sulphone-N,N'-Dextrose Sulphonate) on Experimental Tuberculosis: a Preliminary Report. *Proc Staff Meetings of the Mayo Clinic*: **15**; 695–699.
5. As 1.
6. Hinshaw HC, Pfuetze K and Feldman WH (1942). Treatment of Tuberculosis with Promin. Progress report, *Am Rev Tuberc*: **47**; 26–34.
7. Hinshaw HC, Pfuetze K and Feldman WH (1944). Chemotherapy of Clinical Tuberculosis with Promin. *Am Rev Tuberculosis*: **50**; 52–57.
8. Feldman WH, Hinshaw HC and Mann FC (1944). Promizole in Tuberculosis. *Am Rev Tuberculosis*: **50**; 418–440.
9. Albert Schatz interviews.
10. Schatz A, Bugie E and Waksman S (1944). Streptomycin, a Substance Exhibiting Antibiotic Activity Against Gram-positive and Gram-negative Bacteria. *Proc Soc Expt Biol and Med*: **55**, 66–69.
11. Julius H Comroe Jr (1978). Retrospectoscope. Pay Dirt: the Story of Streptomycin. *Am Rev Resp Dis*; **117**: 773–781.
12. I have taken this from the Schatz interviews. A similar account has however been published: Schatz A (1965). Antibiotics and Dentistry – Part 1. Some Personal Reflections on the Discovery of Streptomycin. *Pakistan Dental Review*: **15**; 125–134.
13. This delightful story was told to me personally by Professor Hinshaw.
14. Hinshaw interviews.
15. Ibid.
16. Feldman WH (1954). Streptomycin: some historical aspects of its development as a chemotherapeutic agent in tuberculosis. *Am Rev Tuberc*; **69**: 859–868.
17. Hinshaw interviews.
18. Waksman SA (1958). *My Life with the Microbes*. Robert Hale (London); 213.
19. Schatz interviews.
20. Schatz A and Waksman SA (1944). Effect of Streptomycin and Other Antibiotic Substances upon *Mycobacterium Tuberculosis* and Related Organisms. *Proc Soc Expt Biol and Med*: **57**; 244–248.
21. Feldman WH and Hinshaw HC (1944). Effects of streptomycin on experimen-

tal tuberculosis in guinea pigs: A preliminary study. *Proc Staff Meet Mayo Clin*; **19**: 593–599.

22. It is uncertain exactly when the final supplies from Schatz ended and those from Merck & Co began. It seems likely there was some degree of overlap. I have tried to piece this together from my interviews with Albert Schatz and H. Corwin Hinshaw. Schatz believes that the very first patients did receive some of his streptomycin. There is also a suggestion from Waksman's books that this was the case. The histories of the first two cases were supplied to me by Professor Hinshaw.

23. I have based this partially on the Hinshaw interviews and partially on the following two accounts: Pfuetze KH, Pyle MM, Hinshaw HC and Feldman WH (1955). The First Clinical Trial of Streptomycin in Human Tuberculosis. *Am Rev Tuberc*: **71**; 752–754.

24. Post-Bulletin, Rochester, Minnesota, Thursday 25 Sept 1969; 24.

25. Cooke RE, Dunphy DL and Blake FG (1946). Streptomycin in Tuberculous Meningitis. *Yale J Biol Med*: **18**; 221–226.

26. Waksman SA (1958). My Life with the Microbes; 189.

15 Hearing God Thinking

See introduction to references in chapter nine. I am indebted to Jorgen Lehmann's son, Orla, to his second wife, Maja and to his friend, Åke Hanngren, for much of this description of his personal life, family difficulties and triumphs at this time. I shall refer to these sources as "Orla Lehmann interview", "Maja Lehmann interview" etc.

I am equally grateful to Mr Karl-Gustav Rosdahl, who supplied me with much original information, both in response to my questions, and in the form of letters, documents, etc. These give invaluable insight into the intimate story at Ferrosan.

I am very grateful to Dr Sven Lindstedt, Director of Clinical Chemistry at the Sahlgren's Hospital, for his help with my Lehmann researches and in particular for the copy of the case notes of the young woman, Sigrid.

For the intimate details concerning Gylfe Vallentin, I am deeply grateful for the help of his son, Gunnar, his daughter Brit Håkansson, and to Dr Erik Berglund (on my behalf, he kindly interviewed Drs Gösta Birath and Lars Öberg, who knew Vallentin and several nurses who worked with him).

In 1990, during my Swedish researches I had the opportunity to interview four representatives of Ferrosan, in Malmö: Stig Nylén, Hans Larsson, Sven Carlsted and Jarl Ingelf. I am very grateful to them for their courtesy and complete honesty. This interview was particularly timely since Ferrosan no longer exists as an independent company, having been incorporated first into Pharmacia and a little later into Kabi Pharmacia. I shall refer to this as the "Ferrosan interview".

1. This letter has been preserved in Gothenburg and a reproduction is included in the illustrations.

2. *Observanda* articles.

3. Ibid.

4. According to Lehmann (see *Observanda* articles) the references are to be found in The *Journal fur Praktische Chemie*, 1900, and *Chemisches Zentralblatt*, 1906. I cannot give further details since I have not searched for these.

5. This emerged from the Ferrosan interview.

6. *Observanda* articles.

7. *Vetandets Värld*.

8. Ibid.

9. Rosdahl, personal communication.

10. Orla Lehmann interview.

11. *Observanda* articles.

12. Orla and Maja Lehmann interviews.

13. Personal communication, Gunnar Vallentin and many others – see above.

14. Copy of her case notes kindly provided by Professor Sven Lindstedt (see above).

15. I have taken these case histories from the *Observanda* articles, which usually refer to more detailed sanitorium case notes, available in Sweden, through the Sahlgren's Hospital.

16. Lehmann J (1964). Twenty-years afterwards. Historical notes on the discovery of the anti-tuberculous effect of para-aminosalicylic acid (PAS) and the first clinical trials. *Am Rev Resp Dis*; **90**; 953–956.

17. Rosdahl, personal communication.

18. Observanda articles.

19. Rosdahl, personal communication. I have a copy of a letter to Rosdahl written by the director, S.O. Ryné, on 17 September 1952, on the occasion of his resignation from Ferrosan. It states: "The intention was also that the paper should be published in the names of Lehmann and Rosdahl. The reason why Lehmann alone was named on the publication resulted from the fact that the company (represented by Rosdahl) considered that point in time inappropriate for the disclosure of the work done by Rosdahl and his co-operators because protection by patenting was not possible."

20. This translation of the discussion was kindly provided to me by Dr Erik Berglund.

21. *Observanda* articles.

22. As 20.

23. Lehmann J (1946). Para-aminosalicylic acid in the treatment of tuberculosis. *Lancet*; **1**: 15–16.

24. Rosdahl, personal communication.

16 Storm Clouds over Gothenberg

I am extremely grateful to Jan Sievers, son of Olof, for the biographical details of his father. I am also indebted to Professor Åke Hanngren, not only for his personal story and the courtesy of allowing me to include his self-portrait in the illustrations to this book, but also for much detailed cooperation on the Lehmann biography and the history of tuberculosis and its treatement with PAS in Sweden.

1. Personal communication, Rosdahl.
2. Ibid.
3. Ibid.
4. The quote is from Lehmann's *Observanda* articles but the story was repeated by Rosdahl and confirmed during the Ferrosan interview. While some may be tempted to criticise Ryné with the advantage of hindsight, would they have behaved otherwise, faced with his responsibilities and potential ruin?
5. *Observanda* articles. The biographical details derive from Jan Sievers.
6. Rosdahl, personal communication.
7. Personal communication, Orla Lehmann.
8. Personal communications, Jan Sievers.
9. *Observanda* articles.
10. The words of the press release are included in the *Observanda* articles, kindly translated for me by Agneta Magnusson.
11. *Observanda* articles.
12. All three lectures were published (1947) in *Nord Med*; **33**: 140–158. I am grateful to Professor Åke Hanngren for a translation of Vallentin's lecture.
13. The comments from the audience are also recorded in the *Nord Med* article, see ref 12, and Lehmann's detailed discussion of the lectures and comments was published in the *Observanda* articles. I also obtained some assistance from Dr Berglund with this aspect.
14. Ferrosan interview.
15. I quote Lehmann's reference from the *Observanda* articles: *Svenska Läkartidningen* (1947); 432.
16. Ibid; 618.
17. Ibid; 823.
18. An example of Lehmann's wit from the *Observanda* articles.
19. From the radio interviews, *Vetandets Värld*.
20. This profound depression was recorded not only by Lehmann in his *Observanda* articles but also noted by friends (Berglund). It is apparent however that it did not stop Vallentin from raising the necessary money to enable the research to go ahead.
21. These two communications are included as illustrations in the *Observanda* articles.
22. Ibid. Illustrations of these patients marching are included in this book.
23. See illustration.
24. Interview with Åke Hanngren.

17 Life and Death

1. Waksman SA (1964). *The Conquest of Tuberculosis*. Univ of California Press; 128.
2. Ibid; 129.
3. Hinshaw interviews (see explanatory note above)

4. Hinshaw HC and Feldman WH 1945. Streptomycin in treatment of clinical tuberculosis: a preliminary report. *Proc Meetings of the Mayo Clinic*: **20**; 313–318.

5. Ibid.

6. Ibid.

7. As 1; 130.

8. Hinshaw HC (1954). Historical notes on earliest use of streptomycin in clinical tuberculosis. *Am Rev Tuberc*; **70**: 9–14.

9. The presentation was published in that same year. Hinshaw HC, Feldman WH and Pfuetze KH 1946. *Amer Rev Tuberc*: **54**; 191.

10. *Streptomycin and Dihydrostreptomycin in Tuberculosis* (1949). Publ National Tuberculosis Association (of America). Edit Riggins H Mc and Hinshaw HC.

11. Hinshaw interviews.

12. As reference 8.

13. Hinshaw interviews.

14. Waksman SA (1958). *My Life with the Microbes*. Robert Hale (London); 215. This child was also mentioned by Hinshaw in our interviews.

15. Hinshaw interviews.

16. Ibid.

17. Ibid. Eleanor's daughter, Anna, was also referred to Professor Hinshaw with suspected tuberculosis but he correctly diagnosed coccidiomycosis, a different infection, which was successfully treated.

18. This letter, together with a photograph of this tragic little girl (see illustrations) is in the collection, "The Streptomycin Babies" in the Special Collections and Archives of Rutgers University of New Brunswick, New Jersey. I am indebted to the archivist, Mr Edward Skipworth, for making it available to me.

19. Dowling HF (1977). *Fighting Infections*. Harvard Univ Press; 163.

20. Hinshaw interviews.

21. Larry Collins and Dominique Lapierre (1978). *Freedom at Midnight*. Tarang Paperbacks, New Delhi; 124.

22. Lehmann J. (1964). Twenty years afterward. Historical notes on the discovery of the antituberculous effect of para-aminosalicylic acid (PAS) and the first clinical trials. *Am Rev Resp Dis*; **90**: 953–956.

23. Pfuetze K H *et al* (1955). The first clinical trial of streptomycin in human tuberculosis. *Am Rev Tuberc*; **71**: 752–754.

24. Dubos R and Dubos J (1953). *The White Plague*. Victor Gollanz; 101.

25. As 1; 90.

26. Ibid.

27. Ferrosan interview.

28. Ibid.

29. Ibid.

30. Ibid. Figures courtesy of Stig Nylén.

31. The doctors involved included Vallentin, Erik Törnell, Allan Beskow, Ragnar Thune, Bo Carstensen and Gösta Helleberg. This was not a placebo controlled trial. The results were presented to the Nordic Congress on Tuberculosis in 1948. (information courtesy of Dr E Berglund).

32. Schatz interviews.

33. Apparently this was a common event. Many of the US customs officials were of German origins so they tended to bestow German names on Russians to make them more acceptable to American society.

34. Vivian was kind enough to allow me to interview her with Albert during the Schatz interviews.

35. Betty Bugie (married name Gregory) lives near to Philadelphia. She was kind enough to allow me a lengthy telephone interview when I was in Philadelphia. From here on I shall refer to this as the "Betty Bugie interview".

36. Schatz interviews.

37. Doris Jones (married name Ralston). Unpublished paper. *A personal glimpse into the discovery of streptomycin.* I have referred to this interesting paper earlier and indicated that it deserves to be published.

38. Schatz interviews.

39. The "Streptomycin Babies" see ref. 18.

40. As 1; 148.

41. As 14; 231–232.

42. As 1; 157.

18   The Order of the Atoms

1. Gerhard Domagk worries over the fate of Wolfgang in his diary. The details of what actually happened to Wolfgang were kindly provided by Götz Domagk.

2. Domagk's diary.

3. It is difficult to obtain figures for the mortality from tuberculosis anywhere in Europe in the immediate post-war years. With regard to Germany in particular this is almost impossible since it was not only in chaos but divided into different zones of military occupation and civic responsibility. The German Red Cross and national statistical organisations have no figures at all. These figures were provided to me by Professor Jahnke, who had direct experience of working on the tuberculosis wards at the Wuppertal and Elberfeld Hospital thoughout this period.

4. Williams HW (1973). *Requiem for a Great Killer.* Health Horizon, London; 92. This delightful book has some very interesting facts and figures.

5. Jahnke, as 3.

6. Domagk's diaries together with the summary of his feelings in: *Chemotherapie der Tuberkulose mit den Thiosemikarbazonen.* Ed Gerhard Domagk. Georg Thieme Verlag, Stuttgart; 85.

7. Domagk G, Behnisch R, Mietzsch F and Schmidt H (1946). Über eine neue, gegen Tuberkelbazillen in vitro wirksame Verbindungsklasse. *Die Naturwissenschaften;* **33:** 1–4. Also Behnisch R (1986). Die geschichte der Sulfonamidforschung Medizinisch Pharmazeutische Studiengesellschaft. Mainz; 62–65.

8. Domagk's diary.

9. Ibid.

10. The many reports of Conteben in these various types of tuberculosis were

presented in considerable detail in a book – see *Chemotherapie der Tuberkulose mit den Thiosemikarbazonen*, in reference 6. This book also lists most of the appropriate journal publications, including the papers on the skin trials.

11. Domagk's diary.
12. Ibid
13. Ibid.
14. Ibid.
15. Ibid.
16. Ibid.
17. As 10.
18. Hoff F (Frankfurt). *Gerhard Domagk – Gedenkrede*. The text of his memorial to Domagk by his longstanding friend was kindly provided to me by Götz Domagk, who also very kindly translated it into English.
19. Jahnke interviews.
20. Ibid.

19 Premature Celebrations

A considerable amount of detail on George Orwell is available from the George Orwell Archive, in the Manuscripts and Rare Books Room, Bloomsbury Science Library of the University of London, WC1E 6BT. I am indebted to the archivist, Jill Furlong, who helped me with these details. I would also like to thank Dr Arnold Bentley, of the Royal British Legion Industries (Preston Hall Incorporated), Royal British Legion Village, Aylsford, Kent, for his kind permission to make reference to the Orwell medical records. The excellent biographies by Fyvel and Crick contain a wealth of medical fact.

1. Fyvel T R (1982). *George Orwell – a personal memoir*. Widenfield and Nicholson, London; 156.
2. Preston Hall medical notes.
3. Bernard Crick (1980). *George Orwell, a Life*. Little, Brown & Co, Boston; 537.
4. Ibid; 538.
5. As reference 1; 163.
6. Steenken W Jr (1949). *Streptomycin and Dihydrostreptomycin in Pulmonary Tuberculosis*. Ed Riggins and Hinshaw. Chapter headed, *Streptomycin and the Tubercle bacillus*; 39.
7. Harry F Dowling (1977). *Fighting Infection*. Harvard Univ Press; 168.
8. Streptomycin treatment of pulmonary tuberculosis: A Medical Research Council Investigation (1948). *Br Med J*; **ii**: 769–782.
9. Florey ME (1961). *The Clinical Application of Antibiotics. Vol II. Streptomycin and other antibiotics active against tuberculosis*. Oxford Univ Press, London; 133.
10. Long ER (1958). *The Chemotherapy of Tuberculosis*. Williams & Wilkins Co, Baltimore; 321.
11. Feldman WH (1954). Streptomycin: some historical aspects of its development as a chemotherapeutic agent in tuberculosis. *Am Rev Tuberc*; **69**: 859–868.
12. Hinshaw interviews.

13. Erik Berglund: personal communication.
14. Carstensen B and Sjölin S (1948). Para-aminosalicylsyra (PAS) vid lung-tuberkulos med sekundar tarmtuberkulos. *Svenska Läkartidn*; **45**: 729–743.
15. Therapeutic trials committee of the Swedish national association against tuberculosis (1950). Para-aminosalicylic acid treatment in pulmonary tuberculosis. *Am Rev Tuberc*; **61**: 597–612.
16. *Observanda* articles: see introduction to references, Chapter Fifteen.
17. Treatment of pulmonary tuberculosis with para-aminosalicylic acid and streptomycin. A preliminary report. *Br Med J* (1949); **ii**: 1521.
18. The veterans statistics come from Dowling (reference 7); 164–165. See also, Tucker (1949). Evolution of the Cooperative Studies in the Chemotherapy of Tuberculosis; 46, 51, 65. Also Veterans Administration, *Minutes of the Eighth Streptomycin Conference, Nov 10–13, 1949* (Washington DC); 343.
19. Waksman SA (1958). *My Life with the Microbes*. Robert Hale, London; 249.
20. Betty Bugie, personal communication.
21. Ibid.
22. Copy of letter provided to me by Schatz. Original in archives of Temple University, Philadelphia.
23. Ibid.
24. Schatz interviews.
25. Ibid.
26. As 22.
27. Ibid.
28. As 22.
29. Lechevalier H and Solotorovsky (1974). *Three Centuries of Microbiology*. Dover Publishers, New York. Chapter heading: *The Search for Antibiotics at Rutgers University*. NB: During an interview with Hubert Lechevalier, who took Waksman's chair in microbiology at Rutgers, he told me he had specifically asked Waksman why he had not simply answered Schatz's questions at the beginning and have the matter sorted out immediately. Waksman's replied that he did not think the questions Schatz was asking were any of Schatz' business. An interesting paper has also been written on this subject by Milton Wainwright, *Society for General Microbiology Quarterly* (1988); **15**: 90.
30. As 19; 253–254.
31. As 29.
32. *Newark Evening News*, 31 January 1951.
33. Hinshaw interviews. This benevolent act by Merck is also recorded in Waksman's books.
34. Karlson AG, Pfuetze KH, Carr DT, Feldman WH and Hinshaw HC (1949). The effect of combined therapy with streptomycin, para-aminosalicylic acid and promin on the emergence of streptomycin resistant strains of tubercle bacilli: a preliminary report. *Proc Staff Meet Mayo Clinic*; **24**: 510–515. Also, Daniels M and Hill AB (1952). Chemotherapy of pulmonary tuberculosis in young adults – analysis of combined results of three Medical Research Council trials. *Br Med J*; **i**: 1162–1168. See also Dowling (reference 7); 167.

35. There is an extensive discussion of the major trials in the US and the UK in Florey ME (reference 9).

36. As 9; 150.

20 The Battle Is Won

I am grateful to GD Schantz, of the Hoffman-La Roche Archives, Basle, Switzerland, and to Miss Caroline Gadsby of the E.R. Squibb and Sons Ltd (UK), who furnished me with information on the American aspects of the isoniazid story. I am equally grateful to the Bayer archivists at Leverkusen for their help with the German aspects of the same. Many thanks also to John Roddom, who arranged for the translation into English of the Domagk/Klee first paper on isoniazid.

1. McDermott W (1969). The story of INH. *J Infect Dis*; **119**: 678–683.

2. Hinshaw interviews.

3. Ibid.

4. Hinshaw HC and McDermott W (1950). Thiosemicarbazone therapy of tuberculosis in humans. *Am Rev Tuberc*; **61**: 145–157.

5. Chorine V (1945). Action de l'amide nicotinique sur les bacilles du genre Mycobacterium. *Compt. Rendu. Acad. Sci.*; **220**: 150–152.

6. I have been unable to acquire this paper, reference to which was made by Fox (see 7) as follows: Huant E (1945). *Gazette des Hopitaux*. Aug 15.

7. Fox HH (1953). The chemical attack on tuberculosis. *Trans New York Acad Sci*; **15**: 234–242.

8. Kushner S, Dalalian H, Casell RT, Sanjurjo JL, McKenzie D and Subbarow Y (1948). Experimental chemotherapy of tuberculosis. I. Substituted nicotinamides. *J Org Chem*; **13**: 834–836.

9. McKenzie D, Malone L, Kushner S, Oleson JJ and Subbarow Y (1948). The effect of nicotinic acid amide on experimental tuberculosis of white mice. *J Lab Cli Med*; **33**: 1249–1253.

10. Domagk's diary.

11. Ibid.

12. Ibid.

13. Ibid.

14. Fox Herbert H (1953). The chemical attack on tuberculosis. *Trans New York Acad Sci*; **15**: 234–242.

15. Domagk's diary.

16. As in reference 1.

17. Ibid.

18. Jahnke – personal communication.

19. Ibid.

20. *The Evening Star*, Washington, Thursday, 21 February 1952. Under headline, 'Two "Wonder" Pills Aid Patients With Hopeless Tuberculosis'.

21. Robitzek EH and Selikoff IJ (1952). Hydrazine derivatives of isonicotinic acid (Rimifon, Marsilid) in the treatment of active progressive caseous-pneumonic tuberculosis. *Am Rev Tuberc*; **65**: 402–428.

22. "Science in Review. New drugs that combat tuberculosis hold out a promise of far more effective control." *New York Times*, 24 February 1952.

23. The story of her return home was covered by the *New York Times*, Saturday, 10 May 1952.

24. *Stadt-Anzeiger*, 1 March 1952. "Die merkwürdige Geschichte eines neuen Tuberkulosemittels."

25. *General Anzeiger*, Wuppertal. This newspaper carried a series of articles, from 12 July to 26 July 1952, under the heading, "Die Wissenschaft im Kampf gegen die Tuberkulose", written by Dr Dieter Muller-Plettenberg.

26. Elmendorf DF, Cawthon WU, Muschenheim C and McDermott W (1952). The absorption, distribution, excretion, and short-term toxicity of isonicotinic acid hydrazide (Nydrazid) in man. *Am Rev Tuberc*; **65**: 429–442.

27. Domagk G and Klee P (1952). Die Behandlung der Tuberkulose mit Neoteben (Isonikotinsäurehydrazid). *Deutsch Med Wschr*; **77**: 578–581.

28. Copy of this correspondence in Domagk's diaries.

29. Meyer H and Mally J (1912). Hydrazine derivatives of pyridine-carboxylic acids. *Mh für Chemie und verwandte teile anderer Wissenschaften*; **33**: 393–414.

30. *New York Times*, Friday 22 February 1952. Headline: "New TB Drugs Are Revealed as Cheap Coal-Tar Synthetics."

31. The script was kindly provided by the Hoffman-La Roche archives.

32. Ibid.

33. As reference 1.

34. As reference 1; also *Time* Magazine, 21 July 1952. Feature headed "Medicine"; 43.

35. Clark CM, Elmendorf DF, Cawthon WU, Muschenheim C and McDermott W (1952). Isoniazid (isonicotinic acid hydrazide) in the treatment of miliary and meningeal tuberculosis. *Am Rev Tuberc*; **66**: 391–415.

36. Steenken W Jr, Meade GM, Wolinsky E and Coates EO Jr (1952). Demonstration of increased drug resistance of tubercle bacilli from patients treated with hydrazines of isonicotinic acid. *Am Rev Tuberc*; **65**: 754–758. Buck M and Schnitzer (1952). The development of drug resistance of *M Tuberculosis* to isonicotinic acid hydrazide. *Am Rev Tuberc*; **65**: 759–760. Pansy F, Stander H and Donovick R (1952). *In vitro* studies of isonicotinic acid hydrazide. *Am Rev Tuberc*; **65**: 761–764. Szybalski W and Bryson V (1952). Bacterial resistance studies with derivatives of isonicotinic acid. *Am Rev Tuberc*; **65**: 768–770. Hobby GL and Lenert TF (1952). Resistance to isonicotinic acid hydrazide. *Am Rev Tuberc*; **65**: 771–774. Suter E (1952). Multiplications of tubercle bacilli within phagocytes cultivated *in vitro*, and effect of streptomycin and isonicotinic acid hydrazide. *Am Rev Tuberc*; **65**: 775–776.

37. Medical Research Council (1952). Treatment of pulmonary tuberculosis with isoniazid. Interim report by the Tuberculosis Chemotherapy Trials Committee. *Br Med J*; **2**: 735–746.

38. Medical Research Council (1953). Isoniazid in the treatment of pulmonary tuberculosis. *Br Med J*; **1**: 521–536.

39. Mount FW and Ferebee SH (1952). Control study of comparative efficacy of isoniazid, streptomycin-isoniazid, and streptomycin-para-aminosalicylic acid

in Pulmonary Tuberculosis therapy: I. Report on twelve-week observation in 526 patients. *Am Rev Tuberc*; **66**: 632–635.

21 Glory and Controversy

1. The Nobel Prize for Medicine saw its first great controversy when they refused to give Koch the prize. He only received it in its fifth year, 1905, after much acrimony. For a detailed dissection of this I can recommend no better source than: Brock T D (1988). *Robert Koch – A Life in Medicine and Bacteriology.* Springer Verlag.
2. The Nobel Committees rules on procedure are standard and rigidly adhered to each year. I have based this description on the procedures as detailed in the Encyclopaedia Britannica and from the testimony of many interviews, especially in Sweden.
3. I have based this on the evidence of many interviews, notably those with Hinshaw and correspondence with Rosdahl.
4. Hinshaw interviews.
5. Personal communication, Karl Rosdahl.
6. Everywhere I travelled in Sweden, including the cities of Stockholm, Gothenburg and Malmö, I was told exactly the same story. The man said to be prejudiced against Lehmann was named, though I would rather avoid naming him in this context. Apparently he had been nominated for an earlier Nobel Prize for a discovery in the anticoagulant field but was refused because it was felt he did not have priority. Animosity between Lehmann and this man was subsequently so strong that neither man would appear at the same medical meeting.
7. Maja Lehmann interview.
8. Waksman SA (1958). *My Life with the Microbes.* Robert Hale, London; 272.
9. Ibid; 272.
10. Ibid; 273–274.
11. A copy of all correspondence was kindly furnished to me by Professor Albert Schatz. The various papers are in the Archives of the Temple University, Philadelphia.
12. Ibid.
13. Ibid.
14. Ibid.
15. Ibid.
16. Letter from Selman Waksman to Prof S. Mudd, Nov 14, 1952; Rutgers Archives. See also, Wainwright M (1991). Streptomycin: discovery and resultant controversy. *Hist Phil Life Sci*: **13**; 97–124. The controversy is also covered in some detail in the Lechevalier reference in the previous chapter.
17. Orla Lehmann interview.
18. As 8; 278.
19. Doris Jones. Unpublished memoir: *A personal glimpse at the discovery of streptomycin.* See reference 7, Chapter 13.

20. As 8; 279.
21. Canetti G (1955). *The Tubercle Bacillus in the Pulmonary Lesion of Man*. Springer, New York; 205. This aspect was also reviewed by Keers RY (1978). *Pulmonary Tuberculosis: a Journey Down the Centuries*. Ballière Tindall, London; 223.
22. The lecture was subsequently published. Crofton J (1960). Tuberculosis undefeated. *Br Med J*; 679.
23. Personal communication. This quote is taken from lecture notes kindly provided to me by Sir John Crofton.
24. Ibid.
25. Ibid.
26. United States Public Health Service Approach to zero tuberculosis (1960). *Public Health Rep*; **75:** 103–106.
27. Communicable Disease Center. The Arden House Conference on tuberculosis. US Department of Health, Education and Welfare, Public Health Service Publication no 784 (1961). Washington, DC: US GPO.
28. A very good modern review of the situation in America. Rieder HL, Cauthen GM, Comstock GW and Snider D (1989). Epidemiology of tuberculosis in the United States. *Epidemiologic Reviews*; **11:** 79–98.
29. Fox W (1970). Advances in the treatment of pulmonary tuberculosis. *Practitioner*; **205:** 502. See also Keers, as in reference 21. This book gives an excellent overall review of this phase of the tuberculosis epidemiology, written for a more scientific reader.
30. Keers (ibid); 236.
31. Shilts R (1987). *And the Band Played On*. Penguin Books; 3.

22 An Alliance of Terror

I am grateful in particular to Dr Jack Adler, formerly of the Bureau of Tuberculosis in New York and latterly of Mount Sinai Medical Center in New York, for his letters, explanations and communications over two years that first alerted me to what is happening in the world today and in keeping me abreast of developments in New York. Walter Ihle, of the CDC, Atlanta, was courteous and helpful in explaining what is now happening countrywide in the United States. I am also indebted to Dr Gisela Schecter for her advice on the situation in San Francisco. Jeff Miller, of *UCSF Magazine*, kindly allowed me unlimited access to his illustrations covering the San Francisco tuberculosis threat. The pharmaceutical company Adria Laboratories (Farmitalia Carlo Erba outside America) was very generous in allowing me access to information on the new trials of rifabutin. Finally, I am grateful to Mario Raviglione of the World Health Organization for his invaluable advice on the modern world situation.

1. This headline was under four-inch letters "TB" on the front page: *New York Post*, 17 October 1990.
2. Taken from U.S. official morbidity and mortality tables, 1953–1989.
3. Statistics kindly provided by Walter Ihle of the CDC, Atlanta, and confirmed

by the detailed bulletin released by the Department of Health and Human Services of the U.S. Public Health Service, dated August 1991.

4. Brown P (1992). The return of the big killer. *New Scientist,* 11 October.

5. Specter M (1992). Neglected for years, TB is back with strains that are deadlier. *The New York Times,* 11 October.

6. Clancy L (1990). Infectiousness of tuberculosis. *Bull International Union Against Tuberculosis and Lung Disease;* **65:** 70.

7. Brudney K, and Dobkin J (1991). Resurgent tuberculosis in New York City. Human immunodeficiency virus, homelessness and the decline of tuberculosis control programs. *Am Rev Respir Dis;* **144:** 746–749.

8. A.P. (1992). Study finds TB danger even in low-risk groups. *The New York Times;* 18 October.

9. As 5. The five articles were published daily in *The New York Times* from 11 to 15 October 1992.

10. Murray JF (1991). An emerging global programme against tuberculosis: agenda for research, including the impact of HIV infection. *Bull Int Union Tuberc Lung Dis;* **66:** 199–201.

11. This was summarised in a bulletin circulated by the Union Internationale Contre La Tuberculose et les Maladies Respiratoires, of 68 Boulevard Saint-Michel 75006, Paris: Murray C (1991). Tuberculosis control and research strategy for the 1990s. Also, leading article, the global tuberculosis situation and the new control strategy of the World Health Organization. *Tubercle* (1991); **72:** 1–6.

12. Murray CJL, Styblo K and Rouillon A (1990). Tuberculosis in developing countries: burden, intervention and cost. *Bull Int Union Tuberc Lung Dis;* **65:** 2–20.

13. Stanford, JL, Grange JM and Pozniak A (1991). Is Africa Lost? *Lancet;* **338:** 557–558.

14. Festenstein F and Grange JM (1991). Tuberculosis and the acquired immune deficiency syndrome. *J Appl Bact;* **71:** 19–30.

15. *Tuberculosis in New York City 1989.* Information Summary. Jack Adler, Medical Director, Bureau of Tuberculosis, Department of Health, 125 Worth Street, New York, NY 10013.

16. Jack Adler, personal communication.

17. Tuberculosis outbreak among persons in a residential facility for HIV-infected persons – San Francisco. *MMWR (USA)* 27 Sept 1991; **40:** No 38.

18. Personal communication, Jack Adler; for review and lead to other references, see 13.

19. Cayla JA, Jansa JM, Plasencia A, Batalla J and Parellada N (1991). Impact of tuberculosis on the new AIDS definition in Barcelona. *Bull Int Union Tuberc Lung Dis;* **66:** 43–45. The first sporadic tuberculosis-AIDS cases in Britain are reviewed in Watson J and Gill ON (1990). HIV infection and tuberculosis. *Br Med J;* **300:** 63–65.

20. Raviglione, MC, Sudre P, Rieder HL, Spinaci S and Kochi A (1992). Secular trends of tuberculosis in western Europe: epidemiological situation in 14 countries. Limited circulation document of the World Health Organization.

21. These figures were taken from a presentation by Professor KPWJ McAdam to the International Congress on Drug Therapy in HIV Infection, 9–12 November 1992.

22. I have researched the accuracy of this despairing remark and can confirm it from two separate sources, both of whom would prefer anonymity. The statistics in this paragraph are updated figures on Sudre P, ten Dam G and Kochi A (1991). Tuberculosis: a global overview of the situation today. Limited circulation document of the World Health Organization. I am grateful to Dr Philippe Sudre, who allowed me access to this global overview.

23. As 10.

24. Keers RY (1978) *Tuberculosis: A journey down the centuries.* Ballière Tindall; 244–250. A very useful summary of the early WHO campaigns and the reasons for their failure.

25. Styblo K and Enarson DA (1991). *Recent Advances in Respiratory Medicine,* ed DA Mitchell, No 5, Chap 9. *The impact of infection with human immunodeficiency virus on tuberculosis.* Churchill Livingstone, Edinburgh, Melbourne, New York and Tokyo.

26. As 20.

27. Murray CJL (1991). Social, economic and operational research on tuberculosis: recent studies and some priority questions. *Bull Int Union Tuberc Lung Dis;* **66:** 149–156.

28. This patient's case is taken from the following, with kind permission of the authors: Iseman MD and Madsen LA (1989). Drug resistant tuberculosis. *Clinics in Chest Medicine;* Vol 10, No 3: 341–353.

29. Iseman MD (1985). Tailoring a time bomb. *Am Rev Respir Dis;* **132:** 735–736.

30. In part this information was kindly provided to me by Walter Ihle of the CDC, Atlanta, and confirmed by *MMWR* 30 Aug 1991/Vol 40/No 34; 585–591. Nosocomial transmission of multidrug–resistant tuberculosis among HIV-infected persons – Florida and New York.

31. As 28. Also with assistance of Jack Adler, Bureau of Tuberculosis, New York.

32. Personal communication, Dr John Stanford.

33. Personal communication, Dr Tony Jenkins.

34. I chased down the information in the *Evening Standard,* with various authorities, including Stanford, Jenkins and the PHLS central information service, which basically confirmed that there are at least a dozen and probably more people at large with tuberculosis resistant to most if not all of the available antibiotics.

35. Personal communication, Dr Pozniak.

36. Rosenthal E (1992). TB, easily transmitted, adds a peril to medicine. *The New York Times;* 13 October.

37. As 34.

38. Specter M (1992). TB carriers see clash of liberty and health. *The New York Times;* 14 October.

39. Rosenthal E (1992). Doctors and patients are pushed to their limits by grim new TB. *The New York Times;* 12 October.

40. Zhang Y, Beate H, Allen B, et al. (1992). The catalase-peroxidase gene and isoniazid resistance of *Mycobacterium tuberculosis*. *Nature*; **358**: 591–593.

41. For a discussion from a very committed British standpoint, read the section on BCG in Keer's wonderful little book. The Styblo reference is to a paper submitted for publication on 19 December 1991 – Styblo K. *Tuberculosis: Where are we now?* The typescript was kindly provided to me by Annik Rouillon of the International Union Against Tuberculosis and Lung Disease. What Styblo actually says is: "Another reason for the difficulty in preventing the vast majority of newly developed smear-positive cases of pulmonary tuberculosis in a population by mass BCG vaccination is the known fact that the protection by BCG vaccination is of limited duration." A similar observation was made in the review Fine PEM and Rodrigues LC (1990). Modern Vaccines: Mycobacterial Diseases. *Lancet*; **i**: 1016–1020.

42. Schulzer M, Fitzgerald JM, Enarson DA and Grzybowski S (1992). An estimate of the future size of the tuberculosis problem in sub-Saharan Africa. *Tubercle and Lung Disease*; **73**: 52–58.

43. Personal communication, John Stanford.

44. Styblo K and Rouillon A. Tuberculosis. Where are we now? Paper submitted for publication in 1992.

45. Rey-Duran R, Boulahbal F, Gonzalez-Montaner IJ, Larbaoui D, McGregor MM, Pretet S and Olliaro P (1991). Role of Rifabutin in the Treatment of Chronic Drug-Resistant Pulmonary Tuberculosis. Abstracts VII International Conference on AIDS, Florence; 33–35. O'Brien RJ, Lyle MA and Snider DE (1987). Rifabutin (Ansamycin LM 427): A New Rifamycin-S Derivative for the Treatment of Mycobacterial Diseases. *Rev Infect Dis*; **9**: 519–530. Rey-Duran R, Boulahbal F, Gonzalez-Montaner IJ, Larbaoui D, McGregor MM, Pretet S and Olliaro P (1991). Efficacy and Safety of Rifabutin in Newly-Diagnosed Pulmonary Tuberculosis. Abstracts VII International Conference on AIDS, Florence; 29–44.

46. (a) Gordin FM. Rifabutin for prophylaxis of MAC bacteraemia in people with AIDS and CD4 less than 200. (b) Cameron W. Clinical impact of rifabutin prophylaxis for MAC. For (a) and (b), see Abstracts: prophylaxis of MAC in HIV-positive people. Satellite symposium held in conjunction with the VIII International Conference on AIDS/STD World Congress, Amsterdam, the Netherlands, 23 July 1992.

Index

450